TOWARDS ADVANCED NURSING PRACTICE
Key concepts for health care

TOWARDS ADVANCED NURSING PRACTICE
Key concepts for health care

EDITED BY

Jane E. Schober MN, RGN, RCNT, Dip N Ed, Dip N (Lond), RNT
Principal Lecturer in Nursing, DeMontfort University, Leicester, UK

Susan M. Hinchliff BA, RGN, RNT
Vice Principal, Continuing Professional Development, Institute of
Advanced Nursing Education, Royal College of Nursing, London, UK

A member of the Hodder Headline Group
LONDON • SYDNEY • AUCKLAND

First published in Great Britain 1995 by
Arnold, a division of Hodder Headline PLC,
338 Euston Road, London NW1 3BH

First edition 1995

Whilst the advice and information in this book are believed to be true and
accurate at the date of going to press, neither the editors, authors nor the publisher
can accept any legal responsibility or liability for any errors or omissions
that may be made. In particular (but without limiting the generality of the
preceding disclaimer) every effort has been made to check drug dosages;
however it is still possible that errors have been missed.

British Library Cataloguing in Publication Data
A catalogue record for this book is available from the British Library

Library of Congress Cataloging-in-Publication Data
A catalog record for this book is available from the Library of Congress

ISBN 0 340 59358 X

1 2 3 4 5   95 96 97 98 99

Typeset in 10/11pt Optima and produced by Gray Publishing, Tunbridge Wells, Kent
Printed and bound in Great Britain by The Bath Press, Avon

CONTENTS

FOREWORD

This is an innovative and readable book with several unusual features. First and most importantly, nursing and the well-being of the patient are firmly at its core. Both the complexity of nursing and the need to recognise and respond effectively to the range of health-care needs underpin the choice of concepts selected and developed. That choice has been shaped by:

1. the insight and understanding of current issues in health and nursing
2. the recognition of the interrelationship between health, the individual, the environment and nursing
3. the need for all nurses to provide sound rationales for their decisions and actions.

The first four chapters take the four major concepts which have influenced the development of nursing theory over the past 20 years. They have been explored, discussed and analysed to highlight issues pertinent to patient care, clinical practice and the development of nursing. The remaining chapters focus on issues which influence the process of care, and are so much a part of national and local initiatives relating to care.

An important feature of the book is the way that the authors have integrated research and knowledge from other disciplines, e.g. social sciences, and have interpreted and applied that research and knowledge to nursing practice.

The book highlights some under-developed concepts commonly used by nurses, though not necessarily with an understanding of their research base and/or theoretical roots. This applies, in particular, to the chapters on environment and humanism, and to a lesser extent to the discussion relating to holism.

Reflective points are found throughout the text which encourage application and analysis and stimulate debate.

The book will be a vital resource for pre- and post-registration students who need literature to support their academic and clinical development and can be used by nurses studying at both levels 2 and 3. The book takes an analytical approach and challenges rationales behind some of the norms in nursing practice, e.g. the way nursing models are used and the contribution of primary nursing.

I think that this is an exciting book which will further develop and shape the art and science of nursing.

Liz Winder, FRCN
Director, Nursing Policy and Practice
Royal College of Nursing

CONTRIBUTORS

Jane Bayliss BSc (Hons), RGN, RM, RHV, NP (dip)
Nurse Practitioner, Birmingham, UK

Gerald S. Bowman MPhil, RN
Research Fellow, Institute of Nursing Studies, University of Hull, Hull, UK

Gosia Brykczyńska BA, BSc, Dip PH, Cert Ed, RGN, RSCN, Onc. Cert
Lecturer in Ethics and Philosophy, Institute of Advanced Nursing Education, Royal College of Nursing, London, UK

Elisabeth Clark BA (Hons), PhD
Distance Learning Co-ordinator, Institute of Advanced Nursing Education, Royal College of Nursing, London, UK. Formerly, Director of Studies, School of Social Work and Health Sciences, Middlesex University, London, UK

Kevin Gournay M Phil, PhD, C Psychol, AFBPsS, RN
Professor of Psychiatric Nursing, University of London. Formerly Professor of Social Science, Middlesex University, London, UK

Sue Hinchliff BA, RGN, RNT
Vice Principal, Continuing Professional Development, Institute of Advanced Nursing Education, Royal College of Nursing, London, UK

Christopher Johns
Reader in Nursing Practice, Faculty of Health Care and Social Studies, Luton College of Health Education, Luton and Dunstable Hospital, Luton, UK

Sally Kendall PhD, BSc (Hons), RGN, RHV
Reader in Nursing, Buckinghamshire College and Associate Senior Research Fellow of Brunel University, London, UK

Siva Murugiah MSc, BSc (Hons), RMN, RGN, Dip N, RCNT, RNT
Lecturer in Science, Institute of Advanced Nursing Education, Royal College of Nursing, London, UK

Judith Reece BA, BA(Hons), MA, RNT, RMN, RGN, Dip Theol (Lond)
Senior Lecturer, DeMontfort University, Leicester, UK

Lynette Rentoul BSc (Hons), MSc, Chart Clin Psychol
Department of Nursing Studies, King's College London, London, UK

Robert Rentoul BSc (Hons), MSc
Department of Psychology, Goldsmiths College, London, UK

Jane Schober MN, RGN, RCNT, Dip N Ed, Dip N (Lond), RNT
Principal Lecturer in Nursing, DeMontfort University, Leicester, UK

Veronica Thomas BSc (Hons), PhD, Dip N RGN, Chart Clin Psychol
Department of Nursing Studies, King's College London, London, UK

David R. Thompson PhD, RN, FRCN
Professor of Nursing, Institute of Nursing Studies, University of Hull, Hull, UK

Greta Thornbory MSc, RGN, OHNC, Dip N (OH), PGCEA
Lecturer in Professional Development and Environmental Studies, Institute of Advanced Nursing Education, Royal College of Nursing, London, UK

1

HEALTH – THE NURSING CONTRIBUTION

Sally Kendall

Introduction

This book takes health as its starting point based on the belief that health is the ultimate goal of nursing. This can be readily traced in the literature and will be reviewed from several nurse theorists' perspectives. However, the introduction of the concept of health immediately raises questions for nurses, many of which will be addressed in this chapter. For example, what does health mean? Does it have the same meaning for everybody or does it vary between groups and individuals? What factors determine health? Can they be created or changed? How do people behave in relation to health? What affects these behaviours? What can nurses do to promote health? What theories and methods will help them? And finally, how do we know that health has been achieved? What methods are available for measuring health? These are just some of the questions which thinking about health raises. This chapter cannot promise to provide all the answers, but it aims to raise many of the issues, to address the theory and research behind them and to appraise critically the relationship between nursing and health on the basis of our current state of knowledge.

The concept of health is evident, either implicitly or explicitly, in the majority of models or theories of nursing, suggesting that there is a synergistic relationship between the two. How the concept of health is defined within the theories does, however, vary according to the underlying philosophy being adopted by the theorist. For example, Nightingale's (1859) model of nursing was based on a philosophy of hygiene. Health was perceived as being the result of putting the person in the best possible environment in terms of both recovery and maintenance. Nursing interventions were focused on the provision of fresh air, light, warmth, cleanliness and nutritional balance. Many would argue that these remain important environmental issues in promoting public health. Later, nurses such as Virginia Henderson (1960) developed the idea that nursing was involved with helping a person to do what they could not effectively do for themselves and a model of nursing based on the activities of daily living was devised. This model and others which developed from it, such as Roper et al.'s (1990), are based on a largely medical philosophy which sees the person as dependent and health is therefore viewed as the absence of disease or disability. The nurse's aim is to help the person to regain health by initially carrying out the activities of living for the person (for example, passive exercising, feeding) and then enabling the person to regain independence by helping the individual to carry out those activities for him- or herself. Later on, other theorists tried to move away from health purely as the absence of disease and other philosophies were introduced. Roy (1984), for example, bases her theory on the concept of adaptation, where health is seen as the ability to adapt to a given situation, be it the loss of a limb, the arrival of a baby or the side-effects of chemotherapy. The nurse's role is to help the person to adapt in whatever way is most appropriate.

Orem (1991) developed a theory which took individualism as a central philosophy so that the concept of self-care and responsibility was central to the approach. Health was seen as the ability to be self-caring in relation to a range of activities which Orem called self-care requisites. The goal of nursing was to help the person towards self-care and therefore health. A completely different philosophy, adopted by Paterson and Zderad (1976), was existentialism. This view totally accepts the subjective experience of nursing and being nursed and therefore sees health as whatever the person experiences it to be. Nursing is helping a person to understand these experiences and to achieve potential as a human being. These authors go further than most others by describing a positive state of health which they call 'more-being', which is seen as a state of becoming as much as is humanly possible within a given situation. None of these theories are without their critics but what this brief overview aims to do is to highlight the issue that health does not have a common meaning even in nursing theory and that meanings change over time according to the context in which ideas are being developed.

Since health does appear to be a central concept for nursing practice, it will be important in this chapter to explore some trends in health and illness and the role of the nurse as a health promoter to enable optimum health to be achieved. This will involve both an exploration of the meaning of health from a number of perspectives in further depth, and also an examination of the nature of health promotion and the methods which nurses can employ to promote health. Whilst prevention of ill-health or the prevention of further pain or suffering is one approach to health promotion, the possibility of promoting positive health will also be explored. This means going beyond the prevention of disease to enabling people to achieve their health potential.

Much of nurses' work in health promotion must be explored within the social and political context. There are many aspects of health policy which are central to the way in which health promotion is defined, analysed and practised. These policies may have implications for the way in which individuals in society are treated in relation to their health and illness and the way in which nurses develop their own philosophies and strategies for health promotion. For example, the NHS and Community Care Act [Department of Health (DoH),

1990] has resulted in shorter hospital lengths of stay, in large institutions, such as psychiatric hospitals, closing down and in more day surgery and technical care being carried out in the primary health-care setting. The implications for patient and family education and for information-giving are obvious. But other aspects of health promotion such as social support, the environment and financial needs must be addressed. The role of the nurse in relation to some approaches to health promotion, which have been described and analysed in the literature, will be explored in the context of health-care policy.

The Health of the Nation (DoH, 1992a) has set out particular targets in relation to changes in mortality and morbidity by the year 2000 which nurses also need to respond to in a variety of ways which will be explored critically in the context of each of the targets defined and in relation to the other issues outlined above.

The aims of the remainder of this chapter are therefore:

- to encourage you to critically analyse the meaning of health
- to stimulate your interest in actively promoting health
- to provide you with some theoretical frameworks within which to practise.

The meaning of health

When we refer to the concept of health, it has to be considered from a number of perspectives as clearly there is no one meaning. Firstly, and most importantly, what do the people we care for mean when they talk about health and being healthy? Secondly, what do policy-makers and managers mean by health and finally what do health professionals mean by health? It is not improbable that there will be some conflict between these groups of people about how health is defined. This can lead to misunderstandings and confusion about how health among populations can be achieved. For example, if the policy-maker sees health in terms of reducing accidental death in childhood by parental education and the parents see health in terms of changing the environment in which they are forced to bring up their children, there will be a direct conflict as to how health can be achieved. The implication is that health can be achieved either through the parents increasing their knowledge of accidents and thereby changing their own behaviour and that of their children, or by making the environment a safer place to play and go to school, which may be outside the power of the parents (but within the power of policy-makers). These conflicting perspectives arise from the different values that people hold about health and the belief systems which create the ideological basis for thought and action. This argument will be explored in greater detail when we analyse the various approaches to health promotion.

Reflective point

It is useful to start by examining our own views on health, so you are asked to write down in one or two paragraphs what health means to you, personally. Later, you can reflect on your own meaning of health in the light of the literature reviewed below.

Let us start by examining some of the research evidence which has informed us about the ways in which ordinary people define and give meaning to health. The discussion will be restricted to research in the western world.

Research in this field goes back to the early 1970s and has more commonly been carried out by sociologists than health professionals. For example, Herzlich (1973) studied 80 middle-class people in France to determine how they viewed health. From her analysis of interviews with these participants, Herzlich identified three dimensions along which the people in her study described health. The first was 'health-in-a-vacuum' which could be described as the absence of disease. Such a view could be argued to be similar to that held by many health professionals. The second dimension was health as a reserve, an inner capacity to maintain wellness. This was seen to be related to two factors – a person's physical strength and a person's potential for resistance to disease. The third dimension was 'equilibrium' which could be seen as the full realisation of an individual's reserve for health. However, this sense of perfect well-being, of which happiness, relaxation and good social relationships were seen to be a part,

was considered rare. Interestingly, Hunt and Macleod (1987) found in their UK study that people did hold similar perceptions to those identified by Herzlich; they also found that all three perceptions could be held by any one person at the same time. For example, one woman described herself as healthy 'except for the asthma' whilst at the same time expressing health as an ability to carry out everyday activities and implicitly referring to a reserve of strength. This study was a small-scale, qualitative study in which 25 people were interviewed. Whilst the authors were interested in the concepts of health which people used, their focus of interest was on how this affected behaviour change. Therefore, all the participants in the study had changed their health behaviour in some way and the majority (22) were women, which may have had some influence on the findings. However, the authors suggest that since their concepts of health were not confined to the idea of health as the absence of disease that their health behaviours were not necessarily related to health in terms of prevention alone. Health behaviours were seen to be an aspect of everyday life rather than intrinsically related to future or present changes in their health status. For example, cigarette smoking was used as a coping mechanism, as a social activity or to relieve boredom and the women in the study were more concerned with immediate weight gain if they stopped smoking than with lung disease at some future time if they carried on.

An American study by Woods et al. (1988) also found that women hold a range of concepts of health. This was a much larger scale study than Hunt's in which 656 women were asked to complete health diaries and respond to a telephone interview, 528 completed the telephone interview. Following content analysis of the data, the authors reduced the data to 12 categories, some of which were more salient for women than others. For example, 56.5 percent saw health in clinical terms, as absence of disease, but many also saw health in terms of positive effect (49.2 percent, well-being, happiness, etc.) and fitness (43.8 percent) which led the authors to conclude that 'clearly, women's images reflected a strong emphasis on exuberant well-being, not merely the absence of symptoms, role performance or management of their environ ments' (p. 42).

Kenney's (1992) study is interesting as its aim was to test out the concepts found in Wood et al.'s study. Kenney starts with an assumption [based on work by Smith (1981)] that there is a hierarchy of perceived health where clinical health would be at the bottom level and well-being and fitness at the top, with concepts related to role performance and adaptation falling somewhere in between. In fact, Kenney's study of 65 adults who completed a questionnaire refuted this hierarchical notion of health, which very much supports Hunt and Macleod's (1987) finding that people can hold several concepts of health at any one time. Kenney concludes that it is important for nurses to acknowledge the very wide range of concepts of health which adults hold.

Perhaps the most important message from this review of just four studies is that health is a complex concept which ordinary people are able to hold views on and articulate. For many ordinary people, health will mean both the absence of disease and will also be described in terms of fitness, strength and well-being. It is not confined to nurses and other health professionals to define health, even though there are many attempts to do so. In order to promote practice in relation to health, nurses do need to take account of the ways in which patients and clients perceive their health as this will have implications for their health behaviour and the approach that the nurse takes to health promotion.

Reflective point

Now reflect on your own account of health and think about what is most important for you and how this fits in with the research cited.

It would also be interesting to ask a selection of people who are not health professionals what they mean by health. How do their views compare with the research findings?

Having recognised that people hold a range of views or concepts of health, it is worthwhile now to explore how some nurse theorists have defined health and the basis for their definitions.

There is a plethora of definitions of health within the nursing literature, indicative of each theorist trying to identify what is unique to her particular theory. Whilst it was suggested in the Introduction that there has been a historical trend in the development of health as a nursing concept, this has not been strictly linear in nature as some of the early nursing theory seems more relevant to the findings on lay understandings of health than theory

emerging in the 1980s and 1990s. For example, Orlando's (1961) work viewed health in relation to human needs such as physical limitations, adverse reactions to a setting and experiences that prevent communication of needs. Orlando's interactional model of nursing therefore emphasises the importance of nurses recognising the needs of the patient and of responding to the need as the patient perceives it, not as the nurse perceives it. Orlando's approach was very much in line with consumerist principles and the values inherent in *The Patient's Charter* (DoH, 1992b) and yet she was writing 30 years ago. Orlando's work was based on her observations of practice and she provides many examples in her writings of how nurse–patient interaction can be used effectively to promote a person's health. Orlando's approach to nursing was not formally constructed as a model and has therefore often been overlooked by nurse educationalists who have introduced nursing theory into the curriculum. Other theories of nursing which emerged later have presented their formal definitions of health and a selection of these are discussed below.

Neuman's (1982) definition of health

Neuman's theory of nursing focuses on the total person who is made up of physiological, socio-cultural and developmental variables. The person is seen as having a range of lines of resistance to stressors which are unique to that person but within a common range with other human beings. When the lines of defence are broken by stressors, then ill-health can occur within any of the systems which have been breached. The nurse's role is to help the person to maintain equilibrium by preventing the lines of resistance from being broken, through primary, secondary or tertiary prevention. Neuman (1982) describes illness as 'variance from wellness' where wellness appears to be equated with the stability of the total system. Her definition of health is given as:

> Health or wellness is the condition in which all parts and subparts (variables) are in harmony with the whole man. Disharmony reduces the wellness state. ... Health, therefore, is reflected in the level of wellness. If man's total needs are met, he is in a state of optimum wellness. Conversely, a reduced state of wellness is the result of needs not met (p. 9).

Neuman appears to view health as a continuum rather than a dichotomy of wellness and illness but nevertheless she does make an assumption about the nature of the person. By adopting a systems theory approach to human development and behaviour she inevitably invites the nurse to break the person down into constituent parts. A holistic practitioner would argue that the whole is much more than the sum of its parts and that isolated systems cannot therefore be considered separately. Whilst Neuman's definition of health would embody some of the meanings of health described by ordinary people, it could not take account of the possibility of a person holding different meanings about health at any one time, as shown by Hunt and Macleod (1987), or for the fact that people can describe themselves as healthy in the presence of disease.

Orem's (1991) definition of health

Orem's theory of nursing is based on the concept of self-care. Self-care is seen by Orem as 'the practice of activities that individuals initiate and perform on their own behalf in maintaining life, health and well-being' (Orem, 1991, p. 117).

Health, then, from Orem's perspective is seen as

that which makes a person human (form of mental life), operating in conjunction with physiological and psychophysiological mechanisms and a material structure (biological life) and in relation to and interacting with other human beings (interpersonal and social life) (p. 180).

In summary, to achieve this state the person must be self-caring in respect of a set of universal and developmental self-care requisites which include such items as maintaining an intake of elements vital to life such as air, food and water, bringing about and maintaining the living conditions that support life processes such as pregnancy and birth and seeking medical assistance in the event of illness. Where these self-care requisites are either missing or weakened, then the person is said to be in a state of self-care deficit requiring help by the nurse to return to a self-caring state. Orem argues that without self-care, integrated human functioning will be disrupted.

The basis for Orem's argument does not appear to have been deduced from research or the literature, but rather was based on consensus agreement among the Nursing Development Conference Group which Orem led. Self-care as a determinant of health relies on an ideology of individualism which assumes that a person has both the will and the capacity to take responsibility for his or her own health. Illich (1992) has argued forcefully against this ideology, reasoning that becoming healthy is more likely to be associated with determinants which relieve poverty and hunger than medical intervention and that the world that human beings have created is polluted by poisons and radiation, which has rendered people powerless. Individuals, he argues, cannot take responsibility for the way in which we have collectively constructed our world. He also argues that the idea of finding health whilst in a state of disease or dying has been constructed by a post-industrial age in which people are afraid to become ill or approach death and that this new ideology has stripped people of their cultural traditions in accepting and finding meaning in death and suffering. Whilst Orem accepts that there are conditions that can affect human development, such as educational deprivation and oppressive living conditions, she also assumes that individuals can provide the care needed to overcome or mitigate the effects of these problems. Health from Orem's perspective, then, may be useful in terms of understanding where a person feels his or her strengths and weaknesses are but it cannot take account of those who perceive themselves to be powerless in relation to their health. We will be returning to the concept of individualism when we look at health promotion strategies, as this has important implications for nursing in the current social and political context.

Benner and Wrubel's (1989) definition of health

Benner and Wrubel discuss health at length from a number of sociological and psychological perspectives. Their view is drawn from the concept of coherence, which they derive from Antonovsky's (1979) work where he defines coherence as

a global orientation that expresses the extent to which one has a pervasive, enduring though dynamic feeling of confidence that one's internal and external environments are predictable and that there is a high probability that things will work out as well as can reasonably be expected (p. 10).

According to Benner and Wrubel, this sense of coherence comes from belonging to a sociocultural group. They draw on research by Durkheim (1951) and Kobasa (1979) which supports their view that health deviation such as suicide and the ability to feel committed, in control and challenged ('hardiness') is strongly related to coherence within a socio-cultural group. Since cultural integration is a major component of this view of health, then understanding the meaning of health for the people who belong to that particular group becomes important. Benner and Wrubel's work therefore differs from many other nurse theorists' work in that they accept health (and illness) as it is lived and experienced by the person or group. In fact, these authors prefer to use the term 'well-being' to health as they suggest that health *per se* is commonly associated with object-ive physiological and psychological measures whilst well-being reflects the lived experience of health. Well-being is defined as:

> Congruence between one's possibilities and one's actual practices and lived meanings and is based on caring and being cared for (p. 160).

The notion that health, or well-being, depends on a reciprocal relationship of caring and being cared for is an interesting one as it raises the question: is it possible to be part of a socio-cultural group and not feel cared for whilst at the same time feeling healthy? Taking nurses as a socio-cultural group, there is considerable research which suggests that nurses do not feel cared for by their profession whilst they are expected to care for others (e.g. Smith, 1990; James 1992; Mackay, 1989). This may explain why some nurses do not feel a sense of well-being but in fact feel under stress and even 'burned out'.

Perhaps Benner and Wrubel come closer to understanding health from the perspective of the ordinary person than other nurse theorists.

Conclusions

What conclusions can be drawn from this discus-sion on meanings of health? One thing is abun-dantly clear, there is no single definition or meaning which nurses can draw on. The research carried out among ordinary people and the theories proposed by nurses demonstrate only too clearly the complex nature of the concept of health. Indeed, Meleis (1989) has argued that this diversity of thought in relation to health is appropriate because of the diverse nature of nursing and nursing clients. As Meleis states:

> Health-care providers tend to have one prominent way of thinking about health; yet, the health care

needs of the client preclude the possibility of focusing only on one level of meaning.

Therefore, it may be important for nurses to consider health from different perspectives with different clients in all their many and varied situations. What is health for the client on the surgical unit will necessarily be very different to health for the woman in the family planning clinic.

Finally, one other issue is uncovered by the above discussion. If health has a diverse range of meanings, what happens when clients and nurses hold different concepts of health? Clearly, it is possible that there may be room for conflict in decision making in relation to identification of needs, planning to meet needs, interventions and even outcomes. For example, if a nurse holds a biomedical concept of health and the patient sees health more in terms of reserves of strength, then advice to change his or her diet to prevent coronary heart disease (CHD) may be falling on stony ground. The patient may be more concerned with the inner strength that he feels he needs to cope with unemployment, which for him may be unrelated to diet. Kleinman *et al.* (1978) have referred to the way we explain health and illness as an 'explanatory model'. These authors advocate that health professionals try to draw out the client's explanatory model of his or her illness or health as this enables the professional to work from the client's perspective rather than his or her own, which may mean that the outcome will be more satisfactory for both parties.

Working for health, then, is concerned with understanding the meaning of health from a range of perspectives and working toward insight into your own explanatory model whilst accepting that it may differ from others.

The context of health

In the previous section, we reviewed some of the ways in which ordinary people and nurses perceive health. These concepts are important for understanding the perceived determinants of health and illness and the approaches that may be taken to health promotion. However it is perceived, health does appear to be related to social, environmental, physiological and psycho-logical factors. Some researchers would emphasise some of these factors more than others. It is important to understand that determinants of health are politically constructed as well so that whilst, as a health promoter, you will be concerned with eliciting the client's explanatory model or concept of health, you will also be acknowledging the social and political context in which this is constructed. To analyse these ideas further, this section of the chapter will explore two broad concepts in relation to health and consider these in relation to two key political documents.

The concepts are individualism and collectivism; the documents are *The Health of the Nation* (DoH, 1992a) and *Inequalities in Health* (Townsend *et al.*, 1988).

Individualism

When the context of health is discussed it suggests a background against which health or well-being can be achieved. It also suggests that there are causative factors which can enhance or hinder health. In the western world, and particularly in the UK and the USA, there are two emerging ideologies which account for the context and or the determinants of health and disease. The prevailing ideology is that of individualism and responsibility for self in respect of health and other aspects of welfare. This ideology presupposes that individual lifestyles and attitudes are the fundamental determinants of health and illness and that individuals have the freedom to choose to change their lifestyle to achieve an improved health status. Lifestyle has been defined by the World Health Organization (WHO, 1986a) as

> a general way of living based on the interplay between living conditions in the wide sense and individual patterns of behaviour as determined by socio-cultural factors and personal characteristics (p. 118).

Whilst this definition takes into account that lifestyle is dependent on the social context, it is interpreted by many as being a purely behavioural concept.

An example of this is in the prevention of cardiovascular disease. Epidemiologists have established that a group of risk factors including smoking, high blood pressure, obesity and raised serum cholesterol levels are determinants of a cardiac event such as myocardial infarction. The individualist assumption is that by giving people information

about these risk factors they will then have the information required to choose to reduce their risk of cardiovascular disease by giving up smoking or losing weight, i.e. changing their behaviour. The responsibility for this change belongs with the individual, if he or she cannot change; then the consequences rest with the individual, an idea encapsulated by McKeowan (1979) as 'victim blaming'. You can observe the results of this approach to health and welfare through reports of significant health-related events in the news media and through the way in which health messages are delivered. For example, recent discussion about whether smokers should be refused cardiac surgery unless they give up smoking implies that they can choose to stop smoking or face the inevitable consequences. It goes further – such individuals will be punished by the medical profession for refusing to make the healthy choice. The drink/driving advertisements which display the consequences of self-indulgent behaviour in graphic detail also suggest that if only the individual had been more responsible for his actions this would not have occurred. There is little or no analysis of the socio-cultural factors which are significant to these behaviours, for example the role of stress or peer pressure. The ideology of individualism is clearly demonstrated in the Department of Health document *The Health of the Nation* (1992a) in which five target areas have been identified for reducing morbidity and mortality within the next decade. The five areas cover reductions in CHD and stroke, reductions in accidents, cancer, sexually related diseases (especially HIV and AIDS) and improvements in mental health (particularly the reduction of suicide). Much of the tone of the document assumes that health professionals will be involved in informing people about the risk factors so that they can change their behaviour. For example, in the opening chapter on health in England it states:

> The way in which people live and the lifestyles they adopt can have profound effects on subsequent health. Health education initiatives should continue to ensure that individuals are able to exercise informed choice when selecting the lifestyles they adopt (DoH, 1992a, p. 11).

What is wrong with individualism? Surely it is up to people to take responsibility for their own health?

One of the problems with this approach is that it focuses on death and disease rather than health or well-being. It is really saying that individuals are responsible for the diseases they contract and their eventual deaths rather than ways in which they promote positive health and well-being. Naidoo (1986) has commented on the ideology of individualism and argues that this approach denies that health or illness are social products, for example the incidence of CHD is much greater among materially deprived social groups (Blaxter, 1990) which invites the question 'why?'. Certainly, *The Health of the Nation* document makes very little reference to inequalities in health, and where it does acknowledge the variations between socio-economic groups it largely accounts for this by variation in lifestyle. This denial of the social context of health and disease perpetuates the victim-blaming approach to health promotion. A key criticism is that it assumes that individuals do have a free choice. Supporters of individualism do not question why people smoke or drink too much alcohol or have many sexual partners, they assume that this choice can be reversed towards a healthier way of living. Milio (1981) has argued that:

> Personal behaviour patterns are not simply 'free choices' about 'lifestyle' isolated from their personal and economic context. Lifestyles are, rather, patterns of choices made from the alternatives that are available to people according to their socio-economic circumstances and the ease with which they are able to choose certain ones over others (p. 76).

This is an important statement because it introduces the idea that choices are not necessarily easy and that often the scope for choice is limited in any case. For example, evidence compiled by Blackburn (1991) on the effects of poverty on health suggests that food choice is influenced by household income, knowledge and attitudes to food, the cost of a healthy diet and the availability of healthy food. The choice is between spending less on healthier foods which children are likely to reject, which is wasteful, or spending more on foods which children will enjoy and at least be satisfied with, despite the evidence that they may already be at risk of CHD. There may also be other factors which make the choice to eat 'bad' foods easier such as ease of cooking in limited facilities, less stress when children are eating what they want and enjoyment of these foods when there is little else in life to enjoy. There is little evidence that people from poorer families have less knowledge

about healthy foods than people from higher-income families. Graham (1984) found in her study of family health that lack of knowledge about healthy diets was not an issue, the problem was more likely to be access to healthy foods. An individualist would argue that people have the power to change the circumstances which they are in and that social problems are caused by over dependence on the state for welfare.

Reflective point

Think about your own lifestyle and focus on one aspect of your health-related behaviour (maybe you exercise regularly or perhaps you are a smoker). What factors do you think most influence this particular behaviour? Think about the key enhancing factors and the key inhibiting factors.

Collectivism

The alternative view argues that individuals are powerless within a society where healthy choices are not necessarily the easy choices and that change is only possible through collective action (self-empowerment) and social policy. For example, the *Ottawa Charter for Health Promotion* (WHO, 1986b) states that:

> Health promotion policy requires the identification of obstacles to the adoption of healthy public policies in non-health sectors and ways of removing them. The aim must be to make the healthy choice the easier choice for policy-makers as well (p. 1).

This view assumes that as a society people want to contribute positively to a health and welfare system which will be for the benefit of all and will help the most vulnerable such as those who are poor, elderly or disabled. The underlying belief is that in many cases individuals do not have the power to change their lifestyles or their circumstances and that they can be empowered through a healthy public policy approach. The view makes the assumption that people are inherently altruistic that; for example, we would be prepared to pay higher taxes to protect those who are poor and vulnerable, as well as providing a welfare system from which everybody benefits. This is difficult to bear out in western societies where people have been encouraged to be responsible for themselves and their families and not necessarily for the wider community. The collective approach has certainly been criticised for its reformist and rather Utopian principles (Beattie, 1991). Nevertheless, there is evidence, at both a political and a community level, that the collective approach can make a positive contribution to determining health and well-being.

On the face of it, it would appear that if healthy choices are limited by socio-economic circumstances then improvements in general welfare will result in overall improvements in health. *The Health of the Nation* and *Inequalities in Health* present us with conflicting arguments.

Inequalities in Health is an edited combination of *The Black Report* (1982, edited by Townsend and Davidson) and *The Health Divide* (Whitehead, 1987). *The Black Report* was commissioned by the DHSS in 1977 in order to review the variations in health across the social classes over the previous four decades. It was researched and written by an expert working group led by Sir Douglas Black, what was then the Chief Scientist at the DHSS. *The Health Divide* was commissioned in 1986 by the then Health Education Council to update *The Black Report* and bring the evidence of other reports on inequalities in health together. For political reasons, both of these reports received very cool receptions from the DHSS. Both reports were consistent in their findings that whilst health for the population as a whole was improving (in terms of age of death, causes of death and morbidity), there were widening gaps between those in the professional classes and those in manual and unskilled occupations. However, the recommendations put forward by *The Black Report* were not considered to be economically viable (these included recommendations for increases in welfare benefits, wider access to child care and nursery education, distribution of resources towards those in greatest need, a greater emphasis on community care and school health, to mention just a few) and ideologically unsound. *The Black Report* was accused of being Marxist in its approach and some politicians refused to accept the evidence produced by the expert working group that poverty and material deprivation were significant in explaining variations in health between socio-economic groups. Edwina Currie, for example, is quoted as saying

I honestly don't think it has anything to do with poverty. The problem very often for many people is just ignorance and failing to realise that they do

have some control over their lives (p. 12, cited by Townsend and Davidson, 1988).

It was also accused of putting forward recommendations for which there was no evidence of success. Naidoo (1986) has put forward the same criticism of the individualist approach – that there is no evidence that people change their behaviour on the basis of education alone.

The Health Divide was published in a general election year at a time when the Health Education Council was being disbanded and was treated with similar derision. Despite criticism from the government of the time, *The Black Report* and *The Health Divide* received strong support from the medical and nursing press. They were reported as being scientifically sound and unbiased accounts of trends in the nation's health which demonstrated undeniable links between poverty and ill-health. Both reports have consistently stated that the causal relationship between poverty and inequalities in health is too complex at the moment to identify, but that this does not deny the significance of the finding. It could be postulated, as has been suggested in the example on children's eating habits, that poverty affects the way in which people behave towards their health as a result of stress, perceived powerlessness and lack of self-esteem but these factors have yet to be statistically proven. The reports do not deny the role of lifestyle in understanding variations in health, but try to explain lifestyle in broader terms than individual behaviour patterns.

The evidence which was presented by *The Black Report* was based on analysis of data from the four previous decades. One example of the evidence is the pattern of mortality for men from all causes of death from the 1930s through to the 1970s. The figures published demonstrate that standardised mortality ratios for men in the professional class have decreased from 90 in 1930–32 to 75 in 1970–72 whilst for the same respective periods the standardised mortality ratio for unskilled men has increased from 111 to 121. Therefore, not only are men from the unskilled occupational groups exposed to a higher death rate than professional men, this situation has actually become worse since the 1930s. A closer analysis reveals that this situation is largely accounted for by age, that it is the older men in the unskilled group who have the highest death rate

The Health Divide reveals similar evidence of

discrepancies between social classes. For example, in 1984 there were significant variations between professional families and unskilled families in terms of numbers of stillborn babies and numbers of infant deaths in the first year of life, which clearly disadvantaged children born to unskilled families. As social class has been criticised as an unreliable method of classifying populations due to changes in the pattern of work (less manual labour) and because Registrar Generals tend to reclassify occupations over time, some researchers have attempted to use other approaches to classification such as housing tenure. This has become particularly important for women's health trends as married women have formerly been classified according to their husband's occupation. *The Health Divide* presents some evidence that when their own occupation as well as housing tenure and car ownership are taken into account, there are wide variations between women from different groups in terms of standardised mortality ratios. Thus, in 1987, according to the report, the death rate for single women with a non-manual job, their own car and owner occupation of a house was 69 compared with married housewives, living in rented accommodation, with no car and a husband with a manual occupation, for whom the death rate was 161. There is no mention of children in this analysis but it could be conjectured that married housewives are more likely to be affected by pregnancy and childbirth than single working women.

The Health of the Nation is a strategic document which provides a framework for improving the nation's health in the five key areas listed on p. 15. The document is responsive to the WHO's initiative on 'health for all' (WHO, 1978) but does not always reflect the spirit of the WHO's work. For example, in the *Ottawa Charter* of 1986, the WHO refers to concepts such as equality and participation which are not emphasised in *The Health of the Nation*. Nevertheless, *The Health of the Nation* provides challenges and opportunities for addressing some of the most prevalent and potentially avoidable health problems of the 20th century and beyond. As has been suggested earlier, and not surprisingly given the history of *The Black Report* and *The Health Divide*, *The Health of the Nation* makes very little mention of the variations in health between socio-economic groups in England. The document refers to overall improvements in health to the whole population, which is largely seen in terms of reductions in infant mortal-

ity and deaths from infectious diseases. Where the document does refer to variations across occupations in terms of present-day health problems, such as cancer and cardiovascular disease, this is seen as a specialist 'at risk' group alongside people from ethnic minorities and people with learning disabilities rather than a fundamental health issue. The document states that:

> People in manual groups are more likely to smoke, and to eat diets containing less vitamin C and beta carotene. There is also a higher proportion of heavy drinkers in non-manual groups. ... There is also evidence of a lower uptake of preventive health services (para. F18, p. 122)

and:

> National mass media health education could be targeted on groups at particular risk (para. F19, p. 122).

Whilst the Secretary of State for Health does acknowledge the role of social policy in reducing the incidence and prevalence of infectious diseases (through improved water and sewage systems, for example), this is almost presented as a historical fact and not as a relevant issue for today's health concerns. There is virtually no reference to the role of poverty in determining health and illness and therefore no political strategy to improve this. The emphasis is clearly on the individualistic, educational approach to mass behaviour change.

Reflective point
Most regional health authorities will have published a public health report. Locate the report for your region (either directly from region or through your college library) and look at the health trends for one aspect of health which interests you. Are there differences in different parts of the region or within different groups? Does the report account for these? What strategies are identified to achieve equity in health?

The effect of public policy on health

Clearly there is historical evidence to support the argument that public policy can improve health. This is evident in relation to the incidence of infectious diseases and infant mortality rates. For example, as the Secretary of State for Health indicates in *The Health of the Nation*, the standardised mortality ratio from tuberculosis decreased from 1500 in 1851–55 to virtually zero in 1986–90. Whilst the discovery of the tubercle bacillus and the development of the BCG vaccine have an important role here, the rate was already rapidly declining before the vaccine was introduced, suggesting that other factors were relevant. Improvements in housing and overcrowded conditions were almost certainly responsible for reducing the spread of infection, but also the National Assistance Act of 1911 helped to reduce poverty and took people out of the workhouses, legislation to increase the age at which children could work and the introduction of the National Health Service (NHS) itself in 1948 have all been significant in improving health. It is only with these retrospective data that patterns can be identified and even then causal significance is difficult to infer as there may be other environmental and physiological factors which have changed and are difficult to control for. Therefore, despite the fact that there do appear to be clear correlations between social deprivation and health problems it is difficult to predict that changes in current public policy would have similarly dramatic effects on today's health problems. Nevertheless, it is argued by some groups of researchers and public health analysts that public policy which has direct impact on social deprivation would contribute to improvements in health status.

The new public health movement is one reflection of the growing trend towards healthy public policy within the medical and nursing professions as well as among other professionals such as environmental health officers and local authority workers. Baum (1990) has suggested that the new public health is

> predicated on the belief that threats to the health of the public are not confined to disease and lifestyle risks. It argues they also emanate from social organisation and structure (p. 145).

This can be observed in the work of the Public Health Alliance, for example, which describes itself as an independent voluntary organisation bringing together individuals and organisations committed to public health. The Public Health Alliance campaigns for:

- equal opportunities for health and access to health services between rich and poor, women and men, people with disabilities and all racial and ethnic groups
- the restoration of Britain's public health heritage

- enhancing individual health by enlarging public and governmental responsibility for the health of everyone
- greater democracy and accountability within national and local government and the health service
- encouraging greater public awareness of health.

The Public Health Alliance remains a relatively small group whose influence is as yet unknown in terms of impact on health policy. However, the organisation remains vociferous in terms of arguing the case for public health ideals and for criticising policies such as *The Health of the Nation* and bringing these criticisms to the attention of the health professions. Whilst the intentions of the Public Health Alliance are honourable, Baum (1990) has also criticised the public health movement for being ostensibly altruistic which may be hindered by a history in the health professions of bureaucracy and control. He suggests that there is a naive expectation that different sectors will come together for the common good and that instead a new form of bureaucracy could be created (consisting of community workers, nurses, town planners and policy-makers, for example). The rhetoric expounded by the new public health movement, Baum argues, does not ensure that the movement will not simply become a different system of social surveillance and control rather than an enlightened approach to health promotion in accordance with people's wishes. Some of these criticisms will be addressed in the next section on health promotion approaches.

Implications for nursing

This section of the chapter has reviewed two health-related documents in relation to the concepts of individualism and collectivism in an attempt to illustrate the social and political context within which health is constructed and in which health promotion approaches are developed. How are these ideas relevant to nurses? In the first section the argument that health is central to the practice of nursing was proposed and a range of nurse theorists' views on health were explored. If this is the case, then it is axiomatic that nursing care has to make a difference to health, and therefore, in order to make professional decisions about health promotion nurses should have an appreciation of the political and social issues. However, the preceding discussion does present a dilemma for nurses. The vast majority of the literature on nursing implies that good practice is predicated on individualised care. This is implicit in the nursing process and in the theories and models of nursing that have been put forward, especially those expounded by the supporters of the so-called 'new nursing' such as McMahon and Pearson (1991). According to the arguments proposed above, individualism can be limiting in terms of lifestyle or behaviour change and in fact makes very little difference to those most at risk from serious illness or premature death. For example, whilst the over-all trend in smoking behaviour has decreased over the past 20 years from 41 percent for women in 1972 to 29 percent in 1990 and from 52 percent to 31 percent for men during the same period (Office of Population Censuses and Surveys, 1992), the health and lifestyle survey (Blaxter, 1990) demon-strated that there are large variations among socio-economic groups where, in her sample, 50 percent of unskilled men were smokers as were 45 percent of unskilled women, compared with 17 percent of men and 14 percent of women in the professional group. Whilst an individualist approach may have had an impact on the professional men and women, there is also the possibility that this trend would have occurred anyway and that this has clearly not had the same effect on those who are underprivileged. Should a nurse continue to give health information and advice on an individual level to a smoker or should she or he take more radical action which will make a difference to the conditions which make smoking the easier choice? It is difficult for nurses to consider the latter approach when the socialisation process into nursing stresses the nurse–patient relationship and the importance of individualised care; the nurse as a political person or an agent of radical change does not reflect the popular image. At the same time, providing high-quality care in a hospital or a community environment clearly does require the nurse to consider each patient and client as an individual within that environment. Clearly, the interrelationships between person, environment and health as stressed by many nurse theorists are a central consideration in the planning and imple-menting of care. Some experts have argued that nurses should be more political in their activities (White, 1986; Clay, 1987) and that as a profes-sional body there is great scope for significant impact to be made on policy and public health.

This requires a high degree of proactivity and a preparedness to take risk through advocating on behalf of vulnerable groups. For example, Gibson (1991) has argued that:

> Nursing practice needs to be defined so that nurses and nursing are oriented towards interventions at the macro-social level to promote health for all. There is a real need for nurses to turn their attention to the conditions that control, influence and produce health or illness in human beings. ... Rather than imposing their expertise on clients, they must use it as a tool for empowerment within the context of equal partnership with clients (p. 357).

Many nurses do not enter the profession with these activities in mind and their intentions are rein-forced by a profession within which the nurse –patient relationship remains the cornerstone of high-quality care.

There is, the writer believes, a middle ground where nurses can remain faithful to the ideology of individualised care whilst at the same time enabling individuals to change the conditions which make healthy choices easier choices. This approach can best be described as empowerment and does not preclude the practitioner who has the skills and competencies to engage in wider politi-cal action also. It does require self-awareness and skills beyond the one-to-one relationship. This empowering approach will form the focus of the next section.

Promoting health as a nursing activity

In the last section it was argued that there are conflicts inherent in the way in which health is constructed socially and politically. Whilst this is certainly true, nurses are nonetheless charged with promoting the health of their patients and clients both through the *Nurses, Midwives and Health Visitors Act* (DoH, 1992c) and through educational directives such as the English National Board Higher Award Framework (ENB, 1992). In the framework for the Higher Award, characteristic six states that the nurse should demonstrate 'Under-standing and use of health promotion and pre-ventive policies and strategies'. In this section, the focus will be on the empowering approach to health promotion as this has been proposed as an opportunity to combine individualised care with the potential for changing the conditions which make healthier choices more available. Through the use of examples and research findings, the empowering approach will be contrasted with other approaches. Despite the critique of *The Health of the Nation* which has been presented, this will be used as a framework for this section for two main reasons. The first is that it is, in fact, the most significant health policy that we have in England, and secondly, using the document as a framework does not preclude exploring the broader possibilities for health promotion.

Approaches to health promotion

Caplan (1993) has proposed a model for approaches to health promotion which encompasses some of the arguments which have been put forward in this chapter. It has been argued here that there is a dualism between individualism and collectivism. Caplan has argued that these can be translated into two theoretical approaches to health promotion – regulation and radical change. He argues that there are two dimensions within this, the objective and the subjective, which then give rise to four approaches to the practice of health promotion. These are represented in the model (Fig. 1.1).

To summarise Caplan's model, each approach is based on a view which a society might hold which will determine the sources of health problems and

therefore the aims of health promotion. This has been argued in the preceding section. I have tried to summarise within the model my interpretation of Caplan's four approaches. Caplan's humanist health education seems to encompass some of the ideas which would incorporate an empowering approach since this view acknowledges the meanings that individuals give to their health and activities and sees health education as improving our understanding of ourselves and others by exploring these meanings through improved communication. It also provides some justification for applying the empowering approach to nursing as Caplan has argued that, whilst collectivist in nature, the radical structuralist approach substitutes the objectivism of individual behaviour change for the objectivism of public policy which is still outside of the control of the individual. The emphasis in nursing on the care of the individual can therefore be embraced by an approach which aims to give the individual some control over his or her health. Tones (1991) has argued that empowered individuals make up empowered communities and it is at this level that political change may occur.

Empowerment

Tones (1986) argues that 'whilst understanding a health issue may be a precursor to action, it is not sufficient'. Thus, health educationists have argued that provision of information should be accompanied by a process of belief and values clarification, which should be followed by development of decision-making skills. The overall aim of the empowerment approach is therefore to foster informed choice, through a process of understanding people's meanings and definitions and enabling decision making. Empowerment is about enabling people to make their own decisions even if the decision which is finally arrived at is not that favoured by the health promoter. It is therefore important to ensure that the perceived healthy option is not the only option and that education for health does not become indoctrination (Campbell, 1990). However, empowerment does not simply aim to make people more skilled in their decision making, but to use those skills to empower themselves and others. In this way it is possible that social change can be brought about which would alter the environment in which people seek to become healthy.

Radical change

Radical health education Community action Self-help	Radical structuralist health education Political change

Subjective ———————————— **Objective**

Humanist health education Empowerment	Functionalist health education Prevention of disease

Regulation

Fig. 1.1. *Theoretical approaches to health education (adapted from Caplan, 1993).*

Tones *et al.* (1990) suggest that such a process involves addressing issues such as self-esteem and self-efficacy as well as social skills. Self-esteem is important as individuals who do not perceive themselves favourably may find it more difficult to change or to take health action. Self-efficacy relates to a person's perceptions of his or her own capabilities, which according to Bandura (1977a) can be influenced by past experience and through self-mastery by accomplishment of specific actions. Self-efficacy is also postulated by Pender (1987) as a determinant of health behaviour and recent research by Gillis (1993) has shown that self-efficacy is the most powerful psychological determinant of health behaviour. The concepts of self-esteem and self-efficacy may be considered to be of particular relevance to underprivileged groups and therefore a starting point for acknowledging the perceived health problems among different social groups.

Thus, the empowerment approach to health promotion involves much more than preventing disease through the provision of knowledge. The health promoter must be able to provide the information which people need to make an informed choice, but she also needs to be able to assess self-esteem and self-efficacy and to appreciate the health beliefs and values of others as well as enabling people to develop skills in decision making and assertiveness. This clearly requires a great deal of ability and initiative on the part of the health promoter and some nurses may not feel that they are prepared for such a role. It implies, for example, partnership between the nurse and the client in order for the client's meanings and self-efficacy to be explored. Research by Kendall (1993) has found that real participation between health visitors and clients can be hindered by communication style and rigid adherence to the professional agenda. Empowerment of individuals or groups is therefore dependent on self-awareness and reflexivity on the part of the health promoter. Salvage (1992) has explored the ideology of partnership between nurses and patients and has cautioned against assumptions being made about whether nurses and patients actually want the kind of therapeutic relationships which have been advocated by nurses such as McMahon and Pearson (1991) and also the extent to which nurses have explored the psychotherapeutic principles which are being advocated. There is a sociological argument that in order to empower clients, nurses

themselves need to have the authority and the autonomy to act, which is not readily obtainable in a system which promotes a hierarchical approach to the provision of care and sustains power relationships which subordinate on the basis of gender, class and race (Salvage, 1992). Empowerment is clearly not a straightforward approach to health promotion and may not present itself as the easy option when constraints such as time and staffing levels are currently high in nursing. Unfortunately, there is very little research evidence which actually compares health promotion approaches, largely because this entails methodological complexities which may be insurmountable – changes in policy may bring about a change in health trends over a long period of time where other factors are uncontrollable, for example. It cannot be assumed, except at a theoretical level, that empowerment is more effective than other approaches.

Application of the empowerment approach to The Health of the Nation

It is not possible within the confines of this chapter to review each of the targets separately in relation to possibilities for health promotion. Examples of a variety of aspects relating to all the targets are provided throughout this section and you are encouraged to read the document for the full details and to make applications for yourself based on the principles described below.

Each of the targets within *The Health of the Nation* were selected by the Secretary of State because they were a significant health concern where it was perceived that demonstrable differences could be achieved, although the government has been criticised for selecting health concerns where downward trends are already observable and the success of the policy will therefore be 'haloed' by this effect (Public Health Alliance, 1992). For example, the document states that 'coronary heart disease accounted for about 26 percent of deaths in England in 1991. It is both the single largest cause of death and the single main cause of premature death. It accounts for 2.5 percent of NHS expenditure, and results in 35 million lost working days each year. Although the death rate for CHD in England has been declining since the late 1970s, it remains one of the highest in the world' (p. 46).

Summary of The Health of the Nation *targets (DoH, 1992, pp. 18–19)*

Coronary heart disease (CHD) and stroke
To reduce the death rate for both CHD and stroke in people under 65 by 40 percent by the year 2000 (Baseline 1990)
To reduce the death rate from CHD in people aged 65–74 by at least 30 percent by the year 2000 (Baseline 1990)
To reduce the death rate for stroke in people aged 65–74 by at least 40 percent by the year 2000 (Baseline 1990)

Cancers
To reduce the death rate for breast cancer in the population invited for screening by at least 25 percent by the year 2000 (Baseline 1990)
To reduce the incidence of invasive cervical cancer by at least 20 percent by the year 2000 (Baseline 1986)
To reduce the death rate for lung cancer under the age of 75 by at least 30 percent in men and by at least 15 percent in women by the year 2010 (Baseline 1990)
To halt the year-on-year increase in the incidence of skin cancer by the year 2005

Mental illness
To improve significantly the health and social functioning of mentally ill people
To reduce the overall suicide rate by at least 155 by the year 2000 (Baseline 1990)
To reduce the suicide rate of severely mentally ill people by at least 33 percent by the year 2000 (Baseline 1990)

HIV/AIDS and sexual health
To reduce the incidence of gonorrhoea by at least 20 percent by 1995 (Baseline 1990), as an indicator of HIV/AIDS trends
To reduce by at least 50 percent the rate of conceptions amongst the under-16s by the year 2000 (Baseline 1989)

Accidents
To reduce the death rate for accidents among children aged under 15 by at least 33 percent by the year 2005 (Baseline 1990)
To reduce the death rate for accidents among young people aged 15–24 by at least 25 percent by 2005 (Baseline 1990)
To reduce the death rate for accidents among people aged 65 and over by at least 33 percent by 2005 (Baseline 1990)

One immediately has to question why the death rates for CHD in England are so alarming and what can be done about it. The individualist response would be to examine the lifestyles of the English population and to suggest ways that individuals could change their lifestyle to reduce the risk factors involved. These are largely held to be cigarette smoking, raised plasma cholesterol, raised blood pressure and lack of physical activity. *The Health of the Nation* supports this view. For example, in relation to diet it exhorts the Health Education Authority to continue to develop nutrition education resources, health and local authorities to maximise opportunities for educating people about healthy eating and the media to give information to the public about diet and nutrition which will encourage healthy eating. It includes recommendations to the food manufacturing industry to improve food labelling and to use marketing policies which are more conducive to healthy foods. This is based on the assumption that people can read, are interested in the nutritional content of food and can afford the healthier food options which would undoubtedly attract higher prices with the overheads from new marketing strategies. It has already been argued that these measures alone are unlikely to produce major changes in behaviour which is socially and economically determined.

In relation to cancers , cervical cancer is seen to be a concern since while the death rate is only 1500 per year (low compared to other causes of death, such as lung cancer at 26,000 deaths per year) it is a preventable form of cancer. The emphasis of *The Health of the Nation* is therefore on screening and the particular benefits of women between 20 and 64 attending the national cervical screening programme. The success of this assumes that all women within this age group will be reminded about screening, will want to attend and will be willing to have the test carried out. There is evidence that this is not always the case (King, 1987).

By using the empowering approach the nurse could:
1. *Explore the meanings, beliefs and values that individuals and small groups (such as the family) assign to health and the implications for them of having a heart attack or getting cancer, for example.* This would take into account the cultural, environmental and social perspectives which contribute to

a person's belief system. For example, a study by Davison *et al.* (1991) discusses the concept of 'coronary candidacy' in relation to lay epidemiology, that there is 'a type of person' who is subject to a heart attack and which is the subject of discussion within the lay community. Understanding whether a person perceives himself or members of his family to be a coronary candidate would be an important aspect of understanding the person's explanatory model in relation to health behaviour and heart disease.

One of the obstacles which prevents women taking up the screening service is their fears and beliefs about the nature of cancer (King, 1987). Accepting screening is an acknowledgement of cancer. Despite the fact that many forms of cancer are now curable, many people equate cancer with certain death and prefer to dissociate from it completely. Susan Sontag (1978) has described how it is the metaphoric invasion and destruction of the body by the advancing army of cancer which seems to differentiate it in people's minds from other diseases. Nurses also may find it difficult to discuss cancer, especially in cases where the client is unaware of her diagnosis. Even the discussion of screening can be hard if both nurse and client are trying to avoid the difficult issue of cancer. Being frank about the purpose of cervical screening brings cancer out into the open. It takes a great deal of skill on the part of the nurse if she is to help the client to overcome her fears. A study by King (1987) has found that generally older women attribute cervical cancer to a 'germ' or 'smoking' and therefore resisted the test on the grounds that it did not apply to them. She also found that older women tended to resist screening as they felt that it reflected on their morality, as cervical cancer was thought to be a 'dirty' disease resulting from 'promiscuity'. Clearly, to enable a woman to feel she can undergo a screening test, these beliefs need to be understood by the nurse who at the same time should be aware of her own response to cancer and related issues. A more recent survey carried out in the United States (Zabalegui, 1994) has also found correlations between perceptions of health and attendance for cancer screening among elderly people, where those having a high perception of their health according to the scale designed by the author, were also more likely to attend for cancer screening. This again suggests that it is important to understand the person's health perceptions when encouraging attendance for screening.

King's (1987) study also found that resistance to cervical screening among older women was often due to fear of the test itself. It was held to be a painful procedure and many were reluctant to be examined internally, particularly by a male doctor. King concludes that beliefs about the test are the strongest indicators of non-attendance. Nurses can use this research finding by helping women, especially in middle age, to understand the nature of the test and reinforcing its benefits to all age groups. This implies that nurses themselves, especially those working closely with women, such as midwives and health visitors, must have a good knowledge of the screening procedure including not only the technical aspects but also what the local policy is for call and re-call and the communication of results. There is also scope, in some settings, for ensuring that a woman's preference for a female doctor is acknowledged and put into practice, even if this means referral to another area.

2. *Provide information about the target area if this is appropriate and likely to be in line with the individual's concept of health.* For example, if the person does not believe him- or herself to be a 'coronary candidate' then advice and information about dietary fat or exercise performance are unlikely to alter this perception over a short period of time.

A review by Towner *et al.* (1993) on the effectiveness of health promotion interventions in relation to accidents found that there have been varying success rates among studies which focus on education and information-giving about accidents in the home [critically important because most deaths for children under 5 years old occur in the home (Department of Trade and Industry, 1992)]. Whilst some of the studies reviewed appear to have concentrated on campaigns and safety inspections with advice-giving, one study is notable in that a mass media campaign was combined with home visits by health visitors (Colver *et al.*, 1982). The study found that 60 percent of the intervention group made some physical change in the home environment, compared to 9 percent of the control group. The conclusion by the author is important:

> Our most encouraging finding is that even the most severely disadvantaged families will respond to health education *if the education is appropriate* (p. 27, cited by Towner *et al.*, 1993, my emphasis).

The participants in this study were given small,

concrete pieces of information which they could realistically respond to in terms of reducing hazards for their children. Although we do not know from this citation how the information was given to the parents, it may be assumed that information which is supportive and acknowledges the value that children have within the family is more likely to be accepted than information which blames parents for bad practices in the home.

3. *Exploring personal control with the person. Health behaviours are associated with the degree of control which people perceive themselves to have over events.* Some research has found that the role of chance in the causation of disease may play a role in people's lifestyle choices (Pill and Stott, 1985). However, the same researchers caution against stereotyping people into 'fatalists' on the basis of social class or educational level as there does not appear to be a clear-cut relationship.

Personal control is also concerned with perceptions of self-efficacy or people's perceptions of what they are capable of achieving. Self-efficacy theory is derived from Bandura's (1977b) work in social learning theory. Social learning theory uses several key concepts to explain and predict behaviour: incentives, outcome expectations and self-efficacy expectations. The concept of self-efficacy expectation is of particular relevance to health promotion.

Bandura (1977a) outlines the role of self-efficacy in the paradigm of a person engaging in a behaviour that will have a consequent outcome (see Fig. 1.2).

When considering self-efficacy, Bandura (1977a) suggests that an important distinction is made between perceived self-efficacy and outcome expectations. Perceived self-efficacy refers to peoples' judgements of their capabilities to execute given levels of performance whilst outcome expectations are judgements of the likely consequences that such behaviour will produce. This may refer, for example, to a person's belief that losing weight will result in less risk of a heart attack (outcome expectation) but their perceived capability of actually carrying out behaviours which

achieve this outcome may be low due to factors such as previous experience of diets not working, perceived lack of exercise facilities or lack of time to prepare special foods. If perceived self-efficacy is low, then the benefits of taking the action will be overridden and the behaviour will not be performed. It is important to remember that perceived self-efficacy refers to a person's beliefs about their perceived capabilities and not necessarily their true capabilities. It therefore becomes important to understand these beliefs before behaviour change can be facilitated.

Equally important in understanding the concept is Bandura's argument that self-efficacy is specific to particular behaviours and particular situations. For example, a pregnant woman may feel she is capable of giving up smoking, but not able to lose weight when she is not pregnant. It is not therefore possible to generalise and label a person as having either 'high' or 'low' self-efficacy without reference to the specific behaviour or situation.

The construct of self-efficacy has been subject to considerable empirical research in relation to its reliability in predicting and explaining health-related behaviour. Strecher *et al.* (1986) have published a comprehensive review of 21 research studies which relate to health behaviours including smoking, weight loss, alcohol misuse and contraception use. For example, in relation to smoking behaviour, Prochaska and DiClemente (1984) found in a survey of 872 smokers that perceived self-efficacy ratings were related to stages in the cycle of stopping smoking. As people progressed from thinking about stopping to maintenance of stopping their self-efficacy increased. An earlier study by DiClemente (1981) found that self-efficacy was predictive of smoking cessation, although this study used a much smaller sample size of 63 heavy smokers.

In relation to contraception use, Gilchrist and Schinke (1983) found that adolescents showed marked improvements in self-efficacy ratings of their own ability to use birth control which was exhibited by more effective contraceptive problem-solving abilities and greater intentions to use contraception. The study used a cognitive–behavioural treatment which aimed to increase self-efficacy through role playing and skills training in relation to contraception. This could be valuable in terms of reducing teenage pregnancy over the next decade as the rate of conception may be more strongly associated with young peoples' perceptions of their

Person - - - - - - - - - - ▶ Behaviour - - - - - - - - ▶ Outcome

Fig. 1.2. Bandura's model of behaviour and outcome.

problem-solving abilities in the face of peer pressure, for example, than with the need for information and education.

Strecher *et al.* (1986) comment that 'self-efficacy appears to be a consistent predictor of short and long-term success' (p. 87). In support of these findings, Gillis (1993), in a review of determinants of a health promoting lifestyle in which 23 studies were examined, suggested that 'the most consistent findings identified self-efficacy as the strongest determinant of participation in a health-promoting lifestyle' (p. 351).

The nature of these studies suggests that perceived self-efficacy can be changed or enhanced, thus enabling an individual to feel more efficacious in carrying out a behaviour. Bandura (1977a) suggests a number of ways in which self-efficacy is informed and which could therefore be drawn on to enhance it. These approaches have been used by Bandura in helping people to overcome phobias, but there is little empirical evidence of their utilisation in health promotion. Nevertheless, they do appear to have clinical relevance to health behaviour and a study by Sturt and Kendall is currently being conducted to evaluate their potential for enabling people to change. According to Bandura, self-efficacy is informed by the following.

Performance accomplishment

This source of efficacy information is especially influential because it is based on personal mastery experiences. Successes raise mastery expectations; repeated failures lower them, particularly if the failures occur early in the course of events. After strong efficacy expectations are developed through repeated success, the negative impact of occasional failure is likely to be reduced. For example, Brown and Harris (1978) in a notable study on the origins of depression among women, found that there were some key vulnerability factors identified as:

1. loss of her own mother before 11 years of age
2. absence of a confiding relationship with a partner
3. lack of employment outside the home
4. presence of three or more children under 15 years of age.

Brown and Harris (1978) and sociologists who have analysed these findings contend that the origins of depression for these women are undoubtedly social and economic ones. However, these very social conditions may affect a woman's self-efficacy in relation to her multiple roles of mother, bread-winner, housewife and partner. Recognition of a possible relationship between social factors and subsequent behaviour could be important in health promotion. In this example, self-efficacy might be increased if the woman feels that she is performing well as a mother. If her experience with the first child is positive in this respect, then it is likely (within Bandura's framework) that subsequent behaviours and outcomes will be more positive. Thus, there may be opportunities for nurses working with women to reinforce the positive aspects of their child-rearing practices. This has yet to be demonstrated through research.

Vicarious experience

Bandura (1977a) also suggests that self-efficacy is influenced not only by personal experience, but also by observation of the experience of others. Thus, if another person is perceived to have mastery over a situation, then this could enhance the belief of the individual that she too could be successful. Using Brown and Harris's (1978) findings, it is possible that if a child loses his or her own mother before 11 years of age, then he or she has not had the opportunity to develop his or her own skills through observation, practice and reinforcement of mothering from this vicarious source of self-efficacy information.

This could provide the theoretical basis for parenthood groups and post-natal groups in which vicarious experience could be gained from other women. On the other hand, observation of another's negative experience can be equally powerful in reducing perceived self-efficacy. For example, if a mother receives positive reinforcement to breast feed which increases her self-efficacy in relation to motherhood, this could be decreased if other mothers are perceived to be having a better nights sleep if they bottle feed – only to find that sleep patterns do not change that dramatically when a baby changes from breast to bottle.

Verbal persuasion

Bandura suggests that verbal persuasion is the most easily available technique for changing self-efficacy but not necessarily the most effective. Although an individual might be verbally persuaded that he or she can cope with an experience, mastery expectations can be readily extinguished by negative experiences. It is thought that the main value of social persuasion is in conjunction with performance mastery. In nursing, the verbal contact is the practitioner's most readily available tool which must therefore be used with some caution if the individual cannot be provided with opportunities to increase self-mastery. Continuing with the example of depression among women, verbally persuading the woman to find a job outside the home is far more easily said than done and where there are one or more children acknowledgement has to be made of child-care issues and the economic balance of working versus staying at home. The study by Kendall (1993) found that advice-giving by health visitors was frequently unsolicited and that this could be implicated in mothers and health visitors having different perceptions about home visits. This would be unlikely to have positive effects on self-efficacy.

Stress reduction

Stressful and taxing situations generally elicit emotional responses which, depending on the circumstances, might have information value concerning personal competence. Therefore, emotional arousal is another source of information that can affect perceived self-efficacy. People rely partly on their state of psychological arousal in judging their anxiety and vulnerability to stress. Because high arousal usually inhibits performance, individuals are more likely to expect success when they are not beset by aversive stimuli or if they are tense and agitated. Thus, stress reduction, Bandura advocates, should be attempted through helping people to develop mastery over aversive situations. Clearly, Brown and Harris (1978) have identified a set of vulnerability factors each one of which could be stressful in its own right and taken together are thought to be the cause of high rates of depression among women. It would be a very complex task for general nurses or even health visitors or midwives to help women to overcome the stress which is self-evident and this role would be more appropriately allocated to the community psychiatric nurse. However, it is often the practice nurse or the health visitor who has initial contact and perhaps simply identifying the factors and using stress reduction techniques, such as relaxation, in some discrete areas may help the woman to increase her self-efficacy in some specific aspects.

These four areas of influencing self-efficacy expectations clearly have implications for those involved with health promotion. Steele *et al.* (1987) suggest that health professionals should assess their patients' self-efficacy perceptions and tailor interventions to those perceptions. Likewise, Barlett (1983) has commented that 'self-efficacy theory provides a theoretical buttress for the notion of the "activated" patient' (p. 547). The concept of self-efficacy does therefore appear to be conducive to the ideology of partnership with clients and patients.

As Steele *et al.* (1987) have proposed:

> Clinicians should therefore actively elicit and try to understand their patients' perspectives and formulate approaches to treatment that are in line with those perspectives (p. 20).

Taking the self-efficacy theory to its logical conclusion may include acceptance that a client's perceived self-efficacy is too low to carry out a behaviour. This could mean working through an experience with them or giving them opportunities to observe others successfully carrying out the behaviour in conjunction with some verbal encouragement and anxiety reduction measures, before it can be realistically expected that the client will carry out the behaviour.

Some detail has been given to the self-efficacy concept as it is potentially this which differentiates an empowering approach from a purely preventive one. This perception of determination over behaviour and subsequent events may be the key to personal decision making about health behaviour. Tones *et al.* (1990) have also argued that positive changes in self-efficacy are healthy in themselves and this could be important in promoting changes in mental health in particular.

Reflective point

As you practise health promotion within your own area reflect on the following key points and try to think about how you could be more effective as a health promoter (you will need to identify a client with whom you have recently used health promotion strategies):

1. Am I considering the client's perception of health and his or her beliefs and values in relation to the health target I am addressing? Make a note of one client's beliefs about health and how different or similar they were to your own.

2. *What information should I be offering to this client? Is it appropriate to their meaning of health and their beliefs? Write down what information you gave to the client identified in (1).*

3. *To what extent did I try to understand the client's perceived self-efficacy in relation to the health behaviour under consideration? How did I try to evaluate or enhance this?*

4. *How can I measure my success as a health promoter? Have I empowered the client? What other approaches could I have used?*

Measuring health

One of the most important questions that nurses in all specialities have to ask themselves is 'How do I know that health has been achieved?'. With regard to the earlier discussion on individual and subjective views on health the simple answer may well be to ask the patient or client. However, whilst this may provide a measure of health for the individual at that moment in time it does not provide the systematic measurement of health outcomes which are necessary if nurses are to maintain their professional position in relation to demonstrating their value in contributing to health promotion. It is therefore imperative that nurses consider a range of possibilities for measuring health which may also be useful in measuring and documenting nursing outcomes. Reynolds (1988) has reviewed a number of approaches to the measurement of health in nursing research. She reviewed the literature in four American journals between 1977 and 1987 in which the concept of health was clearly operationalised. Reynolds excluded qualitative reports at this stage because it is not usually considered appropriate to define the concept of health at the outset of a qualitative study. However, this does mean that the review is limited to quantitative measures. She found that 17 articles met these criteria and that of these physical measures were most widely used (16). These included measures such as physical examination and assessment of prescribed drug use. Clearly such measures on their own cannot give a reliable measure of health, as the label of 'healthy' or 'unhealthy' is a purely diagnostic one. Reynolds found that mental health measures were used in

eight studies, most often in the form of a scale to measure depression, and subjective/self-report measures in 14 studies. Many of the self-reports included reports of physical health. It was more likely that single measures (10) were adopted than multiple measures (7). Reynolds critiques these studies for their generally low reports of reliability and validity. This is significant because whilst the measures may have been useful for the particular populations within the reported studies, there is no scientific merit in using the same measures either in other research studies or in practice. In addition she found that the concepts and measurement of health were rarely based on theoretical constructs:

> The literature examined did not support the plethora of ideas to which so many nurses claim to subscribe, nor did it reflect a holistic stance. Despite literature urging the contrary, it appears that health continues to be understood by nurse researchers mainly in the context of polar opposites (p. 28).

Clearly it would be unwise to assume that one limited American review of the literature covers the extent of our knowledge in measuring health. It does provide a very interesting insight, however, into the current situation which can be considered in the light of further discussion on specific approaches to the measurement of health.

Approaches to measuring health

Mortality and morbidity rates

Mortality and morbidity rates include measures such as perinatal mortality, standardised mortality ratios and maternal mortality. These measures are most often used by epidemiologists to determine the incidence and prevalence of disease in populations. As discussed in the previous section, such indices underpin *The Health of the Nation* policy and have been most widely criticised as measures of death and disease rather then health (Hunt and McEwan, 1980). Some such measures are used in crude terms (e.g. crude mortality rate = number of deaths per year) which means that specific groups at risk or age-related factors cannot be identified from the data whilst others are known as refined indices and include incidence and prevalence rates for specific diseases, absence from work, episodes of illness, type and duration of disability. Clearly these data are important to our understanding of health and illness trends within populations and also provide indicators of where we should target preventive work. They do not, however, provide a holistic measure of health but look at only one aspect which is related to medical diagnosis.

Functional ability

These measures focus on clinical symptoms, or ability to function in one's role or the effect of illness or disability on activities in social, domestic and personal life. They are closely related to the definition of health described by Parsons (1981) and discussed earlier in the chapter. An example would be the activities of daily living index (Katz *et al.*, 1963). Again, such measures have limited application when one considers health from a holistic stance

Psychological well-being

Measures of mental health or psychological well-being are useful when one is specifically trying to measure specific symptoms or attributes such as depression or anxiety. They are more disease oriented than health oriented and are perhaps most usefully employed when it is important to determine rates of psychiatric disturbance within populations. Examples of these measures include the General Health Questionnaire (GHQ) (Goldberg and Williams, 1988) and the Hospital Anxiety and Depression Scale (Zigmond and Snaith, 1983).

Subjective health indices

These focus on how people feel about their illness/disability and how they perceive it to be affecting their lives. Whilst they do have the overall intention to gather data about individuals' perceived health status, they tend to focus on the negative aspects. The Nottingham Health Profile (Hunt and McEwan, 1980), for example, uses statements such as 'the days seem to drag' and 'I lose my temper easily' as indicators of subjective health. The Health Measurement Questionnaire (Centre for Health Economics, York University, 1991) has introduced quality of life indicators into its format but these themselves are derived from data on illness and disability.

Physical fitness indicators

These indicators focus more on positive health and fitness as indicators of health. For example, the Allied Dunbar Fitness Survey (Sports Council and the Health Education Authority, 1992) reported on sports activities and ability to perform a range of physical fitness tests. Whilst the emphasis is on positive health rather than illness, the measure is a purely physical one and takes no account of subjective accounts.

Social support

Research in this area is quite limited but work has been done to develop a measure of health in terms of a person's social support mechanisms, known as the Social Support Questionnaire (Sarason *et al.*, 1987). Whilst this may be a very useful adjunct to assessing health status it is important to recognise that the instrument is an indirect measure of health as it was designed to measure the social support construct.

Some of these measures will now be addressed in more detail and their application for practice explored.

The Nottingham Health Profile (Hunt and McEwen, 1980)

The Nottingham Health Profile (NHP) was developed from a need to complement objective, empiricist measures with subjective, existentialist measures:

> It is a more fruitful approach to regard the two aspects as being essential to our knowledge of human beings and their reactions – the one view enriching the other (Hunt and McEwan, 1980, p. 235).

The scale was developed in two phases. Phase one involved interviews with 768 individuals with varying degrees of acute and chronic illness. From this the researchers derived 2200 statements describing typical effects of ill-health and this was refined to 82 items covering 12 domains such as sleeping, eating, mobility, emotional reactions, etc.

In Phase two the tool was developed as an evaluative tool and instrument for population survey. The instrument is divided into six 'packages', each having its own weighted score out of 100. The overall score is therefore a profile rather than a summated score. The higher the score, the greater the perceived dysfunction.

The profile was found to have discriminant validity between patients with different health statuses and sensitivity to changes over time in people with severe conditions.

However, the instrument has been criticised by Bowling (1991) on a range of grounds:

- it is a limited measure of function, for example sensory defects are not accounted for
- it lacks an index of mental distress
- it has a highly skewed distribution. This means that the nature of the questions results in a high percentage of zero scores and therefore the interpretation of scores within a population has to be understood in this context
- it is a negative measure of health.

The NHP may be useful in specific situations where you need to make an individual assessment of perceived health status. Students who have tried this scale almost invariably have scored zero and feel it is most applicable to elderly or chronically sick or disabled people. With such client groups it should be theoretically possible to measure their subjective health status using the NHP and to measure the effect of nursing care by using it as an evaluative tool, but no such research has been identified in the literature.

The Health Measurement Questionnaire (Kind and Gudex, 1991)

The Health Measurement Questionnaire (HMQ) is a self-report scale from which a disability/distress rating can be derived on the Rosser Classification of Illness States. The Rosser scale (Rosser and Kind, 1978) is used as an indicator of quality of life and ranges from no distress/no disability which scores 1 to severe distress/confined to bed which scores–1.486, where 0 = dead. Therefore, in terms of quality of life the Rosser scale indicates states which can be perceived to be worse than death. The HMQ attempts to ascertain a person's quality of life by asking a range of questions which relate either to distress or to disability and translating the findings into a Rosser score. The authors of the HMQ suggest that a self-report scale is more appropriate than an observer-rated scale when measuring the health of the community.

The HMQ was developed in a study in Wolverhampton where 430 randomised individuals were interviewed at home during October/November 1986. A battery of questionnaires collecting information on health behaviour, life events, medical history and socio-demographic variables were administered. This was known as the 'core data set'. All participants completed the HMQ, half the NHP and half the GHQ and results were compared to the core data set. There were few inconsistencies between the HMQ and the core data set, but where these did exist it raised the question of the reliability of the respondent and the schedules.

Among people identified as being in poor health, the HMQ was found to have discriminant validity as they were found to have significantly lower Rosser-derived scores than those classified as healthy.

Can the HMQ be applied to practice? Clearly, it does provide some indication of how people might perceive their quality of life which is closely related to health. However, it does raise some dilemmas. What is the role of the nurse if a person's score is less than zero, for example? Is it possible to promote a person's health so that their quality of life is better than being dead? Does the instrument enable the nurse to identify sources of distress which she may be able to alleviate or modify? These questions are beyond the scope of this chapter but are important to consider within the overall debate on health promotion.

Physical fitness (Lamb *et al.*, 1988). Physical fitness and health-related fitness as indicators of a positive health state

These authors focus on the need for a measure of positive health defined as 'the potential of the human condition' and 'concerned with thriving rather than mere coping' (Nutbeam, 1986). It extends the health continuum from ill- to normal health to a state of above normal or 'superhealth'.

Fitness is seen as a relative attribute, the indicators of positive health for an elderly person exercising regularly would be lower than for those of an athlete, but both may be considered to be fit within their groups.

Measures of fitness include:

- agility
- flexibility
- power
- speed and reaction time
- strength
- cardiovascular and respiratory capacity

- maintenance of correct body composition
- posture.

The authors advocate the measurement of health-related fitness to be combined with a subjective health questionnaire which focuses on positive health in order to explore the relationship between physical fitness and self-perceived health. Unfortunately, as we have seen, there does not yet exist a reliable and valid subjective indicator of positive health.

Little work has been carried out using the concept of fitness to measure health, but one major UK study which is of interest is the Allied Dunbar Fitness Survey (Sports Council and the Health Education Authority, 1992)

In this study a random sample of 4316 people completed a home interview and 70 percent of these took part in a physical appraisal. The interview included measurement of behaviour, attitudes and beliefs towards:

- levels of participation in sport and active recreation, past and present
- physical activity at work or home
- other lifestyle and health-related behaviour, e.g. smoking
- current health status and history of illness
- sports-related injuries
- knowledge about exercise and attitudes towards physical activity, fitness and health
- psychological variables including well-being, social support, stress and anxiety.

Fitness measures included:

- body composition – height, weight, skinfold
- blood pressure – to screen those at risk of CHD
- muscle function – in terms of strength and power
- flexibility – shoulder abduction
- aerobic capacity – treadmill exercise.

An activity scale was devised to determine people's activity levels based on their reports:

Level	Activity of 20 min duration in the previous 4 weeks
Level 5	12 or more occasions of vigorous activity
Level 4	12 or more occasions of a mix of moderate and vigorous activity
Level 3	12 or more occasions of moderate activity
Level 2	5 to 11 occasions of a mix of moderate and vigorous activity
Level 1	1 to 4 occasions of a mix of moderate and vigorous activity
Level 0	None

where activities are defined as:

- light, e.g. long, slow walks, light DIY, golf, bowls, fishing
- moderate, e.g. long walks at brisk pace, football, swimming, tennis, cycling if not out of breath or sweaty, heavy DIY or housework
- vigorous, e.g. hill-walking, squash, running, football, swimming, tennis, cycling, aerobics if out of breath or sweaty, heavy manual work.

Significant findings

- The proportion of women of all ages who are active at levels 4 and 5 is very low.
- Overall, 1 in 6 people fell in activity level 0.
- Activity levels varied according to social class.
- Men who smoked were less active at levels 4 and 5 than non-smokers.
- Forty-eight percent of men and 40 percent of women were overweight.
- Estimated that one-third of men and two-thirds of women would find it difficult to sustain walking at a reasonable pace up a 1 in 20 slope.
- Estimated that if everyone overweight or obese lost 22 lb, the number having problems rising from a chair unaided would decrease by over one-third and the percentage having difficulty in walking up a 1 in 20 slope would decrease by 37 percent in men and 19 percent in women.
- Eighty percent of men and women of all ages believed themselves to be fit and the majority incorrectly believed that they did enough exercise to keep fit.
- Sixty-one percent of men and 69 percent of women in activity level 0 believed themselves to be very or fairly fit.
- Eighty percent expressed a strong belief in the value of exercise to health and fitness while only a minority actually engaged in physical activity of a moderate or vigorous level.

These findings are of significance in relation to identifying individuals at risk from CHD, for example. They are also useful in identifying the factors that do facilitate a positive approach to health and fitness and could be helpful in determining lifestyle factors which protect from risk factors such as obesity and hypertension. To use this approach to health in practice, a nurse would have to be skilled in a number of physical fitness tests and would have to have particular items of equipment available. This may not be a practical proposition in most circumstances. However, where particular interventions were being tried out, then it may be appropriate to use these measures. An example might be a programme within a primary health-care team to raise awareness about stroke prevention.

What conclusions can we draw about the idea of measuring health and promoting health in nursing practice?

On the basis of this brief review of approaches to measuring health, it would appear that Reynolds' (1988) contention that there are no holistic measures of health which incorporate the theoretical constructs which nurses claim to espouse holds true. There is little evidence of positive health measures existing at all and where they do they are limited to specific attributes, as in the case of fitness. There is clearly room for research here both in the development of new measures and in the further testing of existing ones.

There is a need for nurses to explore the possibilities for measuring health as part of current practice and to develop practice in the future. A recent survey carried out by the DoH (1993) found that whilst there was a great deal of evidence of good practice in relation to nurses' contributions to *The Health of the Nation*, few of the practices were research-based and few used evaluative tools to demonstrate their effectiveness. The qualitative elements of health promotion need to be carefully documented. Building up databases of evidence about how people feel about their health and how they respond to interventions is invaluable. Such data would enable theories of health promotion and nursing to develop and from this nursing outcomes can be identified through the testing of theory in practice. Whilst there is tremendous potential for nurses to develop their role and scope in the promotion of health, there remains a need to demonstrate that nursing does make a difference to health.

Reflective point

How do you measure health in your area of practice? Select a sample of your care plans or case notes from the last three months of your work and review them in terms of:

- *how health was assessed;*
- *what nursing interventions were carried out and why;*
- *how health was evaluated.*

What did you find?
Is there scope for change in the future?
What are the key changes you would make in relation to measuring and evaluating health?

You could work with a group of colleagues to identify the most appropriate ways of measuring health for your area of practice.

Conclusions

The preceding sections of this chapter have attempted to analyse the concept of health to examine a number of issues which arise from this in relation to the practice of health promotion. The discussion has been broad-ranging in that it attempts to cover many aspects of health from the social and political to the personal. The author makes no apology for this. Nursing is a practice-based discipline and as such it has to inform its knowledge base from a wide range of sources. If health, as has been argued, is central to nursing practice, then as a profession we need to appreciate both sociological and psychological perspectives in addition to our long-standing medically based knowledge. However, hereby hangs a dilemma for nursing. Whilst health has become the subject of much debate and discussion amongst nurse scholars, little attention has been paid to how we can bring perspectives together to become more effective as health promoters whilst at the same time retaining that which is most valued by nurses, the nurse–patient relationship. Thus, the section on the context of health was a polemic on the ideologies of individualism and collectivism which aimed to raise some of the serious issues about health which nurses need to be aware of in their practice of health promotion. It was implicit in this section that health is largely politically constructed and that to have any demonstrable effect on the health of the nation, nurses would need to be more proactive at the macro-social level. In order to try and overcome some of the dissonance which may be caused for nurses by raising their consciousness of political issues, but at the same time valuing the one-to-one relationship, the section on promoting health has focused on the empowering approach. Using Caplan's (1993) model of health promotion, this approach has been identified as one which may be the most appropriate for nursing practice as it seeks to move away from a purely preventive approach in which advice and education are the main aim, towards an approach where the nurse can enable the person to feel more able to deal with the conditions which make changes in health behaviour difficult. This empowering approach will not result in immediate political change and may be seen by some as ducking the issue of social reform. However, like Tones (1991) the author contends that by empowering individuals, communities may become more able to recognise their own health needs and take action which may eventually result in political change. To make any serious impact on the major determinant of ill-health – poverty – there has to be complete ideological and cultural reform which nursing alone cannot achieve. This is not a defeatist attitude, it is a realistic one. By raising awareness among nurses of the social and political factors affecting health it might be realistic to expect that this will raise the level of debate among nurses and within the multidisciplinary team. Nurses, doctors, therapists and community workers together may have some impact, but the real impact will come from the individuals and communities we are trying to help. To bring the argument full circle, perhaps we can only really help those people through practising the fundamental principles of nursing such as trust, mutual respect and partnership. *The Health of the Nation* (DoH, 1992a) has been referred to as a framework for health promotion because it is the current health policy and it does provide fodder for critical debate. Examples from research have been cited as to where nurses may be able to contribute to the targets and much emphasis has been placed on the concept of self-efficacy as a way forward within the empowerment approach. Future research needs to consider seriously the contribution of self-efficacy to practice, as to date it has largely been examined as a theoretical construct in psychological research.

A crucial debate for nurses has to be

demonstration of effectiveness. Increasingly, the purchaser–provider contract will be taking account of what nurses can really contribute to health gain within the trust community. Nurses can no longer rely on the rhetoric of nursing theory regarding the centrality of health to their practice; they have to be able to demonstrate that they can make real changes which are both effective and efficient. This means that nurses have to examine more closely how health is measured and be prepared both to challenge the *status quo* and to explore valid alternatives. The section on measuring health raised some issues about the range of approaches which are available and their limitations. There appears to be scope for developing new measures which take account of both objective and subjective factors and which can be readily applied in practice. It is important that nurses themselves develop these indicators so that quality of nursing care can be readily defined. Standards for health promotion in practice settings are equally as important as standards for wound care or pain management. Through a process of standard setting and monitoring procedures it may be possible for a range of indicators of health outcome to be developed.

Important professional issues are at stake here. In order to be accountable for practice, the nurse has to be able to make informed decisions about health and health promotion and she has to be able to select knowledgeably from a range of theories and skills in order to practise. This implies a degree of autonomy in practice where quality of care will depend on effective independent decision making and communication of actions and intended actions to colleagues, relatives and the person concerned. Advocacy is also an important element of the professional nurses' role and will certainly be implemented in health promotion, especially when empowerment is the focus of action. This, in turn, will involve the nurse in assertiveness, risk-taking and a high degree of commitment to both client and goal. These elements of professionalism are key components of the UKCC Code of Professional Conduct (UKCC, 1992). Their true value, and ultimately the worth of professional action to the client, lies with the nurse being assigned the authority to act professionally. Marie Manthey (1992) has argued that currently nurses are being given responsibility to achieve quality of care without authority, and that until nurses are themselves empowered to practise the high quality care they know they can achieve, then it is difficult, if not impossible, for nurses to empower their clients and patients. We need to know more about the styles of leadership and management which enable nurses to practise professionally and autonomously and which produce high quality care from both nursing and patient perspectives, especially in relation to health promotion which has traditionally been seen as an added extra rather than an intrinsic part of practice.

In the Introduction it was stated that the author believes health is the ultimate goal of nursing. This remains the case although it is clear from the issues raised in this chapter that promoting health is not a simple process and that there are still many areas which need further refinement and research. *The Health of the Nation* claims that there will be subsequent health targets for future national interest. Perhaps nurses could become key players in identifying the targets for the future and determining the approaches which may be most beneficial to the nation's health.

References

Antonovsky, A. (1979). *Health, Stress and Coping.* Jossey-Bass, San Francisco.

Bandura, A. (1977a). Self-efficacy: towards a unifying theory of behaviour change. *Psychological Review,* 84, 191–215.

Bandura, A. (1977b). *Social Learning Theory.* Prentice-Hall, Englewood Cliffs, NJ.

Bartlett, E. (1983). Educational self-help approaches in childhood asthma. *Journal of Allergy and Clinical Immunology,* 72, 545–553.

Baum, F. (1990). The new public health: force for change or reaction? *Health Promotion International,* 5(2), 145–150.

Beattie, A. (1991). Knowledge and control in health promotion: a test case for social policy and social theory. In Gabe, J., Calnan, M. and Bury, M. (eds) *The Sociology of the Health Service.* Routledge, London.

Benner, P. and Wrubel, J. (1989). *The Primacy of Caring.* Addison-Wesley, California.

Blackburn, C. (1991). *Poverty and Health – Working with Families.* Open University Press, Buckingham.

Blaxter, M. (1990). *Health and Lifestyles.* Tavistock Routledge, London.

Bowling, A. (1991). *Measuring Health.* Open University Press, Buckingham.

Brown, G. and Harris, T. (1978). *The Social Origins of Depression: A Study of Psychiatric Disorder in Women.* Tavistock, London.

Campbell, A. (1990). Education or indoctrination? The issue of autonomy in health education. In Doxiadis, S. (ed.) *Ethics in Health Education.* John Wiley, Chichester.

Caplan, R. (1993). The importance of social theory for health promotion: from description to reflexivity. *Health Promotion International,* 8(2), 147–157.

Centre of Health Economics (1991). *The Health Status Questionnaire.* York University.

Clay, T. (1987). *Nurses, Power and Politics.* Heinemann Medical Books, London.

Colver, A., Hutchinson, P. and Judson, E. (1982). Promoting children's home safety. *British Medical Journal,* 285, 1177.

Davison, C., Smith, G. and Frankel, S. (1991). Lay epidemiology and the prevention paradox: the implications of coronary candidacy for health education. *Sociology of Health and Illness,* 13, 1–19.

Department of Health (1990). *The NHS and Community Care Act.* DoH, London.

Department of Health (1992a). *The Health of the Nation.* HMSO, London.

Department of Health (1992b). *The Patient's Charter.* DoH, London.

Department of Health (1992c). *Nurses, Midwives and Health Visitors Act.* DoH, London.

Department of Health (1993). *Targeting Practice: The Contribution of Nurses, Midwives and Health Visitors.* DoH, London.

Department of Trade and Industry (1992). *Home and Leisure Accident Research. 1989 Data.* Consumer Unit DTI, London.

DiClemente, C. C. (1981). Self-efficacy and smoking cessation maintenance: a preliminary report. *Cognitive Therapy Research,* 5, 175–187.

Durkheim, E. (1951). *Suicide: A Study in Sociology.* Free Press, New York (originally published 1897).

English National Board for Nursing, Midwifery and Health Visiting (1992). *Framework and Higher Award,* ENB, London.

Gibson, C. (1991). A concept analysis of empowerment. *Journal of Advanced Nursing,* 16, 354–361.

Gilchrist, L. and Schinke, S. (1983). Coping with contraception: cognitive and behavioural methods with adolescents. *Cognitive Therapy Research,* 7, 379–388.

Gillis, A. (1993). Determinants of a health promoting lifestyle: an integrative review. *Journal of Advanced Nursing,* 18, 345–353.

Goldberg, D. and Williams, P. (1988). *A User's Guide to the General Health Questionnaire.* NFER-Nelson, Windsor.

Graham, H. (1984). *Women, Health and the Family.* Wheatsheaf Books, Sussex.

Henderson, V. (1960). *Basic Principles of Nursing Care.* ICN, London.

Herzlich, C. (1973) *Health and Illness.* Academic Press, London.

Hunt, S. and Macleod, M. (1987) Health and behavioural change: some lay perspectives. *Community Medicine,* 9(1), 68–76.

Hunt, S. and McEwen, J. (1980). The development of a subjective health indicator. *Sociology of Health and Illness,* 2(3), 231–246.

Illich, I. (1992). Health as one's own responsibility: No thank you! *The Ellul Studies Forum,* 8, 3–7.

James, N. (1992). Care, work and carework: a synthesis? In Robinson, J., Gray, A. and Elkan, R. (eds) *Policy Issues in Nursing.* Open University Press, Buckingham.

Katz, S., Ford, A. B. and Moskowitz, R. W. (1963) Studies of illness in the aged: the index of ADL – a standardised measure of biological and psycho-social function. *Journal of the American Medical Association,* 206, 1249.

Kendall, S. (1993). Do health visitors promote client participation? An analysis of the health visitor–client interaction. *Journal of Clinical Nursing,* 2, 103–109.

Kenney, J. (1992). The consumer's view of health. *Journal of Advanced Nursing,* 17, 829–834.

Kind, P. and Gudex, C. (1991). *The HMQ: Measuring Health Status in the Community.* Centre for Health Economics, University of York.

King, J. (1987). Women's attitude towards cervical smear. *Update,* 34(2), 25–27.

Kleinman, A., Eisenberg, L. and Good, B. (1978). Culture, illness and care. *Annals of Internal Medicine,* 88, 251–258.

Kobasa, S. (1979). Stressful life events, personality and health: and inquiry into hardiness. *Journal of Personal and Social Psychology,* 37, 1.

Lamb, K., Brodie, D. and Roberts, K. (1988). Physical fitness and health related fitness as indicators of a positive health state. *Health Promotion,* 3(2), 171–182.

Mackay, L. (1989). *Nursing a Problem.* Open University Press, Buckingham.

Manthey, M. (1992). *The Practice of Primary Nursing.* King's Fund, London.

McKeowan, T. (1979). *The Role of Medicine: Dream, Mirage or Nemesis.* Princeton University Press, New Jersey.

McMahon, R. and Pearson, A. (1991). *Nursing as Therapy.* Chapman & Hall, London.

Meleis, A. (1990). Being and becoming healthy: the core of nursing knowledge. *Nursing Science Quarterly,* 3(3), 107–114.

Milio, N. (1981). *Promoting Health Through Public Policy.* Davis, Philadelphia.

Naidoo, J. (1986). Limits to individualism. In Rodmell, S. and Watt, A. (eds) *The Politics of Health Education.* Routledge & Kegan Paul, London.

Neuman, B. (1982). *The Neuman Systems Model: Application to Nursing Education and Practice.* Appleton-Century-Croft, East Norwalk, CT.

Nightingale, F. (1969). *Notes on Nursing.* Dover, New York (originally published 1859).

Nutbeam, D. (1986). Health promotion glossary. *Health Promotion,* 1(1), 113–127.

Office of Population Censuses and Surveys (1992). *General Household Survey.* HMSO, London.

Orem, D. (1991) *Nursing: Concepts for Practice,* 4th edn. Mosby Year Books, New York.

Orlando, I. (1961). *The Dynamic Nurse–Patient Relationship.* Putnam's, New York.

Parsons, T. (1981). Definitions of health and illness in the light of American values and social structure. In Caplan, A., Englehart, H. and McCartney, J. (eds) *Concepts of Health and Disease: Interdisciplinary Perspectives.* Addison-Wesley, Reading, MA.

Paterson, J. and Zderad, L. (1976). *Humanistic Nursing.* John Wiley, New York.

Pender, N. (1987). *Health Promotion in Nursing Practice.* Appleton & Lange, Norwalk, CT.

Pill, R. and Stott, N. (1985). Choice or chance: further evidence on ideas of illness and responsibility for health. *Social Science and Medicine,* 20(10), 981–991.

Prochaska, S. and DiClemente, C. (1984). Self change processes: self efficacy and decisional balance across five stages of smoking cessation. In Liss, A. (ed.) *Advances in Cancer Control: Epidemiology and Research.* Alan R. Liss, New York.

Public Health Alliance (1992). *The Health of the Nation: Challenges for a New Government.* PHA, Birmingham.

Reynolds, C. (1988). The measurement of health in nursing research. *Advances in Nursing Science,* 10(4), 23–31.

Roper, N., Logan, W. and Tierney, A. (1990). *The Elements of Nursing,* 3rd edn. Churchill Livingstone, Edinburgh.

Rosser, R. and Kind, P. (1978). A scale of valuations of states of illness: is there a social consensus? *International Journal of Epidemiology,* 7, 347–358.

Roy, C. (1984). *Introduction to Nursing. An Adaptation Model,* 2nd edn. Prentice-Hall, Englewood Cliffs, NJ.

Salvage, J. (1992). The new nursing: empowering patients or empowering nurses? In Robinson, J., Gray, A. and Elkan, R. (eds) *Policy Issues in Nursing.* Open University Press, Buckingham.

Sarason, B., Shearin, E., Pierce, G. and Sarason, I. (1987). Interrelations of social support measures: theoretical and practical implications. *Journal of Personality and Social Psychology,* 52(4), 813–832.

Smith, J. (1981). The idea of health: a philosophical inquiry. *Advances in Nursing Science,* 3(3), 43–50.

Smith, P. (1990). *The Emotional Labour of Nursing.* Macmillan, London.

Sontag, S. (1978). *Illness as Metaphor*. Penguin, London.

Sports Council and the Health Education Authority (1992). *The Allied Dunbar Fitness Survey*. HEA, London.

Steele, D. *et al.* (1987). The activated patient: dogma, dream or desideratum? Beyond advocacy: a review of the activated patient concept. *Patient Education and Counselling,* 10, 3–23.

Strecher, V., Devellis, B., Becker, M. and Rosenstock, I. (1986). The role of self efficacy in achieving health behaviour change. *Health Education Quarterly,* 13(1), 73–91.

Tones, B. K. (1986). Health education and the ideology of health promotion: a review of alternative approaches. *Health Education Research,* 1(1), 3–12.

Tones, K. (1991). *Health Promotion, Self-empowerment and the Concept of Control*. Leeds Polytechnic Health Education Unit, Leeds.

Tones, K., Tilford, S and Robinson, Y. (1990). *Health Education: Effectiveness and Efficiency*. Chapman & Hall, London.

Towner, E., Dowswell, T. and Jarvis, S. (1993). *Reducing Childhood Accidents*. Health Education Authority, London.

Townsend, P. and Davidson, N. (eds) (1982). *The Black Report*. Penguin, London.

Townsend, P., Davidson, N. and Whitehead, M. (eds) (1988) *Inequalities in Health*. Penguin, London.

UKCC (1992) *The Code of Professional Conduct*. UKCC, London.

White, R. (1986). *Political Issues in Nursing: Past, Present and Future*. John Wiley, Chichester.

Whitehead, M. (1987) *The Health Divide*. Penguin, London.

Woods, N., Laffrey, S., Duffy, M., Lentz, M., Mitchell, E., Taylor, D., *et al.* (1988). Being healthy: women's images. *Advances in Nursing Science,* 11(1), 36–46.

World Health Organization (1978). *Primary Health Care: report of the International Conference on Primary Health Care held at Alma-Ata, USSR, 6–12 September 1978,* WHO, Geneva.

World Health Organization (1985). Health promotion, a discussion document on the concepts and principles. *Journal of Health Education,* 23(1), 431–435.

World Health Organization (1986a). Lifestyles and health. *Social Science and Medicine,* 22(2), 117–124.

World Health Organization (1986b). *Ottawa Charter for Health Promotion*. Drafted by participants in the First International Conference on Health Promotion, 17–21 November 1986, Ottawa, Canada.

Zabalegui, A. (1994). Barriers to health. *Nursing Times,* 90(1), 59–61.

Zigmond, A. and Snaith, R. (1983). The Hospital Anxiety and Depression Scale, *Acta Psychiatrica Scandinavica,* 67, 361–370.

2

ENVIRONMENT AND HEALTH

Greta Thornbory and Siva Murugiah

The aim of this chapter is to consider the environment and its effects on the health and well-being of individuals, their community and vice versa. The chapter will include consideration of the following issues and topics:

- what is the environment?
- what is happening to the environment?
- the greenhouse effect and global warming
- pollution
- the Earth Summit in Rio 1992
- Agenda 21
- what has the environment to do with health?
- why is it happening?
- the ozone layer
- the world population
- sustainable development
- international and national strategies.

What is the environment?

We have all heard of the hole in the ozone layer and global warming; we are aware of pollution and that it affects health but how much of what we know has been gleaned from the mass media rather than from scientific study or published research? Environmental health problems are often called to the attention of governments in a blaze of media publicity with complex horror stories. Aldrich and Griffiths (1993, p. 6) and Hynd (1990) refer to brief paragraphs in newspapers or short items on the television or radio, précised by reporters without scientific or background knowledge, resulting in the public receiving incomplete information taken out of context. This chapter on the environment and its influences on health and nursing aims to correct this situation so that nurses are able to apply this knowledge to their practice and their everyday lives.

Einstein is reputed to have said that the environment is everything that is not me whilst others have said that the environment is everything including me. Labonte (1991) enlarges on this and says that the environment surrounds or encircles and therefore exists beyond humans. Therefore the environment is part of the human ecosystem as this is a concept which implies 'a systems approach to understanding relationships'. An ecosystem encompasses the physical environment in which plants, animals and microbes live within a defined zone. Most ecosystems are extremely complex. Porteus (1992, p. 120) gives the example of a deciduous forest which can support over 100 species of birds as well as flowers, grasses and shrubs, each depending on the other for survival. It would be wise to assume that the environment has some influence on 'me' and has some influence on my well-being.

The environment is dynamic and in a continuous state of flux; therefore the human ecosystem has to adjust to changing circumstances. It is for this reason that environmental issues have become so important towards the end of the 20th century because the environment is changing quicker than man can adapt. This is one theory and only one part of the problem.

Raymond (in Hinchliff *et al.*, 1993) says that 'Health can be viewed as a state of dynamic equilibrium between the individual and his environment'. It is not part of this chapter to discuss definitions or meanings of health but to consider the influence the environment has on the well-being of the individual and the influence the individual has on the environment. Melvin Howe (1977) describes this as follows:

> The environment is a matrix of physical, biological and social circumstances surrounding man and affecting his well-being. It is the sum total of his

habitat, economy and society and as such embraces not only his life support systems of air, water, food and shelter, but also the multiplicity of provocative forces bearing down on him.

This is demonstrated in the model for environment and health (see Fig. 2.1) that fits into the Roper *et al.* (1990) diagram of the model of living under 'factors influencing activities of living' (see Fig. 2.2). Roper *et al.* have a similar focus in their activities of living and if the environment affects health it will also affect nursing practice, particularly with regard to the nurse's role in

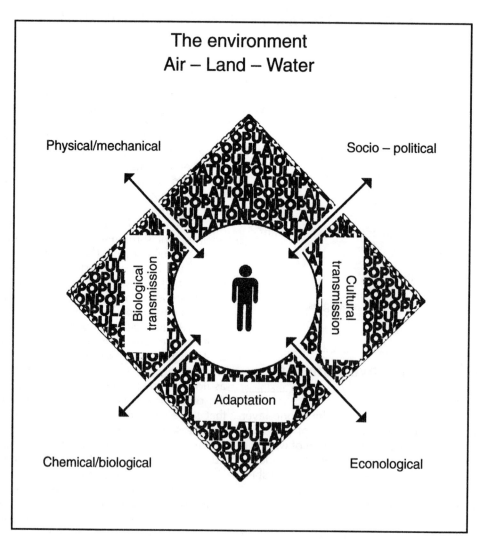

Fig. 2.1. *Thornbory model of the environment and health.*

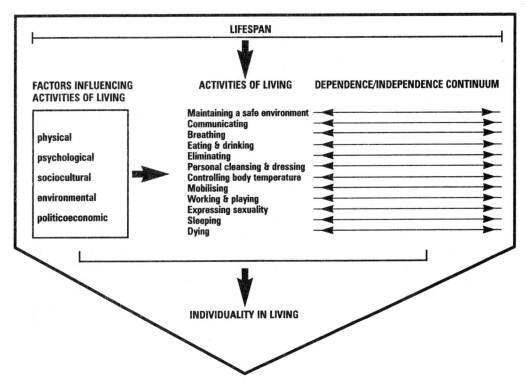

LIFESPAN

FACTORS INFLUENCING ACTIVITIES OF LIVING	ACTIVITIES OF LIVING	DEPENDENCE/INDEPENDENCE CONTINUUM

physical

psychological

sociocultural

environmental

politicoeconomic

Maintaining a safe environment
Communicating
Breathing
Eating & drinking
Eliminating
Personal cleansing & dressing
Controlling body temperature
Mobilising
Working & playing
Expressing sexuality
Sleeping
Dying

INDIVIDUALITY IN LIVING

Fig. 2.2. The Roper et al. *model of living.*

primary health care and the effects nursing practice will have on the environment in secondary and tertiary health care.

The model for the environment and health sees the individual as part of the world population and having some impact on the environment (and vice versa) under the six headings and which results in one or more activity such as biological transmission, adaptation or cultural transmission. A classic example of this is the development of computers. Silicon, from which the chips are made, is a basic element mined from the ground and as such is a chemical substance; it is put into machinery which becomes a computer. Computers (and mining) affect the physical environment in which we live. They have brought about social and financial changes in society and in all aspects of our lives. However, these changes may adversely affect the health or well-being of individuals.

Indeed, most nursing models mention the environment as part of the human ecosystem and in particular the need to maintain a safe environment whatever that means or however it can be

achieved. This indicates that nursing interventions are required if individuals are unable to do this for themselves. However, do individuals have control over their environment? Roper *et al.* (1990) suggest that it is a shared responsibility through action and legislation, yet legislation is only really required when people do not do things as a matter of course. Morally, humankind has a duty to take care of the world provided for them and for others and for future generations, yet people's own behaviour is destroying it. International and national legislative intervention is necessary to halt the advancement of destruction and to allow people time, if necessary, to adapt to the changes.

Roper *et al.* point out (1990, p. 30) that 'the environment is conceptualised in a broad dimension and includes all that is physically external to people', yet their explanation of the environment is very superficial. They talk about light rays with no mention of the electromagnetic spectrum which would encompass many harmful aspects. They mention botanical aspects only from the point of view that they should not be contaminated and regard them as decorative. The Joseph Banks House at the Royal Botanic Gardens, Kew is dedicated to demonstrating the part plant life plays in our lives by producing such things as food, paper, clothing, drugs, furniture, housing, etc. It is not enough that plant life should not be contaminated, it should not be destroyed completely and when used it should be replaced.

Buildings are an essential part of the environment, helping both to protect people from the elements and to protect items they need. When Roper *et al.* consider the environment of buildings no mention is made of the purpose of the building, only that the internal thermal environment should not affect body temperature. Yet buildings may be designed to house substances which require storage or use under specific thermal conditions, some of which are extreme, e.g. frozen food. People have to work in all sorts of environments and spend two-thirds of their life at work; little consideration is given to the primary health-care needs of these workers.

Activity 1

Make a list of all the occupations you can think of where people have to work in extremes of temperature. It may be necessary to do some reading to come up with a list but it should be quite long.

You may have listed such occupations as Arctic explorers, mountaineers and farm workers who may work in cold conditions but you also have to remember people such as those who work outdoors, e.g. milkmen; postmen; and people who work in food storage or any form of cold storage such as in supermarkets, research and laboratories. People who work under extremes of heat include those who work abroad in hot climates, in the oil industry, foundries and workers who operate boilers and incinerators.

In Roper *et al.*'s explanation of their model they stress radiation as an environmental problem. Part of this chapter will discuss the hole in the ozone layer and the associated effects from radiation. Radiation occurs naturally, partly in the electro-magnetic spectrum, partly as a mineral and partly in living organisms in the form of radon, cosmic,

thoron, gamma and internal radiation and this accounts for 87 percent of people's annual exposure to radiation. Artificial radiation accounts for the remaining 13 percent, of which medical usage accounts for 12 percent (National Radiological Protection Board, 1989). It is important not to get the risks to safety from man-made radiation out of proportion. Godlee and Walker (1992), in their review of the literature and research, say that if there is a risk from environmental radiation it is likely to be extremely small and that it inspires anxiety because it is beyond the individual's control.

The concept of 'risk' is introduced here because although a hazard may be identified, the important factor to consider is the 'risk' that it may affect the activity of living. A hazard describes the potential for harm, whilst 'risk' is the chance or probability that a hazard will result in that harm (Holt and Andrews, 1991). When a hazard causes harm it is called an 'accident' and contrary to what Roper *et al.* say, accidents are not always avoidable. They go on to say that accident prevention must not be regarded only in terms of eliminating hazards. Indeed, all the hazards in the world could not be eliminated but the risk of each hazard causing harm can be quantified using statistical data often in the form of epidemiology or inductive analysis using logic diagrams. For clarity a definition of 'accident' is given here:

> An accident is any unplanned, unwanted, unexpected event which causes injury or ill health or damage to physical assets or the environment' (Health and Safety Executive, 1992).

It is important to note that accidents do not necessarily result in injury or ill-health. After all, if you hit a tree in a car you may not be injured but the car will be damaged (physical asset) and the tree may be damaged (the environment) and this is regarded as an accident. To return to the thesis that accidents are avoidable, anyone considering this should read the Royal Society's report *Risk Analysis, Perception and Management* (1992), which is a study of risk assessment. This report considers work in a variety of areas including toxicology, nutrition, engineering, epidemiology, risk perception and management. There is also a considerable amount written on accident causation theory and no matter how safe something is made there is always the 'human element'.

Reflective point

'A thing is safe if its risks are judged to be acceptable'. Consider this statement in relation to examples of hazards from both work and leisure.

How you have answered this reflective point will be entirely personal and may have something to do with how much control you have over the hazards. Radiation, and in particular nuclear energy, is seen as unsafe because people feel they have no control over it, yet they happily travel daily in cars which are responsible for several thousand deaths from accidents each year as well as polluting the environment.

Lastly Roper considers pollution as one dimension needing to be controlled in order to maintain a safe environment. Sweeping statements about air pollution being brought under control by legislation for clean air are made, yet the use of energy and the resultant carbon dioxide and particulate levels are the main contributors to the problem of global warming. It is worthy to note here that Godlee and Walker (1992) say the only effective long-term solution to modern air pollution is to reduce road traffic.

Noise is also discussed by Roper as a pollutant but no link is made between sound as energy transmitted through the atmosphere and noise as an abuse of sound, mainly because no definition is given for noise. Noise is frequently described as unwanted sound, but what is 'wanted' sound to one person may well be 'unwanted' by another and music is a clear example of this. Noise can cause harm, not only because it is excessive but also because it has a nuisance value which may result in stress and affect our well-being. Exposure to excessive noise may cause temporary hearing impairment or, if exposed repeatedly, permanent hearing loss often accompanied by tinnitus (Humphrey and Farmer, 1990).

In considering the environment as a factor influencing activities of living, Thornbory's environment and health model fits Roper *et al.*'s model and should help to enhance discussions on maintaining a safe environment.

One aspect of the environment and health model not considered is the cultural transmission which has been evident in the recent past as people have become more aware of their impact on the environment. New political parties have sprung up and the

last quarter of this century has seen candidates for the Green Party standing for election to Parliament. Pressure groups such as *Greenpeace* and *Friends of the Earth* have been instrumental in bringing environmental issues to the forefront of the media. Developed countries are taking on board environmental issues and beginning to change their behaviour in small ways to improve the situation. But is this enough? Later in the chapter, when considering remedial strategies such as sustainable development, these issues will be discussed.

Activity 2

Think about the environment around you now. Make a list of how you could be affected by your immediate environment. Keep it until you have read all of this chapter.

The quality of our life depends on good health and this depends in part on a quality environment. As already stated the environment is everywhere, so home life, work and leisure all depend on the environment and the environment is affected by our activities within it. In some circumstances the affects will be short term and in others long term; sometimes we have a choice and at others not. A simple example of this is the temperature of the room you are sitting in as you read this. If you are at home and it is too hot or too cold you have a choice and are able to control the environment by turning on the heating or air conditioning, by opening or closing doors and windows, providing you have the equipment and economic provision to do so. At work you may not have the same choice if the temperature is controlled centrally or there are other employees to consider or the work you do either requires, creates or takes place in a specific thermal environment.

We do not always have a choice: we may not have the equipment, money or control. In the short term healthy adults can tolerate fluctuations in thermal conditions, but if the conditions are extreme then homoeostasis is affected (Gould, 1993). For small babies or those who are sick and the elderly, homoeostasis is affected more readily by the thermal environment. They may be unable to control their environment or they may have little choice. In the long term humankind's activities on earth have brought about climatic changes through such initiatives as the use of energy from fossil fuels to heat or cool our environment or drive machinery, and this has resulted in adverse affects on the environment.

Activity 3

Make a cup of tea or other hot drink and think about and list the effects this action has on the environment.

Making a hot drink involves a number of actions which impact on the environment:

1. Having potable (fit to drink) water available is something we take for granted in the UK, but in other countries water may be at a premium or not available at all.
2. A kettle or other similar vessel is required to boil the water. Electric kettles are often made of man-made materials which are not bio-degradable.
3. Electricity or gas is required to heat the water. Using energy increases the use of fossil fuels at the power station and therefore adds to the greenhouse effect.
4. Hot drinks are generally based on plants, tea leaves, coffee and cocoa beans. These plants require huge areas to be cleared for plantations and are worked by poorly paid local workers. Rain forests may have been cleared for the plantation and over-cultivation leads to barren wastelands, soil erosion, etc.

Not only is the environment all around us and we are part of it, but also we know that it can affect us and the quality of our life in both the short and the long term. It can affect us at home, at work and at leisure and we may have little or no choice or control over how it affects us. It is complicated and complex and as nurses we should know more about the environment and its affects on health in order to be proactive carers and to support the World Health Organization's (WHO) global strategy for the 21st century, which will be discussed later in the chapter. After all a healthy environment is not only a need; it is also a right enshrined in the Universal Declaration of Human Rights and everyone shares the responsibility for ensuring this.

The ecological issues which make up the earth and our environment, or in other words the human ecosystem, need to be considered and discussed.

Activity 4

Before embarking on the next section it is suggested that you revise your knowledge of the 'electro-magnetic spectrum', perhaps in *Fundamentals of Science for Nurses* (Harris, 1988) or the leaflet 'Non-ionising radiation' from the National Radio-logical Protection Board.

Ecological issues

In recent years there has been a greater emphasis on the relationships between living organisms and the living and non-living factors in the environment. A dynamic equilibrium has been maintained over the years, however this has been destabilised by human activities. Destabilisation of the equilibrium has resulted in increased health risk to humans. This section will emphasise the effects of atmospheric pollution on health status, and the effects of water and land pollution will also be touched on. To understand the impact of eco-logical changes on human health it is essential to have an overview of the dynamic ecosystem of the atmosphere, water and land.

Atmosphere

About 99.99 percent of the mass of the atmosphere is within 80 km of the Earth's surface and consists of 78 percent nitrogen (N); 21 percent oxygen (O_2); 0.04 percent carbon dioxide (CO_2); water vapour; argon; methane; ammonia; neon; xenon; krypton; solid and liquid particulates. The atmosphere is divided into four shells or zones called the tropo-sphere; stratosphere; mesosphere and thermo-sphere (see Fig. 2.3). Varying amounts of the concentration of the constituents mentioned above are found within each of the zones.

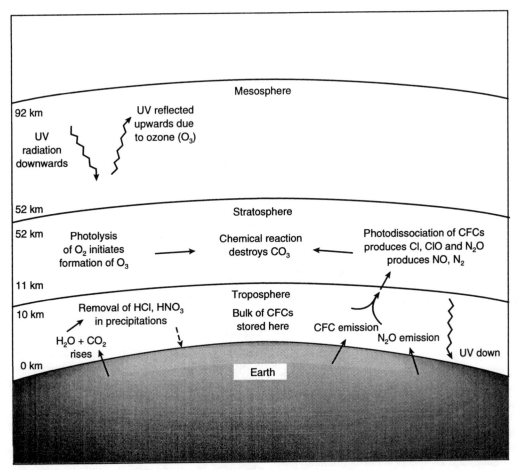

Fig. 2.3. *The various reactions that occur in the atmosphere which have resulted in the destabilisation of the dynamic equilibrium by anthropogenic activities.*

The troposphere

The troposphere stretches from the entire surface to 11 km above on average. In the regions around the poles the troposphere stretches 6–8 km while at the equator it stretches to 17 km. In the troposphere the temperature decreases with altitude, hence water vapour precipitates and storm clouds are formed. There is vertical air movement and life as we know it is supported within this. The upper limit of the troposphere is called the tropopause.

The stratosphere

The stratosphere stretches from the troposphere to 52 km above the Earth's surface. In this zone the temperature increases with altitude and air circulates horizontally as buoyancy forces suppress upward air movement. Water vapour is transformed into stratus clouds which block the shorter wavelength solar radiation. In this zone ozone is formed by photodissociation and this has been associated with protecting life from the damaging effects of ultraviolet (UV) rays. Other processes such as luminescence, photosensitisation and photoionisation occur in this zone. The upper limit of the stratosphere is called the stratopause.

The mesosphere

The mesosphere stretches from 52 to 92 km and the temperature declines with altitude through vertical air movement. Atmospheric substances that reach the stratopause continue to move upwards into the mesosphere until they reach the upper limit of the mesopause. Photoionisation occurs in this zone and is associated with radiation of heat outwards into space.

The thermosphere

This zone stretches from 90 km and beyond and movement of molecules is limited to horizontal flows from buoyancy forces. There appears to be limited photochemical activity in this zone and solar heat is allowed to radiate downwards to the mesopause.

Photochemistry

A brief overview of basic photochemistry is included to highlight the effects that pollutants have on the atmosphere. A variety of chemical reactions occur in the atmosphere that do not occur in the chemical laboratory and health carers need to be aware of these. These reactions are driven by light, and catalysed by the pollutants present. The pollutants are modified by chemical reactions and have environmental consequences.

In the presence of UV radiation, atoms present in the atmosphere become excited and more reactive. Reactions of molecular oxygen (O_2) will be used as an example. In the presence of strong sunlight O_2 becomes electronically excited ($O_2 \overset{UV}{\to} O_2^*$; the asterisk denotes excited state). This excited O_2 has several fates:

1. it can simply decay and airglow or 'luminescence' occurs
2. it can react with some adjacent molecule leaving a photosensitive or excited molecule, a process called 'photosensitisation'
3. it can break down and lose an electron, a process called 'photoionisation', or finally
4. it can dissociate to give atomic oxygen, a process called 'photodissociation'.

The influence of light changes the chemistry of the atmosphere. This mainly relates to the stratosphere, although it can be related to the troposphere. It can be estimated that about 2000 million years ago, before plant life started, there was no oxygen in the troposphere and no ozone in the stratosphere. The process of photosynthesis by plants enabled O_2 to be produced and accumulate in the troposphere. The stratospheric ozone (O_3) is estimated first to have occurred around 2000 million years ago.

The process of photosensitisation does not occur naturally in the troposphere because UV light necessary to drive the photochemical process is absorbed by the ozone in the stratosphere. A cyclic reaction occurs in the stratosphere, where ozone is converted to atomic and molecular oxygen in the presence of UV light and at the same time molecular and atomic oxygen are combined to adjacent molecules to produce ozone. Thus there is a dynamic equilibrium.

Ozone

About 4.2 billion years ago there was no ozone in the stratosphere or oxygen in the troposphere. Ultraviolet radiation in the sunlight would have reached the surface of the Earth, making it sterile (Gribbin, 1988a). Ultraviolet light of 200–350 nm wavelength is a powerful sterilising agent; however, scientists believe that UV light would have provided the energy to induce chemical reactions which were the precursors to life.

About 2.5 billion years ago there were large quantities of oxygen in the atmosphere and it is suggested that oxygen was initially a by-product of carbon dioxide breakdown by organisms which used carbon for their cellular structure. The oxygen once present absorbed UV radiation which enabled oxygen-breathing species to colonise the land surfaces. Oxygen is also reactive and combines with carbon to form food from which energy could be liberated. This enables the energetic lifestyle observed in many terrestrial animals.

Ozone (O_3) is a form of oxygen which has three atoms in each molecule. It is basically the combination of molecular oxygen (O_2) and atomic oxygen (O^*) and is found in both the stratosphere and in the troposphere. Stratospheric ozone will be considered initially, followed by tropospheric ozone.

Stratospheric ozone

Sunlight warms the air, the water and landmass. Warm air including oxygen, carbon dioxide and nitrogen rises. The passage through the troposphere is fairly rapid; however, because of the temperature difference between the troposphere and stratosphere movement becomes slow. There is slow diffusion of gases from the troposphere to the stratosphere. The oxygen that reaches the stratosphere undergoes photochemical changes and ozone is produced. It is also important to remember that ozone is constantly broken down to molecular oxygen and reformed into ozone.

Until recently there was a state of dynamic equilibrium. The depletion of ozone has been happening for a number of years and was first predicted around 1970 in the USA. It was predicted that the action of the exhaust emissions of transport planes that cruised the stratosphere would cause depletion of stratospheric ozone.

Molina and Rowland (1974) suggest that atomic chlorine originates from chlorofluorocarbons (CFCs). CFCs are man-made, synthetic and liquefy under pressure. They were commonly used in refrigeration (30 percent), as aerosol propellants (60 percent) and for making foams. As CFCs are synthetic, there are no natural microbial catalytic pathways, thus they remain in the atmosphere for very long periods. Freon 11 ($CFCl_3$) has a half-life of about 10 years and freon 12 (CF_2Cl_2) has an even longer half-life of about 30 years. Freons diffuse into the stratosphere slowly and participate in photochemical reactions which results in the release of atomic chlorine.

In 1974 a paper by Stolarski *et al.* suggested 'that atomic chlorine will react with ozone and deplete the ozone layer, leading to its total destruction'. The reaction Stolarski suggested was that atomic chlorine (Cl) will react with ozone (O_3) to form chloride (ClO) and molecular oxygen (O_2). Chloride will react with atomic oxygen (O), forming chlorine and molecular oxygen (O_2). Therefore in the presence of atomic chlorine, molecular oxygen is produced, resulting in depletion of ozone. Gribbin (1988a) indicates that 'the majority of the chlorine will be converted to form HCl (hydrochloric acid) and Cl_2 or ClO' over the Antarctic in winter. In summer when the sun returns chlorine will participate in the reactions described by Stolarski *et al.* (1974), thus the hole in the ozone layer during the Antarctic summer.

In the stratosphere, ozone is able to absorb UV-B light of 290–320 nm wavelength. UV light ranges from 1 to 380 nm wavelength and is not in the visual spectrum of the sunlight. The lack of stratospheric ozone is letting even greater amounts of the dangerous UV light through to the Earth's surface. UV-B light is shown to cause sunburn and some forms of skin cancer. Cook (1993) suggested that the second most common cancer in Britain is melanoma and this could be attributed to the effects of UV radiation. In Australia where the problem is severe, Dayton (1993) introduced Rayosan, an UV-absorbent cloth which can protect the skin from the effects of UV light. The effects of Rayosan have yet to be assessed in widescale trials. Direct exposure to UV light is associated with eye problems such as cataracts (Gribbin, 1988a; Cook, 1993). Beardsley (1992) insinuated that the UV radiation causes genetic damage to organisms at the base of the food chain which has implications for the health of higher animals. Horgan (1992) indicates that UV radiation damages DNA and weakens the immune system in animals and humans. If ozone absorbs UV light in the stratosphere, then it reduces the amount of dangerous UV light reaching the Earth's surface. As stated earlier, stratospheric ozone depletion increases the amount of dangerous UV light reaching the Earth's surface and thus enhancing its deleterious effects. It is essential that health-care workers are aware of their role in educating the public about the responsibilities in the maintenance of this delicate ecosystem.

Ground-level ozone

Fishman and Crutzen (1978) suggest that ozone can be formed at ground level from the oxidation of methane (CH_4), carbon dioxide (CO_2) and nitrogen oxides (NO_x). They also postulated that in spring and summer, in the presence of bright sunlight, ozone can be formed, hence the seasonal fluctuations. The Department for the Environment (1987) suggests that the ozone levels have doubled in the past 10 years from 20 to 50 ppm. Harrison (1990) suggests that ozone levels of 100 ppm, with levels reaching 250 ppm in southern England, are not uncommon.

The formation of ground-level ozone is dependent on the prevalence of certain conditions, namely high light intensity, temperature above 20°C, and still air or low wind speeds.

The physiological effects of ground-level ozone have mainly been investigated in plants. Exposure to ozone has shown visual areas of necrosis or flaking of the upper surface of the leaves. It appears that amino acids such as methionine, cystine, tryptophan, histidine, tyrosine and phenylalanine become oxidised and the main damage occurs to the structures of membranes. The effects are the loss of selective permeability and functional action of the cells which results in poor crop yields. Is there a similar reaction in animal cells? What are the effects of these reactions in the animal?

Beardsley (1992) has intimated that ground-level ozone can cause respiratory damage but he does not state the nature of this damage. Josep (1995) suggests that there is a link between NO_x levels, ozone levels and asthma. Haemoglobin has an affinity for oxygen and the question that arises is its affinity for ozone. If the affinity for ozone is the same, then what are the effects and how does it dissociate in comparison to oxygen? Godlee (1992) suggests that low levels of ozone cause coughs, nausea, headaches and irritation of the nose and throat. The article does not, however, state what low-level ozone is.

Global warming: the greenhouse effect

The atmosphere is changing, trapping heat from the sun, altering the climate, the ecosystem, agriculture and the level of the sea. These changes in temperature are termed 'global warming' or 'the greenhouse effect'. The problem was first reported about 30 years ago by Roger Revelle, who stated that 'humans are conducting a geophysical experiment, the results of which will not be known immediately'. Bolina in the 1970s reawakened interest in the greenhouse effect and since then it has become of world-wide concern (Bolina *et al.*, 1986). This section will explore the cause and effects of this phenomenon, the sequence of events that has led to the current state of affairs, and consider some predicative models.

Causes of global warming

Nuclear fusion deep within the sun releases a tremendous amount of energy which is radiated into space. The Earth intercepts solar radiation which includes X-rays, UV and infrared (IR) radiation, radio emissions and visible light. The driving energy for weather and climate comes from the sun. About a third of the solar radiation is reflected by ozone in the stratosphere and clouds in the tropopause, while the rest is absorbed by components such as the atmosphere, ocean, ice, landmass and biota of the climate systems. Part of this absorbed energy is re-radiated to the atmosphere as long-wave IR radiation from the Earth, the ocean and biota. The atmosphere is not completely transparent to this long-wave radiation, because it contains carbon dioxide and water vapour, which absorb a considerable portion of the long-wave radiation before partially re-radiating it back to the Earth's surface. Thus, although a large portion of short-wave solar radiation is transmitted through the atmosphere to the ground a large portion of the re-radiated long-wave radiation is trapped by the atmosphere and does not escape directly back into space. This cause the troposphere to reach a higher temperature than would otherwise be the case.

In the long-term climatic changes on the Earth will result, as the greenhouse effect is intensified due to human activities, substantially increasing the atmospheric concentrations of greenhouse gases within the troposphere and stratosphere. These enhanced levels of greenhouse gases, mainly carbon dioxide and water vapour (precipitates), would increase further in response to global warming. Aerosols (small particles) in the atmosphere can also affect the climate and temperature because it can reflect or absorb radiation. Natural perturbation, such as explosive volcanic eruptions which affect the natural equilibrium, can also contribute to global warming. Horgan (1992) suggests that when Mount Pinatubo erupted in 1991, the particulates from the volcano, which contained sulphur particulate, eroded stratospheric ozone even in the tropical regions.

Precipitates and greenhouse gases

Precipitates

The Sun's energy heats the Earth, water evaporates and ascends, and as it rises into the atmosphere it cools and condenses, forming various types of clouds. Clouds are precipitates of tiny crystals of water. The high-level clouds found in the lower stratosphere are called **cirrus** clouds, the middle-level clouds found in the tropopause are the **cumulus** clouds and **nimbus** clouds are found in the upper levels of the troposphere. The clouds that are of concern are the cirrus and cumulus clouds. The cirrus clouds enable UV rays from the Sun to reach the Earth and warm it; besides this they also reflects the re-radiated IR rays back to the Earth. The cumulus clouds, on the other hand, reflect the incoming UV rays back to the atmosphere before they reach the Earth. Model climate predictions (Russell-Jones and Wigley, 1990) indicate that there would be an increase in cirrus clouds by the year 2010 and a decrease in cumulus clouds which in itself would increase global warming. (**Please remember it is only a prediction based on climate models.**)

Carbon dioxide (CO_2)
The main greenhouse gas is the odourless, colourless and non-toxic gas – carbon dioxide. Man has made carbon dioxide for hundreds of years by burning wood and breathing. Production and the absorption of carbon dioxide (maintained by the carbon cycle) has been in balance. About half of the carbon dioxide produced was absorbed by the top layers of the oceans for plankton growth, the other half being utilised by plants, and the organic carbon being trapped into plant cell structures, while oxygen was released into the atmosphere. Some of the trapped organic carbon was released by decomposition of leaves but most was trapped in trees, which over the centuries became coal.

Since the Industrial Revolution the demand for energy has been growing, and this has led to the increased combustion of fossil fuels like coal, oils and natural gas. This, in turn, has led to the increase in the levels of carbon dioxide in the atmosphere (Harrison, 1990). Mowerlower Laboratories in the Pacific recorded carbon dioxide levels in 1948 as 315 ppm and by 1990 the levels had increased to 415 ppm. The blame cannot be placed just on fossil fuel combustion alone. Deforestation for agriculture, homesteads, etc., has led to the imbalance in the carbon cycle. This has partly contributed to the current state of affairs. Carbon dioxide, which has a long half-life, is emitted into the atmosphere and is trapped there. The carbon dioxide allows UV rays to reach the Earth's surface and re-radiates the long-wave infrared back to the Earth, thus contributing to global warming.

Methane (CH_4)
Methane is mainly emitted from agricultural activities. Cattle produce methane when they digest food. Methane is also produced by methanogens in the world's rice fields. As the demand for food grows, so has the increased concentration of this gas. Many factors influence the production of methane; these include temperature, pH, electron acceptors and availability of carbon dioxide. Under a warmer climate, decreased pH due to acid rain and increasing levels of carbon dioxide have increased the rate of methane production, thus leading to higher levels of methane. Methane is a hydrocarbon and will act in a similar fashion to carbon dioxide and contribute to global warming.

Nitrous oxide (N_2O)
This is produced as a result of hot combustion of car engines, boilers as well as nitrogen fertilisers used in agriculture. With a rapid increase in traffic and a greater demand for increased crop yield per hectare, man has increased the levels of nitrous oxide in the atmosphere. This gas acts in a similar way to carbon dioxide in the troposphere but also depletes the ozone layer in a similar way to CFCs.

Predictions of global warming
It has been suggested that climatic changes would produce a spectrum of health effects. These effects are very much dependent on the actual rise in temperature. If the Smith and Warr (1991) prediction is true, then the temperature will rise by 2 to 4°C by the year 2050 and if Hall's (1990) predictions are true, then the temperature will rise by 1.5 to 5°C by the year 2060.

Effects of global warming
Global mean surface temperature (ambient) has increased by 0.3–0.6°C over the last 100 years, with the five warmest years being in the 1980s (Gribbin, 1988b). Over the same time global sea levels have increased by 20 cm. This increase has not been smooth with time nor uniform over the globe. Ecosystems will effect climate and will be affected by the changing climate, temperature and increasing levels of carbon dioxide concentrations. Rapid changes will alter the composition of the ecosystems; some species will benefit while others will be unable to migrate or adapt fast enough and may become extinct. Enhanced levels of carbon dioxide may increase productivity and efficiency of water usage by vegetation.

Brown (1992) estimates that the amount of land

at risk by a rise of one metre in sea levels would result in a loss of 5 million square kilometres. This is equivalent to 3 percent of the Earth's total land-mass. Smith and Warr (1991) indicate that London would be extensively flooded, extensive areas of East Anglia would be flooded while the polder land of The Netherlands would be vulnerable to floods. Further from home one-third of Bangladesh would be reclaimed by the sea with a rise of only 50 cm (Seager, 1990).

Smith and Warr also suggest that there would be migration of crops and loss of species. The grow-ing season will become longer in England but the types of crops would be different from those grown now. The cereal growing belts of North America might shift northwards by several hundred kilo-metres for every degree rise in temperature. How-ever, some ecosystems may break down and there will be loss of species. Trees adapt over many thousands of years and if the temperature rise is dramatic then many species of plants, trees and animals would be lost.

Emmanuel (1987) argues that tropical cyclones are particularly sensitive to sea surface tempera-tures. For example, a rise of 3°C in the sea surface temperature gives a rise of 30–40 mmHg in baro-metric pressure. Climatologists agree that global warming results not only in heat waves and droughts, but also in more frequent cyclones and sea surges (Smith and Warr, 1991).

The effects on health of climatic changes

Some vulnerable people such as those who are elderly, very young or sick are not efficient at dealing with extremes of temperature. Mortality from coronary heart disease and cerebrovascular accidents increases when the average temperature exceeds 25°C. It is estimated that at above 33°C mortality from all causes increases, mainly owing to deaths from cardiovascular and respiratory diseases (Godlee and Walker, 1992). Warmer climate will lead to a rise in urban air pollution. In the USA in 1988, 76 cities had extended air stag-nation periods and high temperatures caused safe ozone levels to be exceeded which resulted in an increased risk of asthma. Leggett (1990) argues that there would be an increase in sandstorms and associates with this an increase in death rates and symptoms of asthma and bronchitis.

Changes in temperature could result in diseases associated with tropical and sub-tropical areas

moving polewards. The American Environmental Protection Agency (EPA) estimates that there will be an increase in vector-borne diseases. The vec-tors are carriers such as ticks or mosquitoes and the diseases include malaria, dengue fever, Rocky Mountain spotted lyme disease (OECD, 1992), yellow fever and Rift Valley fever (Godlee, 1992). There is little literature about the effects in Europe.

In addition, water supplies would be increasing-ly saline, and during the summer months, the amount and quantity of available fresh water would fall (Godlee, 1992). There would be significant public health risks and diseases such as typhoid, cholera and hepatitis would be rife. There would also be an increase in other diarrhoeal infections (Leggett, 1990). A growth in the rat population, due to the warmer weather, would intensify the risk of diseases such as Weil's disease and plagues. This has implications for nursing and nurse education as nursing would need to adapt aspects of the curricula to place greater emphasis on infectious diseases management.

Leggett (1990) suggests that there is an increased rate of premature births and peri-natal mortality in very hot summers, associated with increased rate of gynaecological infections. Elmsworth (1990) suggests that there would be an increase in dis-eases associated with malnutrition. The loss of arable land and crops would cause even greater famines. Nations would take up arms to secure their share of the scarce food and water resources, resulting in wars. This has implications for the health and health status of the nation and thus for nursing.

Particulates

The term 'particulates' applies to all particles that are present in air in suspension. These can be either organic or inorganic substances which can vary from 100 μm to smaller than 0.01 μm. The main source of anthropogenic particulate pollutants is the combustion of fossil fuels, especially coal.

Smoke is the major particulate pollutant. There is no universally accepted definition of 'smoke' although it is generally taken to mean fine suspended particulates (<15 μm) arising from incomplete combustion of fuels (Harrison, 1990).

It can be seen from Fig. 2.4 that smoke emissions from coal combustion have been reducing since 1960, following the introduction of the Clean Air Act of 1956. Although particulate

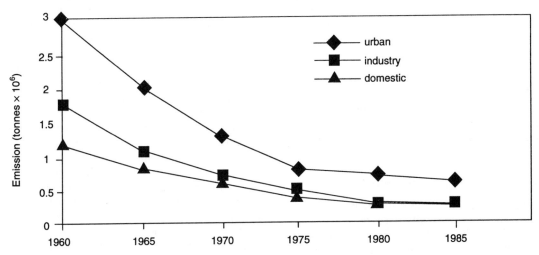

Fig. 2.4. *Smoke emission from coal combustion in the UK (1960–85).*

pollution from smoke has reduced by about 85 percent in the past 30 years (Holman, 1989), other forms of particulate pollution have increased (Godlee, 1992). Other anthropogenic particulate pollutants are ammonium sulphate, lead, hydrocarbons (benzene), ammonium, nitrates, etc. There are, of course, particulate pollutants from natural causes, for example, salts from the crust of waves are found in the troposphere. Volcanic ash is another example of a particulate pollutant. Biological materials, for example spores, bacteria, viruses, pollens, are also present. Dust and sand from soil settle quickly but finer particles can remain in the atmosphere for long periods.

Anthropogenic materials

When fossil fuels are burnt fly-ash is produced which contains soot, silicon, nickel, iron calcium, and carbon. Industrial processes, such as steel works and power stations, contribute to particulate pollution but the level of pollutant depends on the process used in the industries. With declining industrial output there has been a decline in this activity, as shown in Fig. 2.4. The increase in road traffic since the 1970s has contributed to other particulate pollutants, such as hydrocarbons, lead, and nitrogen oxides.

The Conference of European Environmental Ministers (1985) set out a programme to achieve the following by the year 2000:

- reduce smoke to 80 $\mu g/m^3$ of air as a daily mean value
- reduce smoke to 130 $\mu g/m^3$ of air as a daily winter mean value.

The daily mean values for the following cities (see Fig. 2.5) in 1986–87 show that the smoke levels were much higher than that set by the Conference.

In London, the value in 1989 was 70 $\mu g/m^3$ and this can be attributed to the Clean Air Act of 1956 which established smoke-free zones where only

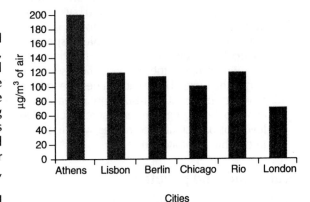

Fig. 2.5. *Smoke levels in 1986–87.*

smokeless fuels could be used. Smoke emissions have reduced by 85 percent, since 1960. However there are a few areas where the levels are higher, mainly in mining regions where miners get free coal. This practice was stopped in 1993 with the closure of many pits.

What happens to the particulates?

Most of them precipitate and settle either in the dry or wet form. The rate at which it precipitates depends on the size or diameter of the particulate (Stokes' law).

What are the effects of the particulates?

1. Act as focus of rain drops resulting in increased rain fall. La Porta, 30 miles downwind of Chicago in the USA, has 31 percent more rainfall and 38 percent more thunderstorms.
2. Soiling of buildings by smoke blackening the walls and following the Clean Air Act of 1956, the pollution and emission are mainly due to diesel fuels from vehicles.
3. Effect on plants. There is a 30 percent drop in yield near brickworks because of the reduction of sunlight for photosynthesis, as particulates refract light rays away from the plants. Stomatal pores can be blocked by fine dust or wedged open by larger particles, resulting in reduced gas exchange or loss of water.
4. Effects on human. The main effect is on the respiratory system. Most inhaled particles of between 10 and 15 μm are deposited in the nose, mouth and throat, where they cause irritation. Particles smaller than 10 μm are more damaging as they can actually enter the lungs. The term used in assessing and quantifying particulate matter is **total suspended particulates** (TSP), which refers to all particles regardless of size and **respirable suspended particulates** (RSP) are those smaller than 3.5 μm, which reach the deepest, most sensitive part of the lungs. These cause a decline in lung function, pre-existing respiratory diseases are exacerbated. Long-term exposure to elevated levels of particulates correlates with increase in chronic respiratory diseases.

Water and land pollution

Although the main emphasis of this chapter is atmospheric pollution and its effects on health, the chapter would be incomplete without mentioning the effects of water and land pollution on health of the population. To this end a brief review of water pollution and land pollution will be considered.

Liquid water is a vital ingredient for all living organisms. Water makes up to 90 percent of the mass of animals and plants. Water from the Earth's surface evaporates due to the sun's heat and rises as water vapour. This water vapour cools at it reaches altitudes and combines with a cocktail of chemical pollutants which have poured into the atmosphere from anthropogenic activities and natural causes (Fig. 2.4). The precipitation returns to Earth as occult, wet (rain) or dry deposits. Rain in an unpolluted environment has a pH of 5.7. The ecological concerns is with acid rain, where the pH is 5.0 or below. In areas where the acid rain is severe a pH of 3.5 has been recorded (Pearce, 1987).

Acid rain occurs when acid is formed from several important air pollutants, mainly sulphur and nitrogen. Sulphur dioxide (SO_2) in the atmosphere, if it remains long enough, is eventually oxidised to SO_3 and dissolves in water precipitates to form sulphuric acid (H_2SO_4). Nitrogen oxides (NO_x) are oxidised to nitrogen dioxide (NO_2) and this dissolves to form nitric acid (H_2NO_3). Additionally hydrochloric acid (HCl) is also formed. These acids that fall as acid rain have untold effects on the environment which have indirect implications for the health of the population.

Effects of acid rain on the environment

Although there are many effects only a few are mentioned as this is an overview of water pollution.

- In the 1970s there were reports from Scandinavia and North America of acidification of soft water lakes and streams and the destruction of the fish population, particularly salmon and trout (Pearce, 1987). In 1971 Sweden complained to the United Nations about Britain being responsible for the acid rain from the emission of air pollutants which were causing the destruction of the fishing industry and spoiling Swedish holiday resorts.
- Acid rain mobilises heavy metals in soils as they are more soluble at a low pH. This causes heavy metals to enter the food chain and presents a hazard to human health. If the soil pH is changed by acid rain releasing the heavy metals,

then this will eventually reach water tables, lakes, and rivers. Many lochs in Scotland and Scandinavia are almost without fish, as are hundreds more in Canada and parts of eastern USA. Fish die or fail to reproduce in acid water; acid *per se* is rarely the cause. The deaths are mainly due to poisoning by aluminium. which has also been implicated in the cause of Alzheimer's disease in humans. Thus there is a possible relationship between acid rain and human health.

- Acid rain has a profound effect on the freshwater ecology. Acid lakes are usually crystal clear with luscious carpets of green algae and moss. When these proliferate they change the 'metabolism' of the lake, providing less energy for life in the lakes, resulting in fewer species of fish and a changed ecosystem.

Population

If world resources are diminishing, then the number of people using them should be reduced in order to preserve sufficient resources for future generations. Yet the world population continues to grow and in 1990 reached 5 billion compared with approximately 1 billion in 1850. At the present rate of growth, statistics indicate that by 2050 there will be 10 billion people in the world (United Nations, 1991; Godlee and Walker, 1992).

It is estimated that 40 percent of the world population is poor and these numbers consist of mainly women and children. Statistics on poverty only cover income and do not relate to standards of living so the poor who are illiterate, have no clean water and/or have environmentally-induced disease are not included in statistics on poverty. (Those people who are exposed to threats of violence or crime do not appear in poverty statistics yet their well-being is threatened also.)

Statistics indicate that where health care exists there is also a lower fertility rate (WHO, 1992). However, in areas where child deaths and infant mortality rates are high, parents may feel the need to replace a child who dies or to have large families to compensate for deaths. Infant deaths also mean that natural contraception by suppression of ovulation is lost. In countries such as China where reducing birth rates and controlling the population is regarded as a civic duty, then substantial reductions in the rate of growth of the population have been made. Such measures in other cultures may pose a problem where religious or other influences predispose to large families.

Population growth makes demands on resources – more goods and services are required and more food. Rural areas become more crowded and waste products from these communities result in further environmental damage and pressure on natural resources. Estimates of population growth include the effects on rural areas, turning them into new cities or being destroyed by the continuation of environmentally destructive practices.

The United Nations Population Fund aims to have family planning available for 59 percent of married women of reproductive age by the year 2000. Availability for all would not be a realistic objective in the time as it relies on contributions from the international community to fund its efforts and funding levels remain pitifully low. Family planning is not high on most countries' agendas. It has been suggested that government departments responsible for health and welfare do not have the same power, strength or voice as those of industry and defence (WHO, 1992). In order to reduce the pressure on the environment, the tide of poverty and promote health, it is essential that the UN objectives relating to family planning are realised.

National and international strategies

The Health of the Nation document (Department of Health, 1992, pp. 2, 12–13) states that its objectives are based on the WHO 'Targets for health for all' and the WHO European Region's targets. The overall message is the prevention of ill-health and the promotion of good health. *The Health of the Nation* document identifies key areas, objectives and targets. Included in these is a reference to the quality of the environment as an important influence on health (p. 29). It goes on to refer to the government White Paper *This Common Inheritance*, which sets targets and other environmental objectives.

The WHO (1992, pp. 1–15) when discussing health says:

Human health should be seen in a physical, social, behavioural and ecological context. In this holistic model, promotion of health plays a prominent part ... health promotion activities should involve other sectors making a contribution to health, such as education, food, nutrition, and *environment*.

Such statements indicate that the quality of the environment is directly related to human health. The WHO has identified areas in the environment which require international remedial action such as the destruction of the ozone layer; global warming; safe and adequate supplies of drinking water; safe disposal of sewage; energy production; air quality; hazardous substances and their disposal; and major disasters.

In their report to the United Nations Conference on Environment and Development in Rio de Janeiro held on 3–14 June 1992, the WHO pointed to three main objectives (WHO, 1992):

1. to achieve a sustainable basis for health
2. to provide an environment which promotes health
3. to encourage all individuals to be more aware of their responsibility for health on an environmental basis.

From this conference the United Nations reaffirmed its declaration on the 'human environment' adopted in Stockholm in 1972 and sought to build on it. They established the goal of a 'global partnership' through the creation of new levels of cooperation between states, key sectors of societies and people – and so an agenda was born for the 21st century with 27 principles, the first being:

Human beings are at the centre of concerns for sustainable development. They are entitled to a healthy and productive life in harmony with nature (United Nations, 1993, p. 3).

Agenda 21 is the basis for action, a blueprint for the 'global partnership'. It has seven themes:

1. Revitalizing growth and sustainability	Prospering world
2. Sustainable living	Just world
3. Human settlements	Habitable world
4. Efficient resource use	Fertile world
5. Global and regional resources	Shared world
6. Managing chemicals and wastes	Clean world
7. Peoples' participation and responsibility	Peoples' world.

These themes are all interlinked and attempt to address the main environmental issues affecting health and the quality of life of the human population.

For revitalising growth and sustainability international and national initiatives are required to develop relevant policies at strategic planning and management level. These will include economic instruments, environmental accounting, legal and regulatory frameworks, whilst the priority actions of sustainable living are combating poverty; changing consumption patterns and consideration of the demographic dynamics and the health problems of different world regions. Consideration must be given to these issues. Developing countries experience different health problems from those of the west. Health problems resulting from hostile natural environments, exploitation of natural resources, poverty and therefore susceptibility to infectious and parasitic disease. This coupled with a lack of the necessary health-care infrastructure needs to be addressed on a partnership basis with the west.

The European Region of WHO has 32 active member states and is unique in the world as it consists of mainly industrialised countries with advanced medical services (Rantanen, 1990). The First European Conference on Environment and Health was held in Frankfurt in December 1989. It resulted in the European Charter on Environment and Health. Amongst other issues the charter identified that, since developing countries are faced with major environmental problems, there is a need for global cooperation.

As well as the European Region of the WHO there is also the European Union (EU). The WHO European region covers countries in the EU as well as non-EU states. The EU has issued a number of directives on health and health and safety matters. Indeed article 129 of the Maastricht Treaty states that part of the community's commitment should be to protect health. Directives issued by the EU to member states on issues to do with health and safety at work have resulted in a series of new UK legislation known affectionately as 'the six pack'. This new legislation is now on the statute book in order that, under the Single European Act, workers may travel between EU member states and find the same standard of health and safety at work in each (Commission of the European Communities, 1993).

The new legislation considers the working environment from mainly the physical aspects and suggests minimum standards for space, lighting, thermal environment, and welfare facilities. It includes all workplace equipment and machinery including computer technology and in particular display screen equipment (DSE). There has been so much printed about DSE and its effects on health that the public is still confused and thus unaware. It will take time and education to improve the situation and convince people that it is the ergonomics of the workstation and the job specification that cause health problems, such as work-related upper-limb disorders (WRULD), and not the display screen itself.

For nurses perhaps the most important new legislation is the Manual Handling Regulations 1992 and it is hoped that these regulations, coupled with the removal of crown immunity from NHS premises, will reduce if not eliminate back injuries to nurses. For the first time legislation requires that an assessment of manual handling is made and where appropriate mechanical means must be used to lift unsuitable loads. The regulations also require that adequate training is given on lifting and handling techniques including the use of mechanical devices. Where patient lifting and handling is required, nurses, and other health-care workers, should now be better prepared for the task. Where failure to comply with this legislation can be demonstrated, then prosecution in a court of law may result.

Besides the new legislation required for the Single European Market, the EU has issued directives on substances hazardous to health, including carcinogens, and these are now on the UK statute book as the Control of Substances Hazardous to Health Regulation 1988 (COSHH) and draft directives being discussed on physical agents such as vibration, thermal conditions and a reappraisal of noise as agreed with the first directive ten years ago.

The UK has had a few problems in adopting and translating the Directives into legislation as the Health and Safety at Work, etc., Act 1974, as an enabling act, provided a suitable basis for updating and improving legislation.

There is therefore a commitment by the WHO, the WHO European region, the EU and the British parliament to improve health by improving the environment.

Sustainable development

Labonte (1991) has developed 12 principles for sustainable development and these provide a basis on which to discuss the concept further. He also coined the term 'econology' which combines ecology and economy, as so much of the health/environment equation depends on the economic issues. Sustainable development is a concept and as such is difficult to define, but most publications which discuss the concept attempt a definition. One such definition is that sustainable development is:

> Development that meets the needs of the present without compromising the ability of future generations to meet their own needs (World Commission on Environment and Development, 1987).

Although Labonte (1991) challenges this definition and simplifies it by saying that the Earth is not growing, he suggests as a global epigram for the 1990s:

> 'Live more simply, so that others might simply live'.

But is it that simple? How are we to do this? Firstly sustainable development needs principle-based decision making based on the concept of 'anticipate and prevent'. Scientific data only describes what exists, it does not predict; an example of this is global warming. As was pointed out earlier global warming is only based on models and cannot be guaranteed. The human ecosystem cannot wait until it happens to change. Some strategies must be developed to control and slow down the process until the population has time to adapt and develop.

If health, environment and economy are inextricably entwined then information must be gathered together and shared. Risk assessments are required to determine environment and health. Already the UK has developed BS7750, which is an environmental risk assessment model based on BS5750, the UK standard for quality systems (Grayson, 1992). Economy and health require equity assessments and economy and environment require full cost accounting. It is no good burying our heads in the sand and saying that health should not depend on financial issues, unfortunately it does and certainly if health is to be considered in future development, then economic issues must be included. It is recommended that where there is any doubt the benefit of the doubt must be biased towards human health.

One of the principles for sustainable development requires that there should be shrinking global inequities; that is, that efforts should be made to lessen the gap between nations which have and those which have not. The WHO (1992) suggests that this involves the transfer of resources, reductions in trade barriers and more generous assistance on the part of richer countries. The WHO goes on to say that good health and good environment do not require high per capita incomes but that all individuals require sufficient income or land to meet their basic needs. This brings us to the fourth principle, that of shrinking national inequities, in other words, a more equal distribution of wealth and the basic human right to participate in the political process. This serves not only to promote action but also to check and prevent abusive action on the environment. Altogether it is empowering people individually to take part in preserving the environment, rather than leaving it to a few others. Empowerment, not only in their social or home environment but also in their working environment, especially as one considers that it is in working that we are being productive or offering a service in order to meet the needs of others. Whether or not such an idealistic political situation will ever exist is debatable. As one political regime is defeated or destroyed, then another flares up and never more so than in the final part of the 20th century when civil unrest in countries throughout the world dominates the news, indicating that there are people who still do not have the basic human right to participate in the political process.

Sustainable development is not just about reducing global warming or the hole in the ozone layer it is also about the life we lead, the social interactions, aesthetic qualities and how to maintain the culture or history of the community. Take, for example, the rain forests, not only has chopping these down had an impact on carbon dioxide levels and in turn on global warming, but also it has affected the lives of the indigenous population of the area. Other ecosystems which inhabit the rain forest have also been affected and much of the plant life which is being destroyed has not been properly researched and valuable resources may be lost forever. Sustaining communities must be part of sustainable development.

Five 'Rs' are suggested as ways of considering sustainable development: replenish; replace; reduce; reuse; recycle. The first two replenish and replace the resources used. These are not new concepts, as Canada apparently noted them as far back as 1915 in their conservation programme. Replenish means putting more back than we take out. At present we take out more than we put back and the most we do is to replace what we take out. It has been said that this is most governments' answer to sustainable development. Reducing is what most people envisage as sustainable development and the developed countries should be reducing the use of natural capital such as fossil fuels. This, of course, includes the reduction of waste products such as toxic waste. Primarily if we reduced production both energy and waste would be cut automatically. Lastly the reuse or recycling of commodities is important but may not be the answer to the whole problem. Until we make a positive effort to cut production, energy and waste, reuse/recycling will remain only the tip of the iceberg in sustainable development.

Reflective point
Think about what you recycle/reuse. Is there anything else you could recycle or reuse? Are there ways you could cut down on buying new things or reduce the use of energy?

Sustainable development is the buzz word for the 1990s. It is more than local effort, it requires governments to make positive efforts to change the consumer society and for consumers to take responsibility for the replacement of natural resources and the costs of doing so. Along with this they need to consider the concept of sustaining diversities so that producers and consumers respect both the human and other ecosystems as well as the human cultural system to ensure that their activities have a positive rather than a negative 'knock on' effect.

In 1993 the Secretary of State for the Environment announced the UK proposals for reducing carbon dioxide emissions as required under the Convention on Climatic Change signed at the Earth Summit in June 1992. These proposals include VAT on domestic fuel and power and an increase on fuel duty. Already the lobbyists have been pointing out to the government the problems of such actions on the health of those who are less fortunate, the elderly and the very young. The government is also relying on voluntary agreements on energy efficiency by industry. Pressure groups such as *Friends of the Earth* are asking is this enough? Would legislation be more effective to curb major sources of carbon dioxide emissions? This together with government plans for deregulation seems highly unlikely.

At the beginning of this chapter you were asked in Activity 2 to identify and make a list of how you could be affected by your immediate environment. Were any of the things on your list included in this chapter? Did you consider air, land and water, thermal conditions, plant and animal life which we rely on for our food and with whom we share the Earth? Did you consider the energy from fossil fuels which we take for granted and the machinery which it drives? Perhaps we should consider Labonte's maxim to

live more simply in order that others might simply live.

References

Aldrich, T. and Griffiths, J. (1993). *Environmental Epidemiology and Risk Assessment*. Van Nostrand Reinhold, New York.

Beardsley, T. (1992). Add ozone to global warming equation. *Scientific American*, March.

Bobak, M. and Leon, D. A. (1992). Air Pollution and infant mortality in the Czech Republic 1986–88. *The Lancet*, 340, 1010–1014.

Bolina, B., Doos, B., Jager, J. and Warwick, R. (1986). *The Greenhouse Effect: Climatic Changes and Ecosystems*. John Wiley, Chichester.

Brown, L. R. (1992). *The United Kingdom Environment*, Department of Environment Government Statistical Service. HMSO, London.

Commission of the European Communities (1993). *European Social Policy: Options for the Union, A Green Paper*. Office for official publications of the European Communities, Luxembourg.

Conference of European Environmental Ministers cited in Harrison, R. (1985). *Pollution: Causes. Effects and Control*, 2nd edn. The Royal Society of Chemistry, Cambridge.

Cook, R. (1993). Sun scream. *Nursing Standard*, 7(49).

Dayton, L. (1993). T-shirts find their place in the sun. *New Scientist*, 28 August, 19.

Department of the Environment (1987). *Ozone in the UK*. HMSO, London.

Department of Health (1992). *The Health of the Nation: A Strategy for Health in England*. HMSO, London.

Elmsworth, S. (1990). *A Dictionary of the Environment*. Paladin Grafton Books, London.

Emmanuel, W. R., Shugrat, H. H. and Stevenson, M. P. (1987). Climatic changes and the broad scale distribution of terrestrial ecosystem complexus. *Climatic Changes*, 7, 29–43.

Fishman, A. J. and Crutzen, R. H. J. (1978). Production of ground level ozone. *Nature*, 274, 855.

Grayson, L. (1992). *What the New Environmental Standard Means for Your Business*. Technical Communications (Publishing), Herts.

Godlee, F. and Walker, A. (1992). *Health and the Environment*. BMA, London.

Gould, D. (1993). Homeostasis. In Hinchliff, S. M., Norman, S. E. and Schober, J. E. (eds) *Nursing Practice and Health Care*. Edward Arnold, London.

Gribbin, J. (1988a). The ozone layer. *New Scientist*, Inside Science, No. 9.

Gribbin, J. (1988b). The greenhouse effect. *New Scientist*, Inside Science, No. 13, 1–4.

Hall (1990). *Health and the Global Environment*. Polity Press, Cambridge.

Harris, C. J. (1988). *Fundamentals of Science for Nurses*. Butterworth, Kent.

Harrison, R. (1990). *Pollution Causes Effects and Control*. Royal Society of Chemistry, Cambridge.

Harrison, R. M. (1981). *Lead Pollution: Causes and Control*. Chapman & Hall.

The Health and Safety at Work, etc. Act. (1974) HMSO, London.

Health and Safety Executive (HSE) (1992). *Successful Health and Safety Management*. HMSO, London.

HSE (1992). *Manual Handling Operations: Guidance on the Regulation*. HMSO, London.

HSE (1995). *Control of Substances Hazardous to Health: Approved Code of Practice*. HMSO, London.

Hinchliffe, S. M., Norman S. E. and Schober, J. E. (1993). *Nursing Practice and Health Care*. Edward Arnold, London.

Holman, C. (1989). *Air Pollution and Health*. Friends of the Earth, London.

Holt, A. St J. and Andrews, H. (1991). *Principles of Health and Safety at Work*. IOSH Publishing, Leicester.

Horgan, J. (1992). Volcanic disruption. *Scientific American*, March, 16–17.

Humphrey, J. and Farmer, D. (1990). *Too Loud: A Guide to Workplace Noise, Its Measurement and Control*. Croner, Kingston-upon-Thames.

Hynd, S. W. (1990). Health promotion in the mass media: discussion. *World Health Forum*, 11.

Josep, M. A. (1995). Nitrogen dioxide and allergic asthma: starting to clarify an obscure association. *The Lancet*, 345, 402.

Labonte, R. (1991). Econology: integrating health and sustainable development. Part 1: Theory and background. Part 2: Guiding principles for decision making. *Health Promotion International*, 6(1/2).

Leggett, J. (1990). *The Greenpeace Report.* Oxford University Press, Oxford.

Linn, S. W. (1993). Respiratory effects of sulphur dioxide in freely breathing heavily exercising asthmatics; a dose responsive study. *American Review of Respiratory Disease,* 127, 234–239.

Melvin Howe, G. (ed.) (1977). *A World Geography of Human Diseases.* Academic Press, New York.

Molina, M. T. and Rowland, F. S. (1974) Stratospheric sink for chlorofluoroethanes; chlorine atom catalysed destruction of ozone. *Nature,* 2(49), 810–812.

National Radiological Protection Board (1989). *Living with Radiation,* 4th edn. NRPB, Chilton.

Organization for Economic Co-operation and Development (OECD) (1992). *Global Warming – The Benefits of Emission Abatement.* OECD, Paris.

Pearce, F. (1989). Acid rain. *New Scientist,* 5 November, 1–4.

Porteus, A. (1992). *Dictionary of Environmental Science and Technology.* John Wiley, Chichester.

Rantanen, J. (1990). *Occupational Health Services: An Overview.* WHO Regional Publications European Series No. 26, Copenhagen.

Raymond, E. (1993). Primary health care. In Hinchliff, S. M., Norman, S. E. and Schober, J. E. (eds) *Nursing Practice and Health Care.* Edward Arnold, London.

Read, C. (1990). *Air Pollution and Child Health.* Greenpeace, London.

Roper, N., Logan, W. W. and Tierney, A. J. (1990). *The Elements of Nursing: A Model for Nursing Based on a Model for Living.* Churchill Livingstone, Edinburgh.

Russell-Jones, P. D. and Wigley, T. M. L. (1989). *Ozone Depletion – Health and Environmental Consequences.*

Seager, J. (1990). *The State of the Earth – An Atlas of Environmental Concern.* Unwin Hyman, Boston.

Smith, P. and Warr, K. (1991). *Global Environmental Issues.* The Open University, Milton Keynes.

Stolarski, R. S., Kruegar, A. J., Schoelerl. M. R., McPeters, R. D., Newman, P. A. and Alper, J. C. (1974) Nimbus 7 satellite measurements of the springtime Antarctic ozone decrease. *Canadian Journal of Chemistry,* 322, 808–811.

The Royal Society (1992). *Risk: Analysis, Perception and Management.* Report of The Royal Society Study Group. The Royal Society, London.

United Nations (1993). *The Global Partnership for Environment and Development: A Guide to Agenda 21.* United Nations, New York.

United Nations Population Fund (1991). *The State of World Population 1991.* UN Population Fund, New York.

World Commission on Environment and Development (1987). *Our Common Future.* Oxford University Press, New York.

World Health Organization (1992). *Our Planet, Our Health: Report of the WHO Commission on Health and Environment.* WHO, Geneva.

Further reading

Many of the books and articles in the list of references are worth reading in greater detail in particular we recommend the following.

Godlee, F. and Walker, A. (1992). *Health and the Environment.* BMA, London. This book is made up of a series of articles previously published in the *British Medical Journal.* Each article is a review of the literature published on environmental topics such as populations, climatic change, air pollution, drinking water, etc.

Labonte, R. (1991). Econology: integrating health and sustainable development. *Health Promotion International,* 6(1/2). These two articles look at how health promotion and education can help with sustainable development.

National Radiological Protection Board (1989). *Living with Radiation,* 4th edn. NRPB, Chilton. This booklet helps people to put radiation into perspective as something which naturally occurs rather than something that is man-made. It is particularly relevant to nurses who have little understanding of radiation.

A new book well-worth reading is *The Global Environment: Securing a Sustainable Future* by ReVelle, P. and ReVelle, C. (1992). Jones & Bartlett Publishers, London. It gives a lot of statistics and historical factors as well as further reading lists.

3

THE INDIVIDUAL AND HEALTH

Elisabeth Clark and Kevin Gournay

Introduction

Health psychology is primarily concerned with the promotion and maintenance of health, the prevention and treatment of illness and the improvement of health-care delivery. This chapter will demonstrate how a knowledge of certain, carefully selected, fairly robust psychological theories can improve the understanding of health and health-related behaviours which are essential for the delivery of individualised, holistic care.

Following a brief account of how the discipline of health psychology has evolved and its underpinning by various psychological theories, we shall focus on the following areas.

1. **Personal control and learned helplessness** – the effects of a belief in self-determination on behaviour are outlined and ways in which a patient's or client's perceived sense of control may be increased. Conversely, it is recognised that people experiencing prolonged, high levels of stress can begin to feel that they are unable to influence what happens to them. As a consequence, the individual may come to believe that they have little or no control over what happens to them and may cease trying to influence the outcome, leading to passivity. The likely consequences of people feeling helpless are considered.

2. When working with patients and clients in a health education context, it is clearly important to try to understand why people act in particular ways in order to nurture and enable health promotion. Attribution is the process by which we seek to identify the causes of others' behaviour by inferring others' traits, motives and intentions from observing their behaviour, and the associated theory about how we do this is known as **attribution theory**.

3. **Information-giving** – the provision of adequate information by health-care practitioners is now widely recognised to be crucial in preparing patients for diagnostic tests, admission to hospital, surgery and discharge into the community. It provides an important means by which a person's sense of control may be increased, promoting better recovery and greater independence.

4. The **health belief model** is an attempt to explain health-related behaviours and why some people continue to do things that can potentially damage their health. In particular, it provides a useful framework to examine how individuals can be assisted to establish behaviours that promote health.

Case studies are used to illustrate how psychological insights can be used in clinical practice.

What is health psychology?

Health psychology is a new discipline which has only emerged in the last 15 years or so. A widely accepted definition of health psychology comes from Matarazzo (1982), who states that:

> Health psychology is the aggregate of the specific educational, scientific and professional contributions of the discipline of psychology to the promotion and maintenance of health, the prevention and treatment of illness, the identification of aetiological and diagnostic correlates of health, illness and related dysfunction and to the analysis and improvement of the health care system and health policy formation (p. 1).

Although health psychology is a way of looking at the individual from a psychological perspective, it also assumes that health and illness involve social, biological and psychological factors which interact; this perspective is referred to as the biopsychosocial model (Schwarz, 1982; Sarafino, 1994).

Health psychology has expanded rapidly over the last decade and health psychologists are now to be found working in a variety of hospital and community settings in many countries in the western world. In the United Kingdom, a specific Health Psychology Section has been created within the British Psychological Society (BPS), thus recognising it as a discrete area, and the BPS has also recently established a register of psychologists who practise in this speciality. Increasingly, health professionals are beginning to recognise that there are many applications of health psychology across hospital and community settings, and that it can also be applied in the educational arena in a whole range of preventative strategies.

Where does health psychology come from?

The idea that various mental and spiritual processes could influence the body, and hence determine health, goes back thousands of years. It has long been known that in ancient cultures people believed that mental illnesses were caused by mystical forces such as demoniacal possession, and there is considerable evidence that attempts were made to 'unlock' these forces (Szasz, 1987). One of the most dramatic examples of this is to be found in skulls that have been unearthed which show evidence that holes were bored in them by a process of trephination, so as to release evil spirits. Even more remarkable is evidence that people survived this process!

Philosophers throughout the centuries have contemplated the relationship between the mind and body. The Greek philosophers regarded the mind and body as being separate. Throughout the middle ages, religious ideas had a great influence on the relationship between mind and body and many illnesses, particularly the more dramatic ones such as epilepsy, were seen as either an indication of demoniacal possession or as punishment. In the 17th century, the French philosopher Descartes continued to propagate the argument that mind and body were separate, but stated that they were connected by the pineal gland and that through this gland some sort of communication could take place. Eventually, the foundations of modern neurology were laid down and for the past 200 years, medicine has been based on a knowledge of what we know today as the sciences of anatomy, physiology and biochemistry. Certainly by the early 19th century, the idea that various emotional states and mental illnesses were caused by physical factors was prevalent, and early textbooks written on psychological medicine stressed how mental conditions could be caused by physical factors, and recognised mind and body as part of a highly complex system.

Perhaps the best-known accounts of how physical manifestations such as pain and paralysis could be caused by mental phenomena were those written by Sigmund Freud. Freud's major writings are to be found in no fewer than 24 volumes, published between 1900 and 1940 – a year after his death (see, for example, Freud, 1901, 1940). However, Freud was but one of many physicians from Britain and Europe who studied this connection. Freud and these other workers formed the school of **psychoanalysis** which continues, in a much modified form, to the present day. This school of thought sees the 'unconscious' as responsible for producing both physical and mental reactions. It is interesting to note that psychoanalysis has developed somewhat in isolation of neurology, and is not generally concerned with making links between unconscious processes and specific brain structures or functions. Despite this, the contribution made by psychoanalysts to the recognition of mind and body as one entity has been considerable.

Contemporary health psychology, however, draws much more on more conventional schools of psychology than on psychoanalysis. In particular, health psychology is underpinned by various theories of learning and thinking. While we are unable, by reason of space restrictions, to detail all these theories, some notable ones are worthy of mention. Specifically, operant learning theory and social learning theory have been important in the evolution of theories of health behaviour and perceptions and beliefs about health.

Operant learning theory

Operant learning theory is a major psychological approach which emphasises the contingency between a person's behaviour (or response) and some event; that is to say, the probability that a given response will occur changes according to the consequences that follow it. The original experiments which led to the formulation of this theory were conducted by the well-known American psychologist B. F. Skinner during the 1930s (see Skinner, 1938). In operant learning theory, two types of consequence are regarded as being particularly important:

- **reinforcement** – the likely occurrence of a particular behaviour tends to be increased if what follows that behaviour is in itself pleasing or rewarding (for example, praise), or if it removes an unpleasant or aversive event (for example, avoidance of unpleasant experiences such as nausea or extreme cold). The process of reinforcement involves either applying a positive stimulus (positive reinforcement) or removing an unpleasant stimulus (negative reinforcement)
- **punishment**, on the other hand, involves the presentation of an aversive stimulus whenever a specific response occurs, thereby weakening or decreasing the likely incidence of that specific behaviour in future

These are merely simple examples to illustrate central aspects of operant conditioning theory which have been studied in detail over the last 60 years.

Social learning theory

Social learning theory developed from operant learning theory. The American psychologist Albert Bandura has been the most notable figure in the development of this movement and much of his work has been carried out over the last 30 years. Indeed, as we shall see, his theories have been refined and are widely used in contemporary health psychology. Bandura (1986) argued that while operant processes such as reinforcement are important, the role of thinking is also important in learning. Previously cognitive psychology (that is to say, the study of mental processes that are involved in making sense of the environment such as perception, learning, memory, language, problem solving and thinking) had largely developed in isolation from operant learning theory. Bandura argued that various thinking processes mediated the process of learning.

Bandura was especially interested in how children learn fear behaviour. In particular, he was concerned with how children imitate others, and learning by imitation (often referred to as **modelling**) became central in his theories. More fundamentally, Bandura believed that human beings are not merely passive recipients of reinforcements and punishments, but are in a much more active, reciprocal relationship with their environment. Much contemporary health psychology is, therefore, construed in terms of behaviour, thinking and perception.

Physiological responses and psychological processes

Another area of psychology that has been important in underpinning health psychology is **psychophysiology**. This area of psychology is concerned with studying the complex relationship between physiological and psychological processes. One of the best-known areas of psychophysiological work is the work concerning lie detection. Equipment developed for lie detection measures respirations, the galvanic skin response (a change in the electrical conductivity of the skin that occurs with emotional arousal), blood pressure, heart rate and muscle tension. A polygraph simultaneously measures and records these various physiological responses. It is claimed that predictable changes in these measures can be identified when a person is lying. As one might imagine, there is an ongoing debate about the accuracy of such measures. Whilst the American Polygraph Association claims 90 percent accuracy, evidence collected by Lykken (1984) suggests that the test is only correct about 65 percent of the time, and, moreover, that an innocent person has a 50–50 chance of failing the test. This is because the equipment will also record arousal due to the stress that an innocent person may experience whilst undergoing the process.

Of considerable relevance to health psychology is the study of physical responses to states of anxiety. As long ago as the 1920s, Jacobson noted that the muscles of anxious people were more tense than those of relaxed individuals (Jacobson, 1929). He subsequently developed deep muscle relaxation training which involves the systematic tensing and relaxing of muscle groups to help people with anxiety achieve states of physical relaxation. As a corollary of this procedure, psychologists have developed ways of feeding back, either by sound or via a visual display, various manifestations of physiological arousal (e.g. muscle tension or electrical resistance in the skin); this is known as **biofeedback**. Indeed, advocates of biofeedback claim that it can help people learn to control their states of physical tension. In the last decade or so, it has been recognised that training people to gain control over their physical state can yield beneficial outcomes (Marcer, 1986). For example, it has been shown that teaching people to control their skin temperature may, for a complex set of reasons, help them to control migrainous headaches. Furthermore, relaxation training may also lead to reduction in chronic pain and help people endure stressful medical procedures (for a detailed discussion, see Pearce and Wardle, 1989).

Psychological factors and the immune system

In the last few years, another exciting area concerning the interaction between mind and body has opened up a new approach, known as psycho-immunology. Several groups of workers noticed that when people are under stress, they are more prone to develop various physical illnesses. For example, Jemmott and Locke (1984) showed that respiratory illnesses increase when people experience high levels of stress.

The study of the relationship between immunity and psychological factors has produced a range of exciting ideas. For instance, researchers are investigating the relationship between the development of certain types of cancer and their relationship to both psychological processes and changes in immune function (see, for example, Temoshok and Heller, 1984; Martin, 1987). While there does appear to be a strong relationship

between immunity and factors such as anxiety and depression, the precise mechanisms involved have not as yet been identified. What has become clear is that individuals react in very different ways, both mentally and physically. So, for instance, high levels of anxiety in one individual may be found in the context of otherwise sound physical and mental health, while in other individuals high levels of anxiety and depression appear to be related to problems such as high blood pressure and to diseases such as ulcerative colitis or, indeed, cancer (Antoni, 1987).

To sum up, health psychology has its roots in several diverse areas of psychology, including learning theories, the psychology of thinking and perception and the study of psychophysiology. In general, health psychology has also been influenced by psychoanalysis, although very few health psychologists would use psychoanalytic principles directly in their day-to-day practice.

In the rest of the chapter, we shall consider a number of areas that have been specially selected to provide an understanding of particular aspects of health behaviour and which can be used by health professionals to deliver more effective individualised care.

Personal control

As we have already seen, people may learn many forms of behaviour through conditioning and may respond to external factors such as positive and negative reinforcement. This, however, suggests a pretty mechanistic view of interaction and one which views behaviour as being largely controlled by various kinds of stimuli in the physical and social environment. Such a view contrasts with the belief that many of us hold that we make our own decisions about how to act and that we exert considerable control over our behaviour. In an attempt to identify the main factors that facilitate operant conditioning, numerous experiments have been undertaken. One of the key issues has been found to be a person's perceived sense of control. Operant conditioning appears mainly to occur when an organism believes reinforcement to be under its control (Seligman, 1975).

According to social cognitive theory, behaviour may also be influenced by internal factors such as complex cognitive matters and personal dispositions as well as by reinforcement contingencies and the physical and social environment (Bandura, 1986). In this section, we shall consider the effects of a belief in self-determination on behaviour and begin to look at the consequences if people feel that they have little or no control over their environment.

Personal control can be defined as feeling that one is able to take effective action in order to produce desirable outcomes and to avoid less desirable ones. Most people like to feel that they do have some control over their lives and over what happens to them, and this has been demonstrated by a number of experiments. For example, in one study, Langer (1975) found that a group of people who were allowed to choose their own lottery tickets, valued the tickets more highly and believed that their tickets were more likely to win, compared with a second group of people who had their tickets allocated to them, even though every ticket had an equal chance of winning a prize. It is interesting to note that it is the **perception** of control rather than actual control that appears to be important.

Levels of stress experienced by individuals in a range of situations can be reduced by the use of specific strategies that increase the perceived sense of control (Cohen *et al.*, 1986). These strategies may be classified into three main types:

- cognitive control
- behavioural control
- informational control.

Each of these will be briefly outlined in turn and an example provided of how it might be used in a health-care context.

Cognitive control involves the ability to use mental strategies to reduce the effect of a potentially stressful event. Such a strategy might involve the use of positive imagery and imagining or remembering a pleasant and relaxing situation, such as lying on a beach or floating in warm water, while undergoing a stressful medical technique such as endoscopy. Research evidence suggests that although all three types of control may be effective in reducing levels of stress, cognitive control has been shown to produce the most consistent beneficial effects (Thompson, 1981; Cohen *et al.*, 1986).

Behavioural control requires an individual to take a particular action to reduce the effect of a potentially stressful event. For instance, during antenatal classes, pregnant women are taught special breathing techniques and muscle relaxation which can be used during childbirth to reduce the pain during the second stage of labour; or a person with diabetes mellitus will be taught how to provide their own medical care such as how to give themselves injections of insulin and to monitor their blood glucose levels using an electronic meter.

Informational control involves the acquisition of knowledge about a potentially stressful event. For example, pregnant women may be provided with descriptions of the physiological processes of childbirth and the procedures and sensations to expect during labour and delivery. A further example is provided by the research of Rodin (1983), who first reviewed the range of methods used to prepare children for hospital and then developed two simple and truthful preparation games which provided clear information about what would happen when they had a blood test and explaining why. She then evaluated the benefits of using the games systematically by observing the anxiety levels of children undergoing venepuncture. Rodin found that the use of the specially prepared material was effective in reducing the anxieties of children at the time of venepuncture when compared with children who did not receive the information, via the games, prior to undergoing the procedure.

The provision of information concerning various alternative treatments or courses of action can also increase a client's sense of personal control over key aspects of decision-making. For instance, prior to giving birth, a pregnant woman is likely to be told about a range of alternative approaches to pain relief. These might include no medical form of intervention, the use of nitrous oxide and oxygen, pethidine, epidural anaesthesia, transcutaneous electrical nerve stimulation (TENS), acupuncture and, possibly, hypnosis. Rodin (1986) suggests that patients try to make decisions and act in ways that will increase the likelihood of desirable outcomes and minimise the risk of less desirable outcomes.

Reflective point

Imagine that you are a patient and have just been admitted to hospital for minor day-surgery. Write a list of all the events in the day over which you could exert real control. For instance, can you control when you are ready for discharge?

Your list may have been fairly short. Whilst patients cannot be given real control over all aspects of their health-care, it is often possible to increase their feeling of control by keeping them fully informed over what is going to happen to them and encouraging involvement in decision-making. Remember, it is the **perception** of control rather than the actual control that is important.

Studies of the effect of personal control on health-related issues

Numerous studies undertaken in health-care settings have investigated the benefits of enhancing people's sense of control. It would appear that one of the most effective ways of helping people to cope with surgery and specific treatments including those that are potentially distressing is to encourage individuals to use one or more types of control (Wilson-Barnett, 1989a). For example, Kendall *et al.* (1979) studied the effects of psychological preparation on the anxiety levels experienced by male patients undergoing cardiac catheterisation. Those who agreed to participate were randomly allocated to one of four groups:

- **Group 1** received training in methods of cognitive control which helped them to recognise and cope with anxiety symptoms
- **Group 2** received preparation to increase their informational control and learned about the procedures and what to expect through printed booklets and discussion with a therapist
- **Group 3** (comparison group 1) only received general conversation with a therapist and if patients asked questions they were told that they had to ask the cardiologist
- **Group 4** (comparison group 2) received the standard preparation, which consisted of a brief verbal account of the catheterisation procedure from the cardiologist during a ward round, together with general reassurance from staff about the procedure.

Behavioural control could not be employed in this study since patients are required to be entirely inactive throughout the procedure. Using three independent measures of anxiety, it was found that subjects in Groups 1 and 2 experienced lower levels of anxiety both before and during catheterisation when compared with the two comparison groups (Groups 3 and 4).

Both Langer *et al.* (1975) and Ridgeway and Mathews (1982) have also reported benefits of cognitive control for patients scheduled to undergo major elective surgery in terms of reductions in pre- and post-operative stress, and less need for medication following surgery. Benefits of increasing the informational and behavioural control of patients undergoing surgery have also been reported (see, for example, Johnson *et al.*, 1978; Anderson, 1987). When considering the practical implications of these findings, it is important to note that all information provided needs to be unambiguous and clearly communicated, otherwise it can lead to misunderstandings and can result in increased anxiety (Wallace, 1986). Particular care also needs to be taken with young children, who may become more anxious if told a lot of detail about potentially distressing aspects of treatment or of surgery. Information regarding sensory experiences, such as the sounds of different types of equipment or the tingling feeling following a local anaesthetic, has, however, been found to be helpful (Miller and Green, 1984).

Carey and Burish (1988) suggest that the use of behavioural control via behavioural intervention techniques (such as deep muscle relaxation training or stress management techniques) provides patients with greater perceived control over their situation because they are able to take a more active role in the intervention, which appears to reduce reported levels of helplessness and thus improve patients' psychological state. Similarly, Johnston (1982) concluded that reductions in blood pressure can be achieved through using behavioural techniques. More recently, Johnston (1989) has argued the case for the use of stress management techniques to reduce coronary heart disease through the lowering of a large number of stress-related risk factors in high-risk groups. He does, however, acknowledge the need for further research in this area to verify his claims.

Taylor *et al.* (1984) studied women with breast cancer and found that those who used cognitive control and those who used behavioural control had adjusted better to breast cancer than those who did not. The former group focused on thinking about their lives differently but positively, whilst those using behavioural control tended to alter their lifestyle and take regular exercise, carry out relaxation programmes and the like. Interestingly, this study did not find that reading books on breast cancer (informational control) affected adjustment. It may be that informational control is more effective when combined with the use of other forms of control.

Reflective point
Think about a patient/client you have cared for who has received a diagnosis of a life-threat-ening illness. Consider both the positive and the negative ways in which the person has handled this information, and how you might have helped him/her cope better by enhancing his/her sense of control.

It is important to tailor different types of activity designed to enhance a sense of personal control to the specific circumstances and needs of the individual. Remember that informational control alone may not be as effective as when it is combined with cognitive and/or behavioural forms of control.

Feelings of personal control and of self-efficacy can also affect individuals' efforts towards re-habilitation. Self-efficacy is the belief that we can successfully achieve something if we want to do so (Bandura, 1986). To investigate the effect of self-efficacy on the achievement of specific goals, Kaplan *et al.* (1984) studied patients suffering from serious respiratory disorders, such as emphysema and chronic bronchitis, who had been given guid-ance concerning exercise programmes. At the same time, they were asked to assess their capabi-lities (their self-efficacy) on a range of physical activities such as walking. Correlational data sug-gested that patients were more likely to comply with the prescribed exercise programme if they had rated themselves highly on their physical capabilities.

Locus of control

Not only are there different types of control that people can use to achieve a greater sense of control over specific events, psychologists have also found that there are important individual differences in the overall amount of control that people believe they have over things that happen in their lives. According to Rotter (1966), indivi-duals develop general expectations about the

effects of their behaviour, and he put forward the concept of **locus of control** to describe a person's beliefs about their control over events in everyday life. During the course of our lives, we use a range of complex sources of information, some of which may not always be objective, to judge the amount of control we have. For instance, we use personal experience and the perception of our own perfor-mance – the successes and failures that we experience in our everyday lives, particularly at important transitions such as starting school, leav-ing school or college, and starting a job. If there appears to have been some relationship between one's actions and the outcomes, we may tend towards a more internal orientation, whereas if the relationship between actions and outcomes appears to be more random (i.e. if a person still continues to perform badly in exams however hard he or she works beforehand), then a more external orientation is likely.

People who think that they have considerable control over both the successes and the failures in their day-to-day lives are described as having an **internal locus of control** orientation. Such people feel responsible for what happens to them. Others who feel that they have little or no control over what happens to them are described as having an **external locus of control** orientation, since they believe that their lives are largely determined by random forces such as fate, luck or chance. Thus, a person's locus of control is determined by the degree to which he or she attributes res-ponsibility for events either to him or herself or to external forces. In an attempt to measure indivi-dual's beliefs about control, Rotter (1966) devised a scale, known as the Locus of Control Scale – a self-administered questionnaire compris-ing a series of pairs of opposed statements such as:

1a. Making a lot of money is largely a matter of getting the right breaks
1b. Promotions are earned through hard work and persistence
2a. Many times the reactions of teachers seem haphazard to me
2b. In my experience I have noticed that there is usually a direct connection between how hard I study and the grades I get
3a. Most of the things that happen to me are a matter of luck
3b. I am in complete control of my destiny.

Individuals are required to indicate which statement from each pair of statements most closely reflects their own beliefs. Their overall score describes their orientation either towards internal or external locus of control. Coefficients of internal consistency were used to assess the extent to which all the items measure the same construct range, and these ranged from 0.49 to 0.76. Meanwhile, the test–retest reliability was found to range from 0.49 to 0.83 (Rotter, 1966). These two measures enable us to feel fairly confident that the scale is both homogeneous and reliable.

Rotter's Locus of Control Scale has been used to assess locus of control orientation and then relate this to specific health or health-care issues. For example, Lowery and Ducette (1976) found that people with diabetes with a more internal locus of control had greater knowledge of their condition than those with a more external locus control.

Unlike many other personality characteristics, locus of control does not necessarily remain fixed over time (Rodin, 1987). Diamond and Shapiro (1973) have shown that participation in an encounter group may increase a person's feeling of control. (An encounter group is a type of group in which participants are encouraged to express and act out their emotions through body contact and structured activities in an environment of mutual trust.) Meanwhile, Lachman (1986) has found that as people grow older, their locus of control may shift more towards external if chance appears to be playing a greater role in what happens. This can result in some older persons being far more prepared than they might previously have been to leave important decisions relating to their health and treatment options up to the 'professionals'.

People who have experienced high levels of stress over long periods of time may begin to believe (whether or not this perception is real) that nothing that they do really matters and that they cannot influence what happens to them. The individual may, therefore, come to feel that the or she has little or no control over events and may even stop trying to strive for particular goals, and this can lead to passivity. More worryingly, individuals may even cease to exert control over situations where success is likely and where they can influence what happens to them. Seligman (1975) has described this condition resulting from lack of control over events as **learned helplessness** which, he believes, is experienced by those suffering from severe depression. Abramson *et al.*

(1978) subsequently revised the theory of learned helplessness to emphasise that what matters is the perception of control (rather than actual control over circumstances).

Much of the early work in this area was undertaken with animals, raising important questions about the generalisability of the findings. It was found that exposure to uncontrollable negative outcomes – unpleasant electric shocks over which the animals had no control – resulted in complete passivity on the part of the animals who eventually stopped trying to escape the electric shocks (Seligman, 1975). Experimental studies, using an unpleasant loud noise rather than electric shocks, have demonstrated similar effects in college students (e.g. Hiroto and Seligman, 1975; Miller and Seligman, 1975), but these studies were carried out in artificial laboratory contexts which, it can be argued, are far removed from everyday life.

However, studies undertaken in more naturalistic settings have also shown that a lack of control over events may result in more negative outcomes including stress-related illnesses and passive behaviour. For example, Schulz (1976) divided a group of residents in an old people's home into two sub-groups. Only one of these groups was allowed to make their own arrangements about who should visit them, whilst the other group was not. The health and morale of the second group were found to be considerably worse than the first. Whilst this study raises obvious ethical concerns, it does highlight the detrimental effects that can result when control over one's environment is curtailed. Another interesting study was that of Greer *et al.* (1979), who undertook a prospective study of women who had undergone a mastectomy following early diagnosis of breast cancer. The women's reactions to cancer were categorised as either an active 'fighting response' or more passive 'acceptance and helplessness'. After five years, 75 percent of those who adopted a fighting response were still alive compared with just 35 percent of those who were more passive.

The health locus of control and the multidimensional health locus of control

To improve the predictive ability of measures of locus of control in health-related settings, Wallston *et al.* (1976) developed an instrument specifically related to health, entitled the Health Locus of

Control which enabled individuals to be categorised as 'health externals' or 'health internals' according to how they rated six externally worded statements and five internally worded statements. This scale was subsequently modified to create the Multidimensional Health Locus of Control (MHLC), comprising 18 items, divided into three scales:

- internal health locus of control
- powerful others' health locus of control, and
- chance locus of control.

Thus, the external dimension has been sub-divided into two distinct components – the powerful others and the chance locus of control (Wallston *et al.*, 1978).

An individual must decide, using a Likert-type rating scale, the extent to which they agree or disagree with each of the 18 statements. The 'internal' and the 'chance' locus of control scales measure the extent to which people believe they are in control of the state of their health. The powerful others' health locus of control scale provides a useful indication of the extent to which people perceive their health to be controlled by health-care professionals rather than by themselves.

A number of studies have investigated whether the degree of externality/internality provides a useful predictor of health behaviours. For example, it has been found, using the MHLC, that patients with serious illnesses, such as cancer, tended to experience less helplessness or depression if they scored highly on both the internal health locus of control and the powerful others' health locus of control when compared with those who scored highly on the chance scale (Marks *et al.*, 1986). In a study of the feasibility of using insulin pumps, Bradley *et al.* (1987) noted the decisions of a group of patients with diabetes when offered three different approaches:

- the continuation of injections of insulin once or twice daily
- intensified conventional treatment, or
- the use of a continuous subcutaneous insulin infusion pump.

They found that those who chose the latter treatment felt that they had less control over their diabetes and attributed more control to the health professionals responsible for their care, when compared with those selecting the other two treatment options.

Several studies have used the MHLC to investigate health locus of control and levels of physical activity. For instance, Dishman *et al.* (1980) found that those who undertook regular physical activity programmes had higher internal health locus of control scores than those who did not. More recently, Slenker *et al.* (1985) administered the MHLC to 123 young people who regularly jogged to keep fit and to 93 people who did not exercise on a regular basis. They also found that the latter group scored significantly lower on the internal health locus of control scale when compared with the joggers.

Whilst the research findings are not always consistent, there is an increasing volume of research evidence to suggest that there may be a relationship between locus of control and people's health behaviours (Wallston and Wallston, 1981). Those who are more internally oriented appear to be more likely to take greater responsibility for their actions and to take active steps to change their lifestyle if needed, compared with more externally-oriented individuals. Hussey and Gilliland (1989) also conclude that internally-oriented individuals are more likely to be health oriented and concerned about their physical well-being, and are also more likely to follow recommended health regimens. Oberle (1991), however, notes that when the locus of control is considered along with other variables, such as a person's health beliefs, the predictive power is further improved. It would appear, therefore, that the locus of control is associated with specific behaviours in a highly complex fashion and merits further investigation.

In the meantime, however, it is important for all health-care professionals to be mindful of the practical applications of research that have demonstrated that encouraging patients and clients to take greater personal control can produce all kinds of positive outcomes including reductions in reported pain in children suffering from severe burns (Kavanagh, 1983), raised morale in elderly people living in institutions (Ryden, 1984) and reduced anxiety levels in critical-care patients (Boeing and Mongera, 1989). Conversely, a lack of control has been found to have a negative effect on the course of tumour growth (Sklar and Anisman, 1979) and on the number of physical complaints a person reports (Pennebaker, 1982). In a paper examining the influence of personal control on health promotion, Peterson and

Stunkard (1989) conclude that greater control – whether this is 'actual' or merely perceived – is associated with better coping, better motivation in relation to health matters and thus improvements in lifestyle, reductions in stress level and more positive overall physical and mental health. There are clearly numerous benefits to be gained by enhancing a person's perception of personal control.

It is important to note that the research evidence relating to personal control and learned helplessness discussed so far describes how many people have been observed to respond in a range of research settings. It is, however, important to note that exposure to negative events, even those that are outside of one's control, does not always lead to helplessness in every individual and on every occasion. In order to begin to understand why some people react differently, it is necessary to focus on the cognitive processes by which we make inferences about a person's actions, motives, feelings or intentions on the basis of observing that person's behaviour. Figure 3.1 summarises some of the main factors that can influence a person's ability to cope with various health states such as chronic disease, medical interventions or childbirth.

Attribution theory

Social psychologists have been concerned for many years with the judgements that people make concerning their own and other people's behaviour and with the way that people explain events. When working with patients and clients in a health education context, it is clearly important to try to understand why people act in particular ways in order to enhance health promotion activities. The process by which we seek to identify the causes of others' behaviour by inferring traits, motives and intentions from observing their behaviour is known as **attribution**, and the associated theory about how we do this is known as attribution theory.

The origins of attribution theory may be traced back to the work of Heider (1958), who was interested in lay people's understanding of causes of behaviour. He suggested that we are not merely happy to observe behaviour, but want also to know the 'why' behind a particular behaviour and provide reasons for it. You will almost certainly have asked yourself similar questions. For example, why does Claire Brown continue to

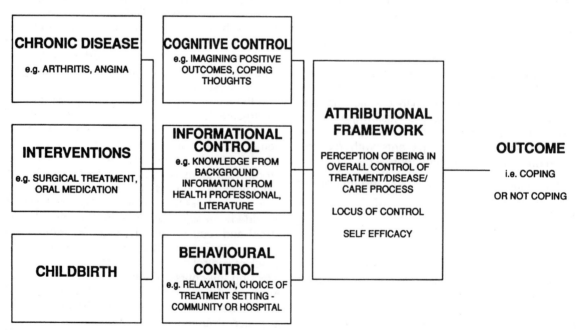

Fig. 3.1. *Factors influencing coping with various health states.*

smoke so heavily and to drink considerable amounts of alcohol regularly when she has been told and appears to understand the likely harm that may be caused to her unborn baby?

According to Heider, behaviour results from the combined effects of factors from within the person (these are referred to as internal factors relating to the disposition of the person) and from the environment (external factors to do with the situation). Thus, a central question is whether we attribute specific behaviours to internal or external factors. Internal attributions explain behaviour in terms of some characteristic of the person (e.g. Mr Jones suffered a massive myocardial infarction because he was overweight, smoked heavily and ignored the advice he was given about the need to change his lifestyle), whilst external attributions explain behaviour in terms of the situation or context (e.g. Mr Jones' heart attack was largely due to the constant pressure he was under at work because of his demanding boss who continually required very tight deadlines to be met).

Since internal factors are located within the person, they are deemed to provide a more reliable basis for making judgements or predictions about that person. Kelley (1967, 1973) suggested that people use three types of information to make judgements about whether behaviour is likely to be the result of internal or external factors. These are:

* distinctiveness
* consistency
* consensus.

If a person behaves in a particular way on a number of different occasions (low on distinctiveness), and also behaves similarly on a number of different occasions (high on consistency), and others tend not to behave in similar ways even when in the same or a similar situation (low on consensus), then it may reasonably be assumed that the cause of the behaviour is within the person (i.e. it is internal), rather than triggered by the situation in which the person finds him or herself (an external cause). So, behaviour that is judged to be low on distinctiveness, high on consistency and low on consensus is likely to lead one to believe that internal causes may be largely responsible for that behaviour. On the other hand, behaviour that is judged to be high on distinctiveness, low on consistency and high on consensus would lead one to believe that external causes may be largely responsible, and that these may well be beyond

anyone's control. Some conditions, however, may be perceived to be externally caused and yet also within a person's control. King (1982) undertook a prospective study in which attempts were made to predict attendance at a blood pressure screening clinic. It was found that people were more likely to attend if they perceived the cause of their condition to be external, yet controllable.

As one might expect, there are potentially differential effects when a particular outcome or condition is attributed to an internal rather than to an external cause. For example, a person undergoing a rehabilitation programme following a serious accident, who fails to make the rate of progress that was expected, is likely to suffer a greater loss of self-esteem if this lack of progress is attributed to internal causes (such as a lack of effort) than if the lack of progress is attributed to some external cause (such as the person running the programme). Even when nothing or no-one can be held to blame for a particular outcome, people often need to attribute blame to an external cause in order to deal with the situation and, indeed, this may provide an important coping strategy, even though an external attribution may not enable individuals to feel in control of their environment. By contrast, a person in similar circumstances who is unable to sustain a belief in an external attribution could suffer a devastating negative effect on self-esteem which could result in a perceived loss of control and a growing feeling of helplessness, and this in its turn would be likely to hinder progress further. It appears that it is not necessarily a real lack of ability, but rather a perceived lack of ability which can reduce an individual's potential to achieve particular goals.

In addition to the attribution of internal and external causes, two further dimensions appear to be used to assess a situation. If a person experiences negative events that are not controllable and these are attributed to a stable, long-lasting cause (as might be the case in a chronic illness or disabling condition), then people are more likely to experience helplessness, or even depression, than if they believe the situation to be only temporary. Finally, people also appear to assess whether a particular behaviour that they are not managing to control (e.g. an inability to stick to a low-fat diet for health reasons) is due to a more general (global) cause such as a lack of will-power, or whether it is attributed to a much more specific issue such as the inability to give up eating chocolate. The more general the attribution, the greater the risk of feeling helpless and depressed compared with more specific attributions.

Whilst it is recognised that many factors play a role in depression, one area that has been investigated in recent years is the difference in the pattern of attributions between depressed and non-depressed individuals, with the former tending to display self-defeating patterns of attributions. It has been noted that people who are depressed tend to attribute negative life events to internal causes that are stable and global, such as lack of ability, while attributing positive events to temporary, external causes, such as luck or the task being particularly easy (Alloy *et al.*, 1990). As you might imagine, this can lead to an individual feeling that they have little or no control over what happens to them; they become depressed and opt out of life. As we shall see, these ideas are similar to Beck's cognitive theory of depression (Beck *et al.*, 1979).

Attribution theory has provided us with some useful insights into the nature of depression in terms of cognitive issues. Crocker *et al.* (1988) reported that individuals who were depressed were more likely to perceive negative events as happening to them whilst believing that positive events happen to others, when compared with those not suffering from depression. Meanwhile, Weary *et al.* (1987) found that depressed people were less confident in their attributions than others, believing themselves to have poorer understanding of other people and of their social world. It has also been suggested that people who are depressed are less motivated to make sense of what is happening in their social world (Marsh and Weary, 1989).

Contemporary clinical psychology has used attribution theory and learned helplessness as the basis for a cognitive behavioural model. This model of treatment recognises that whilst depression is often complex in its cause, the patient's main problem is, nevertheless, an essentially negative view of themselves, of present experiences and about the future – what Beck (1991) has called the 'cognitive triad'. A person who is depressed expects to fail rather than to succeed, with the additional tendency when evaluating their performance to maximise failures and to minimise any successes. Moreover, when something does go wrong, this is often blamed on personal inadequacies or deficiencies (internal causes) rather than on other people or events (external causes). Even in ambiguous situations when others may see that there are obvious alternative explanations for what has happened, the person who is depressed is likely to blame him/herself. Thus, negative perceptions and thoughts tend to dominate the person's consciousness.

Cognitive behavioural treatment of depression is summarised in Figure 3.2. Treatment focuses on identifying and correcting an individual's distorted

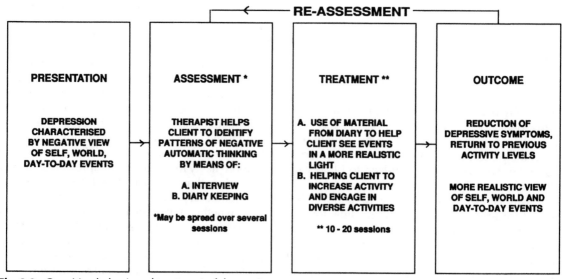

Fig. 3.2. *Cognitive behavioural treatment of depression.*

perceptions and thinking which have become automatic, by training clients to view their lives in more positive and realistic ways. Clients are interviewed by the therapist to identify patterns of negative thinking and are encouraged to employ self-monitoring by using a diary to keep a written record of specific events in their lives and their reactions to those events. The therapist will then utilise the diary entries to discuss alternative viewpoints. As a corollary to this, the therapist will encourage clients to engage in diverse and increased levels of activity, thus providing them with a sense of achievement and greater personal control over their lives. In this way, the earlier pattern of learned helplessness may be broken (Beck *et al.*, 1979; Brewin, 1988). Treatment commonly takes between 10 and 20 sessions (Hawton *et al.*, 1989).

As yet, studies of attribution continue to raise many more questions than are answered, but then this typically happens in the early stages of research in any new field. Attribution research is likely to continue to generate a number of interesting insights in future years and there are many important avenues to be explored, including how attitudes and personality affect attributions, and also the fundamental question of why people use attributions to explain behaviour. You may have identified questions of your own as you read this section.

In the next section, we shall consider the important area of providing adequate information to patients and clients so that they can make informed decisions regarding health-related matters and feel more in control of their lives.

Information-giving and compliance in a health-care context

Everyone needs sufficient, accurate information in order to make important decisions, whether buying a car or deciding whether or not to take up whooping cough immunisation for a young baby. However, when a person is seeking advice about lifestyle issues related to health, or is unwell and has to make decisions about different treatment options, it becomes all the more crucial to ensure that the provision of information is adequate to enable a fully informed choice to be made.

Indeed, one of the seven existing rights listed in *The Patient's Charter* (Department of Health, 1991) is the right 'to be given a clear explanation of any treatment proposed, including any risks and any alternatives, before you decide whether you will agree to the treatment'. This shift towards self-empowerment rests on the ideological concept of autonomy and is related to recent initiatives for client advocacy and partnership in care, whereby the relationship between client and health-care professional is redefined, and the sense of control experienced by the health services consumer is increased. Wherever possible, doctors, nurses and other health-care staff should aim to provide patients and clients with the knowledge and skills needed to care for themselves, rather than encouraging the assumption that they will be 'cared for' which can initiate passive responses, greater dependence and the adoption of the 'sick role' (Wilson-Barnett, 1989b).

An important skill when giving information is to select the facts that are the most relevant and useful to the individual concerned. To start with, the health-care practitioner will need to find out just how much a person already knows about his condition and possible treatment(s). Figure 3.3 highlights the vast array of sources of information available to patients and clients. Only when you have identified what is known and understood any misconceptions and concerns is it possible to plan what, if any, additional information may be deemed necessary. This has several important implications for the health-care practitioner, who clearly needs good communication skills and to be aware of the range of strategies available for imparting information, including one-to-one inter-action, small group sessions, visual displays, provision of leaflets and booklets, audio- and video-tapes, etc. It also requires health-care professionals to keep up to date with new developments and knowledge and be aware of relevant research evidence.

Despite recognition that the provision of information is a central part of the nurse's role and of total nursing care of the patient/client (Wilson-Barnett, 1983), and despite numerous studies providing sound evidence of the benefits of good information-giving (e.g. Wilson-Barnett, 1979; Engstrom, 1984; Hathaway, 1986; Corney *et al.*, 1992), lack of information continues to be high-lighted as being one of the greatest sources of dis-satisfaction among patients, clients and carers

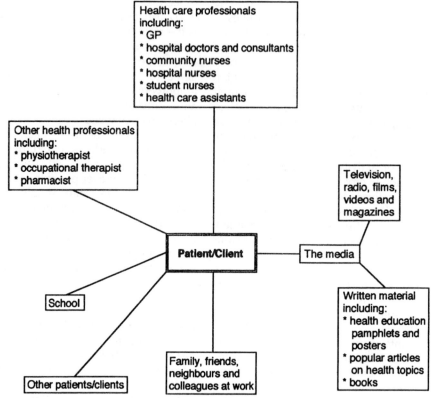

Fig. 3.3. *Sources of information available to patients and clients (adapted from Hall, 1982).*

(Moores and Thompson, 1986; Ley, 1988; Dimond, 1990; Health Service Commissioner, 1993).

Reflective point

What is your experience of patients who have been told that they are about to undergo an unpleasant medical procedure? How well do you think the information was delivered by the health-care professional(s) concerned? Think of an instance where you felt that the information could have been more effectively communicated and identify ways in which this might have been improved.

Wilson-Barnett (1991) recommends that when a patient or client is told about a specific diagnostic test, he or she should be provided with details that are likely to be most relevant and to have the greatest meaning, including:

- the name and purpose of the test
- the time it will take to carry out the procedure
- when it will be carried out
- what preparation, if any, is required (e.g. starvation, bowel preparation)
- an account of the procedure, including details of the anaesthetic or analgesia
- sensations involved (e.g. pressure, bloating)
- guidance on how to cope with the sensations
- any after-effects
- when the results will be available.

The health-care practitioner should aim to provide patients and clients with a realistic account of what will happen so that they can form their own 'mental map' of events which should correspond closely with what they actually experience at the time of the test.

Whilst the benefits of information-giving are well documented, it is important to be aware that some individuals may prefer not to be given prior information about a potentially stressful event, and it is important to be equally sensitive to their needs as to the needs of those who wish to be well informed. Some patients may use denial as a temporary coping strategy and need, therefore, to be given the choice about whether they are provided with information. Thus, it is necessary for every health-care practitioner to be aware of the relevant research findings in this area but these should not be used prescriptively. Rather, they should be regarded as just one of several factors that should be taken into account when planning and delivering care that is truly individualised.

Rapid turnover and early discharge from hospital into the community means that preparation for discharge to aid recovery outside of hospital is becoming increasingly important. A study by Vaughan and Taylor (1988) of the problems faced by surgical patients following discharge highlights the fact that many of the difficulties that were reported could have been either removed or at least alleviated had patients been given better information prior to discharge. Information was needed about subjects such as bathing, diet, when to resume driving and about sexual activity following surgery, suggesting that some hospital staff were not in touch with the range of everyday concerns that are likely to be experienced after major surgery.

Compliance

Continuing concern about patients' levels of understanding of medical information and their compliance with agreed courses of action has stimulated a considerable amount of psychological and medical research. Research evidence has indicated that a number of factors improve the likelihood of compliance. These include a good relationship with the person concerned (Baekeland and Lundwall, 1975) and the credibility of the person offering the advice (Hovland and Weiss, 1951). According to Berscheid (1966), credibility is further enhanced if the information and advice are being given by someone who has had a similar experience to the patient or client. The effects of using one-sided as opposed to two-sided messages has also been investigated (Skilbeck, 1977; Ley *et al.*, 1979). It has been found that presenting one side of the argument is likely to produce greater change in situations where a person is unlikely to be exposed to counter-arguments, but that presentation of both sides of the argument for and against whatever is being suggested provides a more effective basis for longer-term change.

Researchers have also studied the effectiveness of fear-arousing communications in encouraging people to change their behaviour (e.g. Janis, 1967). Sutton (1982) reviews the results of over 30 studies of the use of fear appeals on people's attitudes and behaviour. He concludes that fear arousal seems to increase the likelihood that people will accept recommendations and follow specific advice, but recognises that this is not always the case. What is interesting is that the growing volume of evidence appears to challenge the frequently cited early work of Janis and Feshbach (1953) which found that fear-arousing messages were less effective than neutral messages: the former would appear to be either more effective or, at worst, equally effective as neutral messages.

Ley (1977) has proposed a useful set of guidelines that aim to increase compliance and produce satisfied individuals in a paediatric context. He suggests that when trying to maximise the likelihood of a child complying with a particular regimen, the health-care professional should:

- be friendly
- talk about some things that are not directly related to the problem
- spend time talking to the child
- discover the parents' expectations about the situation, and if these are not being fulfilled, explain why not
- discover any concerns that the parents might have and take appropriate action
- give information as well as ask questions.

To be persuasive, it is important to give reasons for the proposed treatment or self-care – how it achieves its effect, how long it is likely to take and what is likely to happen during the interim period so that an individual can weigh up the risks (costs) and benefits of complying with the proposed advice. Thus, a pregnant woman may decide to continue to smoke even though she understands the risks because she feels that she needs to smoke in order to cope with all the stressors in her life (a perceived important benefit). To increase the other person's sense of control over key decisions to comply with advice, it can be helpful to encourage ownership of the ideas so that the individual feels it was his or her own idea. It is also important to check whether advice being given conflicts with a person's ideas and beliefs about his or her situation or illness and what has been learned about their condition from other sources such as the media, friends and relatives, and other health-care professionals.

According to Sarafino (1994), a range of specific techniques may be used to help ensure effective presentation of health-care information; these include:

- simplification of instructions by using clear language and straightforward sentences
- the use of concrete and specific statements such as 'you should eat at least five pieces of fruit each day' rather than 'you need to increase the amount of fruit you eat'
- breaking down complex procedures that need to be mastered into smaller segments to help individuals achieve mastery of these, step-by-step
- emphasis on key information highlighting why it is important and presenting it early on
- the use of written instructions
- requesting patients/clients to repeat instructions in their own words to check understanding.

However, it has been suggested that such techniques are likely to be more effective in improving compliance with short-term interventions than with those that are longer term (Haynes, 1982), when it is necessary to be more mindful of the factors discussed previously, including the issue of perceived control. House *et al.* (1986) were interested in the level of compliance with dietary advice for people with diabetes. Whereas the patients themselves tended to attribute reasons for non-compliance to external factors or to physiological factors (both of which they felt to be out of their control), the doctors were far more likely to attribute lack of compliance to problems with motivation (an internal cause).

Social support

If a recommended treatment programme requires a change in lifestyle (such as increasing the amount of exercise taken or altering one's diet to reduce the intake of saturated fats), it can be helpful to involve others who can provide social support (Rosenstock, 1985). Such support may be provided by family, friends, colleagues, a health-care worker, or may come from self-help groups, patient groups or organisations offering assistance with particular health issues. One such organisation is Cancer Link. Let's take the example of Jane, a 35-year-old woman, who has chosen to have a mastectomy following the discovery of a malignant breast tumour and who decides to approach Cancer Link. First, she is put in touch with someone who has had a mastectomy (high credibility) and who will explain what will happen, and thus provide accessible information in an informal setting. This should help to reduce the level of fear concerning the actual operation, the pain following surgery, and possible feelings of loss of femininity. This person will also provide an important source of social support throughout Jane's illness and treatment by keeping in touch with Jane's family over the telephone whilst she is in hospital, encouraging them to voice their fears and by providing appropriate reassurance.

Following the recognition of the important contribution of social support for those undergoing stressful experiences, four different types of support have been identified (Cohen and McKay, 1984; Wills, 1984). These are:

- **emotional support** involves expressing care and concern to another so that he or she feels comfort and a sense of belonging
- **esteem support** involves encouragement and the expression of respect which serves to increase a person's self-esteem and sense of self-worth
- **instrumental support** involves the provision of practical assistance, such as helping with child-care arrangements or providing transport to and from hospital, during stressful periods
- **informational support** includes making suggestions and giving advice.

A recent meta-analysis of the social support literature, undertaken by Schwartzer and Leppin (1989), suggests that when people are in stressful situations, the presence of some form of social support can provide a buffer effect and reduce the risk of physical and/or mental illness. Conversely, a lack of social support may result in an increased likelihood of ill-health, particularly mental health problems in women. Also, perceived lack of social support in individuals suffering from chronic illness tends to result in a perception of being in a poorer state of health compared with those who feel that they receive adequate or good social support. Wherever possible, therefore, health-care practitioners should encourage individuals actively to seek out one or more forms of social support and even help them to make contact with the relevant groups and organisations. In this way, the impact of highly stressful experiences can be moderated so that potential health problems may be minimised and recovery from illness is not further hindered.

Reflective point
Consider the four types of social support listed above and identify which ones might be most helpful to (a) a lone parent who has lost his job and who is finding it difficult to pay the bills, (b) an elderly person who is seriously ill in hospital, and (c) the forms of social support that were provided for the woman described above who was due to have a mastectomy and who approached Cancer Link.

The lone parent described in (a) would almost certainly benefit from all four types of social support; in order to maximise his chances of finding a job, esteem support is likely to be particularly crucial.

(b) Emotional and informational support may be especially important for someone who is seriously ill and is being cared for in hospital.

(c) From the brief description of the support provided for Jane by Cancer Link, all four forms of support were available to her and her family.

The beliefs and attributions that a person holds can influence his or her health by affecting behaviour. When trying to empower an individual to make informed decisions concerning health issues, such as taking regular exercise, eating a healthy diet, immunisation, taking prescribed medication or attendance at a screening programme, it is important to be alert to that person's beliefs and values. To be effective, health promotion activities need to be grounded in a clear understanding of how individuals conceptualise their own health. As we will see in the next section, the health belief model (Becker et al., 1977) provides one important means of understanding a person's health behaviours and their relationship to health beliefs.

The health belief model

The health belief model evolved from a series of studies which looked at people's beliefs and perceptions in states of health and illness. This evidence led researchers to try to explain why people behaved in certain ways with regard to health. The

model was put forward in the late 1970s and early 1980s (Becker, 1979; Becker and Rosenstock, 1984) as an attempt to predict the degree to which an individual is likely to play an active part in his/her own health-care.

The health belief model, shown in Fig. 3.4, centres on a process of appraisal by the individual comprised of four sets of components. As a background to taking action regarding one's health, the health belief model recognises that individuals are very different and that factors such as race and culture are extremely important. It also accepts that individuals place different values on aspects of health. For example, Jehovah's Witnesses have specific beliefs about the transfusion of blood, Roman Catholics may not believe in artificial contraception, Jews and Moslems have specific dietary restrictions. As further background, the health belief model sees as important the background knowledge of health possessed by the individual. This background knowledge may come from schooling and health education, from media information and such diverse sources as television, books, films and poster campaigns and also the information received from health professionals such as doctors, nurses, midwives and health visitors. Given this background of individual variation and differences in knowledge, the person then goes through a process of appraisal consisting of the following four components:

- perceived benefits of taking action (to achieve health)
- perceived barriers to taking action (to achieve health)
- perceived threat of illness
- perceived seriousness of illness.

The following case history will help to illustrate how the model works in practice.

Case history

Background

Paula is a 25-year-old data-processing clerk who lives in a council flat in a large city. She is in her 25th week of pregnancy and intends working as late as possible before the baby is born. She lives on her own, having broken up with her partner soon after she found out that she was pregnant. She has a number of money worries but nevertheless is overall a fairly cheerful person. Her parents

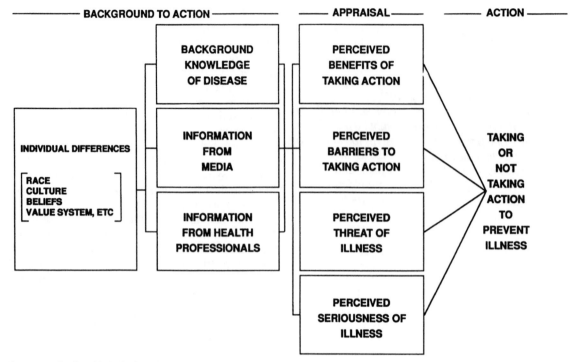

Fig. 3.4. *The health belief model (after Becker and Rosenstock, 1984).*

live close by and although she gets on well with her mother, her relationship with her father has been difficult since Paula was a teenager and they have had long periods without talking to one another. Her parents are both in their 60s and retired and are both heavy smokers.

Apart from smoking, there are no other health problems: Paula drinks very little alcohol, is normally within the healthy range of weight and has put on 7 kg during the pregnancy.

Problem behaviour

Paula smokes at least 20 medium-tar cigarettes per day and at times, when feeling particularly under pressure, she smokes up to 30 cigarettes a day.

Cues to action

1. Her general practitioner (GP) has told her repeatedly that smoking will probably lead to her baby being born with a low birthweight and hence susceptible to complications.
2. She has received more detailed advice from her midwife at the ante-natal clinic who has discussed the whole range of problems associated with smoking and pregnancy.
3. Several posters in the ante-natal clinic and GP surgery put across the message of smoking leading to complications in pregnancy.
4. Paula has come across a number of leaflets about smoking and pregnancy in her GP surgery and the ante-natal clinic.
5. Paula has recently seen a programme on television about the dangers of smoking.
6. Paula passes a large advertising billboard each morning on her way to work, which has an anti-smoking message.
7. One of her friends, who is a heavy smoker, recently suffered a miscarriage at 12 weeks.

To consider these components in more detail, we will now look at each of the four components and how they affected Paula.

Perceived benefits of taking action
As far as Paula is concerned, the perceived benefits of taking action were pointed out by her midwife. These included reduction of risk of complications to her unborn baby, the immediate financial sav-

ings which would help her in her particular situation and, more long term, the reduction of the risk of various serious diseases which are known to be linked to smoking. For example, carcinoma of the lung and coronary heart disease.

Perceived barriers to taking action

Although Paula recognised that smoking was bad for her health and that of her unborn child, she faced a number of considerable barriers to doing anything about stopping smoking. Paula's strong belief was that smoking was helpful in reducing her 'stress'. She also believed that if she tried to stop smoking, she would then suffer withdrawal symptoms. Previously, when she tried to give up smoking, she felt very nervous and edgy and had difficulty sleeping. Although Paula has only put on 7 kg during the pregnancy and is still very much within the normal, healthy range of weight, she believes that if she stops smoking, she will inevitably put on a lot of weight and that after the baby is born, she will continue to be overweight. Paula also suffers considerable pressure from her friends who tell her that smoking a few cigarettes won't do her any harm and all that she really needs to do is to cut down. One of the most obvious barriers to taking any action is the fact that Paula still feels physically very well and does not seem to suffer any adverse effects of smoking. For example, she does not have a cough and she is able to swim several lengths of the local swimming pool without getting too breathless.

Perceived threat of illness

Paula realises that smokers have a considerable risk of developing certain diseases such as heart disease and respiratory disease, but still has considerable problems in believing that she personally will succumb to these smoking-related illnesses. Simply put, this is a case of 'it will never happen to me'. In addition, because Paula feels so well, it is difficult for her to believe that there is a real threat of complications to her unborn child.

Perceived seriousness of illness

Paula realises that low birthweight is a factor associated with problems in newly-born babies and her midwife has told her that such babies are more prone to illness and to longer-term developmental problems.

The overall appraisal process

In order for Paula to take action to stop smoking and hence prevent illness in herself and complications in her unborn child, she must believe that she is personally at risk and that there are significant and serious consequences for both herself and her baby. In summary, she needs to feel that the benefits of taking action outweigh the barriers to taking action. This appraisal process is, therefore, complicated and depends on a large number of factors.

The challenge for Paula's midwife

As stated above, Paula already has a good relationship with her midwife, who has spent a considerable amount of time discussing the nature of the problems associated with smoking and pregnancy. The midwife could help Paula deal with the challenge in several ways.

The midwife can reinforce the benefits of taking action and remind Paula of the financial savings she will make, remind her of the long-term health benefits and remind her of aesthetic factors, such as being able to wear clothes that do not smell and being able to taste the full flavours of food.

The midwife can do several things to help break down some of the barriers to action. With regard to Paula's belief that smoking is stress reducing, the midwife should be able to explain that the intake of nicotine can actually make a person more anxious and that there are other ways of dealing with stress. For instance, the midwife may encourage Paula to use one of the widely available relaxation cassettes so that Paula can deal with some of the withdrawal effects of smoking by systematically trying to relax. Paula can also be reminded that she does not necessarily have to put on weight if she stops smoking. Although there may be an increase in appetite, the weight gain she fears can be prevented by ensuring a plentiful supply of fruit and salad items so that when she becomes hungry she can eat foods which will not cause a weight problem. With regard to the peer pressure she experiences, Paula should be encouraged to discuss her smoking behaviour with other women attending the ante-natal clinic who do not smoke or, better still, those who have successfully given up the habit.

One of the biggest barriers that Paula will face is that she feels physically very well. The midwife can help in this regard by asking Paula to use one of the widely available monitors which measure levels of carbon monoxide in a person's breath. She can thus be given instant feedback about how much carbon monoxide is present in her breath; this feedback should then be followed by information about how carbon monoxide displaces oxygen in the blood and hence leads to problems with the blood supply to the baby.

With regard to the perceived threat and the perceived seriousness of the consequences, the midwife should be able to use much of the readily available health education material to reinforce the wide range of illnesses and complications which can affect people in general and unborn babies in particular. The midwife should not alarm or frighten Paula unduly but she must give her realistic information which will help Paula to make a judgement.

Generally speaking, the application of the above principles by the health professional will help many people to take action and so lead to healthy outcomes. Nevertheless, Paula may well find that smoking is a difficult habit to give up and if the above strategies do not work, the midwife should consider referring Paula to a psychologist who may well be able to give more specialist advice regarding smoking cessation methods.

We shall end with a case history to demonstrate how some of the key concepts outlined in this chapter may be used in a specific context. The case history concerns the nursing management of a young girl, called Sarah, who has been newly diagnosed as suffering from diabetes. As you read the following account, consider how some of the concepts might be used to understand Sarah's needs and her care.

Case history

Sarah is an active, 10-year-old child with one older brother and a younger sister, living with her parents. Her father works as a maintenance engineer and her mother has a part-time job as a clerk. She is doing well at the local junior school, has a wide circle of friends and is very keen on a range of sports; she has already shown indications of being an all-round sportswoman and has competed in county trials.

Over recent months she has often complained of feeling thirsty, she has lost weight and has been feeling generally tired and unwell. In the past

month, her GP has confirmed that she is suffering from diabetes mellitus and has referred her to the diabetic unit at the local hospital. There is a family history of diabetes – her maternal uncle has severe, poorly controlled diabetes and, despite being relatively young (35), is in poor health.

Sarah has seen the consultant physician who specialises in diabetes in children, who has referred her to the clinical nurse specialist attached to the unit.

There are a range of issues that will need to be addressed to help Sarah to adjust to the diagnosis and to ensure satisfactory management of her diabetes in both the short and the longer term. These include:

- information about her condition for both Sarah and her parents
- information about the management of diabetes mellitus for both Sarah and her parents
- training in blood glucose monitoring, injection technique, dietary management
- involvement of parents in the management of Sarah's condition
- information about exercise and its role in maintaining good health
- information about, and training in, the management of hypo- and hyperglycaemic attacks
- information about general health-care because of increased susceptibility to infections and injury.

Reflective point
Before reading on, stop to think about how the clinical nurse specialist might address each of these areas.

Sarah can be given information about her condition in several ways. The nurse may simply tell Sarah about diabetes, its management, complications, etc., and she could also use a widely available range of leaflets and books. She might use a number of videos produced by health education agencies. Although of no relevance to Sarah, the clinical nurse specialist also needs access to interpreting services so that information can be given to people whose first language is not English.

Ideally, Sarah's parents should also be involved in the process of information-giving and should join Sarah in these sessions. Sometimes, the clinical nurse specialist will wish to see groups rather than individuals and this, of course, may help both Sarah and her parents to feel that they are not alone in their problems.

Likewise, information about the management of diabetes can be transmitted verbally and by the use of leaflets and books and by videos.

With regard to training in blood glucose monitoring and injection technique, Sarah can be shown videos of children of a similar age to herself undertaking these procedures and this modelling effect will be important. Ideally, Sarah should also be introduced to other children in the clinic and should watch them giving themselves injections and undertaking blood glucose monitoring. This process of learning by imitation (modelling) is the most effective method of learning a complex behaviour and using both videos and 'live' models is the preferred approach (Wessler, 1984).

It is important to involve Sarah's parents in the process of management, emphasising that they are there to help and encourage Sarah rather than 'take over'. It is most important for Sarah to feel in control of what is happening to her. Her parents may need to be offered counselling to help them deal with the impact of the diagnosis. This counselling may be carried out by the clinical nurse specialist and will be helpful in three ways:

- parents need to be reassured and to see the problem as serious but manageable
- they may express, and this is common, guilt that they may have contributed to the onset of the disease by, for example, allowing too many sweets
- the nurse may need to give considerable information about prognosis and management and help the parents begin to gain a feeling of control, via increased knowledge of the disease.

With regard to diet and exercise, Sarah and her parents need to be given a range of written information and also some practical help with monitoring this. The clinical nurse specialist may well ask Sarah to use a diary so that Sarah can record what she eats, what fluids she drinks, what exercise she takes, what her blood glucose levels are, what doses of insulin she administers and generally how she feels. The nurse may also ask Sarah to record her levels of anxiety on a scale, say from 0 to 10, where 10 is used to indicate the worst possible anxiety and zero represents complete relaxation.

The nurse needs to provide general information that is realistic and informative and while it should warn Sarah of the seriousness of her illness, and her increased risk from injury, it should not provoke too much anxiety.

Reflective point
Now consider how the following concepts from health psychology could be used in the nursing management of Sarah:

- *personal control*
- *social support* and
- *the health belief model*.

---

1. **Personal control**: the clinical nurse specialist should aim to provide Sarah with a sense of personal control by first of all giving her informational control via the process of information-giving described earlier. Second, she can provide Sarah with behavioural control by helping her acquire the necessary skills to give herself injections of insulin and monitor her blood glucose levels. The clinical nurse specialist will also help Sarah gain cognitive control by introducing her to other children whose diabetes is being successfully managed and, therefore, help her to consider positive outcomes in her eventual management of the condition. Likewise, Sarah's parents can be helped to gain a sense of personal control in the same way, although the extent of their behavioural control should be less than Sarah's, since the ultimate objective is to make Sarah the manager of her own condition. Similarly, with regard to locus of control, Sarah needs to be helped to attribute personal responsibility for what happens to herself and this can be achieved by teaching her to monitor the effects of eating sensibly, exercising appropriately and giving herself the correct dose of insulin.

If Sarah is provided with accurate and clear information about her condition, given a sense of control over the total management and involved from an early point, compliance need not be a problem. As we saw previously, the credibility of the information given is much enhanced by exposure to someone who has had a previous experience and therefore in Sarah's case, the introduction to other children in the diabetic clinic will be most helpful. It is important also to consider the details of how information should be presented verbally by the nurse and you may recall that the presentation of information will be most effective if a range of specific techniques are used. Consider what has been said earlier about the effective presentation of health-care information and bearing this in mind, write down some examples of how the clinical nurse specialist may present the information to Sarah.

2. The case history also highlights the necessity for all four types of **social support**: emotional, esteem, instrumental and informational support. Emotional and esteem support can be provided within the context of a good nurse–patient relationship. This relationship will need to be built up gradually and the clinical nurse specialist will need to get to know Sarah as a person to understand her likes and dislikes and to understand where she may feel vulnerable. The nurse is also faced with the challenge of providing support for Sarah's parents by establishing a good relationship with them. They in turn can provide additional emotional and esteem support for Sarah. Instrumental support may be facilitated by the clinical nurse specialist who will help Sarah and her parents in facing the practicalities of obtaining the necessary equipment (needles, syringes, blood glucose monitoring devices) and in giving her access to more general sources of help such as the British Diabetic Association. Informational support is provided by the education and training programme associated with the giving of insulin and the monitoring of blood glucose.

3. With regard to the **health belief model**, the nurse will need to show Sarah that there are considerable benefits to taking healthy action. These benefits will include a sense of well-being and a minimisation of side-effects. However, there may be considerable barriers to Sarah taking action and these may include the temptation to give in to peer group pressure, to accept sweets or to avoid exercise. The nurse should pre-empt these difficulties and discuss how Sarah may resist peer group pressure, what alternatives there may be to eating sweets and how exercise may be most usefully built into her routine. The clinical nurse specialist will always need to ensure that Sarah feels that the benefits of taking healthy action are greater than any barriers to taking effective action.

In summary, from the time of diagnosis of Sarah's diabetes, the clinical nurse specialist needs to consider several important issues which derive from health psychology. Sarah needs to be given a sense of personal control over her problem, principally via several different processes of information-giving and skills training. This in turn will help with her compliance. Diabetes is a serious problem and there is the necessity for providing various types of social support. Throughout Sarah's treatment programme, the nurse must try to ensure, as an overriding principle, that Sarah always feels that the benefits of taking healthy action are worthwhile and in excess of any barriers.

Summary

1. Health psychology is concerned with promoting and maintaining health, preventing and treating illness, and improving health-care delivery.
2. Contemporary health psychology draws on psychoanalysis, operant learning theory, social learning theory and psychophysiology.
3. Levels of stress experienced by individuals in a range of health-care contexts can be reduced by the use of specific strategies designed to increase a person's perceived sense of control, including cognitive control, behavioural control and informational control.
4. People who experience high levels of stress over long periods of time may come to believe that they can do little to influence what happens to them and become passive. This condition has been described as learned helplessness and may be experienced by those suffering from severe depression.
5. Research findings suggest that there may be a relationship (albeit a complex one) between a person's locus of control and his or her health behaviours: more internally-oriented individuals tend to take greater responsibility for their health compared with those who are more externally oriented.
6. Enhancing a person's perception of personal control can produce a range of benefits and positive health outcomes.
7. Attribution theory has provided some useful insights into the nature of depression which have been used, together with an understanding of learned helplessness, to develop a cognitive behavioural model of treatment.

This approach to treatment aims to correct the depressed person's negative perceptions and encourage the individual to take part in activities designed to provide a sense of achievement and greater personal control over his or her life.

8. To improve the effectiveness of information given to patients and clients, health-care practitioners should aim to provide a realistic account of what will happen during specific health-care events. This will facilitate the empowerment of individuals to make informed choices regarding treatment options and to take greater responsibility and personal control for their health and for their care.

9. Research has highlighted a range of factors that can improve the likelihood of a patient or client complying with an agreed course of action, including a good relationship with the person concerned, a credible source of advice, presentation of both sides of an argument, the provision of reasons for a proposed treatment or self-care, and the encouragement of ownership of ideas.

10. Forms of social support (emotional support, esteem support, instrumental support and informational support) can provide an important buffer and reduce the risk of physical and/or mental illness in people undergoing stressful situations. Health-care professionals should, therefore, encourage patients and clients to seek out one or more forms of social support.

11. The health belief model attempts to explain why people behave in certain ways with regard to their health. An individual will appraise the options by assessing the perceived benefits and barriers of taking particular actions, the perceived threat of illness and the perceived seriousness of the illness.

References

Abramson, L. Y., Seligman, M. E. P. and Teasdale, J. D. (1978). Learned helplessness in humans: critique and reformulation. *Journal of Abnormal Psychology*, 87, 49–74.

Alloy, L. B., Abramson, L. Y. and Dykman, B. M. (1990). Depressive realism and nondepressive optimistics:

the role of the self. In Ingram, R. (ed.) *Contemporary Psychological Approaches to Depression: Treatment, Research and Theory*. Plenum Press, New York.

Anderson, E. A. (1987). Preoperative preparation for cardiac surgery facilitates recovery, reduces psychological distress, and reduces the incidence of acute postoperative tension. *Journal of Consulting and Clinical Psychology*, 55, 513–520.

Antoni, M. H. (1987). Neuroendocrine influences in psychoimmunology and neoplasia: a review. *Psychology and Health*, 1, 3–24.

Baekeland, F. and Lundwall, L. (1975). Dropping out of treatment: a critical review, *Psychological Bulletin*, 82, 738–783.

Bandura, A. (1986). *Social Foundations of Thought and Action: A Social Cognitive Theory*. Prentice-Hall, Englewood Cliffs, NJ.

Beck, A. T. (1991). Cognitive therapy. *American Psychologist*, 46(4), 368–375.

Beck, A. T., Rush, A. J., Shaw, B. F. and Emery, G. (1979). *Cognitive Theory of Depression*. Guilford Press, New York.

Becker, M. H. (1979). Understanding patient compliance: the contributions of attitudes and other psychosocial factors. In Cohen, S. J. (ed.) *New Directions in Patient Compliance*. Heath, Lexington, MA.

Becker, M. H., Maiman, L. A., Kirscht, J. P., Haefner, D. P. and Drachman, R. H. (1977). The health belief model and prediction of dietary compliance: a field experiment. *Journal of Health and Social Behaviour*. 18, 348–366.

Becker, M. H. and Rosenstock, I. M. (1984). Compliance with medical advice. In Steptoe, A. and Mathews, A. (eds) *Health Care and Human Behaviour*. Academic Press, London.

Berscheid, E. (1966). Opinion change and communicator–communicatee similarity and dissimilarity. *Journal of Personality and Social Psychology*, 4, 670–680.

Boeing, M. H. and Mongera, C. O. (1989). Powerlessness in critical care patients. *Dimensions of Critical Care Nursing*, 8, 274–279.

Bradley, C., Gamsu, D. and Moses, J. L. (1987). The use of diabetes-specific perceived control and health belief measures to predict treatment choice and efficacy in a feasibility study of continuous subcutaneous insulin infusion pumps. *Psychology and Health*, 1, 133–146.

Brewin, C. R. (1988). *Cognitive Foundations of Clinical Psychology*. Lawrence Erlbaum, London.

Carey, M. P. and Burish, T. G. (1988). Etiology and treatment of the psychological side effects associated with cancer chemotherapy: a critical review and discussion. *Psychological Bulletin*, 106(3), 307–325.

Cohen, S. and McKay, G. (1984). Social support, stress and the buffering hypothesis: a theoretical analysis. In

Baum, A., Taylor, S. and Singer, J. (eds) *Handbook of Psychology and Health*. Erlbaum, Hillsdale, NJ.

Cohen, S., Evans, G., Stokols, D. and Krantz, D. (1986). *Behaviour, Health and Environmental Stress*. Plenum Press, New York.

Corney, R., Everett, H., Howells, A. and Crowther, M. (1992). The care of patients undergoing surgery for gynaecological cancer – the need for information, emotional support and counselling. *Journal of Advanced Nursing*, 17(6), 667–671.

Crocker, J., Alloy, L. B. and Kayne, N. T. (1988). Attributional style, depression and perceptions of consensus for events. *Journal of Personality and Social Psychology*, 54, 840–846.

Department of Health (1991). *The Patient's Charter*. Department of Health.

Diamond, M. J. and Shapiro, J. L. (1973). Changes in locus of control as a function of encounter group experiences: a study and replication. *Journal of Abnormal Psychology*, 82(3), 514–518.

Dimond, B. (1990). *Legal Aspects of Nursing*. Prentice-Hall, London.

Dishman, R. K., Ickes, W. and Morgan, W. P. (1980). Self motivation and adherence to habitual physical activity. *Journal of Applied Social Psychology*, 10, 115–132.

Engstrom, B. (1984). The patient's need for information during a hospital stay. *International Journal of Nursing Studies*, 21, 113–130.

Freud, S. (1901/1960). *Psychopathology of Everyday Life* (The Standard Edition of the Complete Psychological Works of Sigmund Freud, Volume 6). Hogarth Press and the Institute of Psychoanalysis.

Freud, S. (1940). An outline of psychoanalysis. *International Journal of Psychoanalysis*, 21, 27–84.

Greer, S., Morris, T. and Pettingale, K. W. (1979). Psychological response to breast cancer: effect on outcome. *The Lancet*, No. 8146, 13 October, 785–787.

Hall, J. (1982). Communicating with the patient. In Hall, J. (ed.) *Psychology for Nurses and Health Visitors*. Macmillan/British Psychological Society, London.

Hathaway, D. (1986). Effect of pre-operative instruction on post-operative outcomes: a meta-analysis. *Nursing Research*, 35, 269–274.

Hawton, K., Salkovskis, P. M., Kirk, J. and Clark, D. M. (1989). *Cognitive Behaviour Therapy for Psychiatric Problems*. Oxford Medical Publications, Oxford.

Haynes, R. B. (1982). Improving patient compliance: an empirical review. In Stuart, R. (ed.) *Adherence, Compliance and Generalization in Behavioral Medicine*. Brunner/Mazel, New York.

Health Service Commissioner for England, for Scotland and for Wales (1993). *Annual Report for the Session 1992–93*. HC764, HMSO, London.

Heider, F. (1958). *The Psychology of Interpersonal Relations*. John Wiley, New York.

Hiroto, D. S. and Seligman, M. E. P. (1975). Generality of learned helplessness in man. *Journal of Personality and Social Psychology*, 31, 311–327.

House, W. C., Pendleton, L. and Parker, L. (1986). Patients' versus physicians' attributions of reasons for diabetic patients' non-compliance with diet. *Diabetes Care*, 9, 434.

Hovland, C. I. and Weiss, W. (1951). The influence of source credibility on communication effectiveness. *Public Opinion Quarterly*, 15, 635–650.

Hussey, L. C. and Gilliland, K. (1989). Compliance, low literacy and locus of control. *Nursing Clinics of North America*, 24, 605–611.

Jacobson, E. (1929). *Progressive Relaxation*. University of Chicago Press, Chicago.

Janis, I. L. (1967). Effect of fear-arousing communications. In Berkowitz, L. (ed.) *Advances in Experimental Social Psychology*. Academic Press, New York.

Janis, I. L. and Feshbach, S. (1953). Effect of fear-arousing communications. *Journal of Abnormal and Social Psychology*, 48, 78–92.

Jemmott, J. B. and Locke, S. E. (1984). Psychosocial factors, immunologic mediation and human susceptibility to infectious diseases: how much do we know? *Psychological Bulletin*, 95, 78–108.

Johnson, J. E., Rice, V., Fuller, S. and Endress, M. (1978). Sensory information, instruction in a coping strategy and recovery from surgery. *Research in Nursing and Health*, 1, 4–17.

Johnston, D. W. (1982). Behavioural treatment in the reduction of coronary risk factors: type A behaviour and blood pressure. *British Journal of Clinical Psychology*, 21, 281–294.

Johnston, D. W. (1989). Will stress management prevent coronary heart disease? *The Psychologist*, 2(7), 275–278.

Kaplan, R., Atkins, C. and Reinsch, S. (1984). Specific efficacy expectations mediate exercise compliance in patients with chronic obstructive pulmonary disease. *Health Psychology*, 3, 223–242.

Kavanagh, C. (1983). A new approach to dressing change in the severely burned child and its effect on burn-related psychopathology, *Heart and Lung*, 12, 612–619.

Kelley, H. H. (1967). Attribution theory in social psychology. In Levine, D. (ed.) *Nebraska Symposium on Motivation*. University of Nebraska Press, Lincoln, NB.

Kelley, H. H. (1973). The process of causal attribution. *American Psychologist*, 28, 107–128.

Kendall, P., Williams, L., Pechacek, T., Graham, L., Shisslak, C. and Herzoff, N. (1979). Cognitive-behavioural and patient education interventions in cardiac catheterisation procedures. *Journal of Consulting and Clinical Psychology*, 47, 49–58.

King, J. B. (1982). The impact of patients' perceptions of high blood pressure on attendance at screening: an attributional extension of the health belief model. *Social Science and Medicine*, 16, 1079–1092.

Lachman, M. E. (1986). Personal control in later life: stability, change and cognitive correlates. In Baltes, M. M. and Baltes, P. B. (eds) *The Psychology of Control and Aging*. Erlbaum, Hillsdale, NJ.

Langer, E. J. (1975). The illusion of control. *Journal of Personality and Social Psychology*, 32, 311–328.

Langer, E. J., Janis, I. L. and Wolfer, J. A. (1975). Reduction of psychological stress in surgical patients. *Journal of Experimental Social Psychology*, 11, 155–165.

Ley, P. (1977). Psychological studies of doctor–patient communication. In Rachman, S. (ed.) *Contributions to Medical Psychology*, Vol. 1. Pergamon Press, Oxford.

Ley, P. (1988). *Communicating with Patients: Improving Communication, Satisfaction and Compliance*. Croom Helm, London.

Ley, P., Pike, L. A., Whitworth, M. A. and Woodward, R. (1979). Effects of source, context of communication and difficulty level on the success of health education communications. *Health Education Journal*, 38, 47–52.

Lowery, B. and Ducette, J. (1976). Disease-related learning and disease control in diabetics as a function of locus of control. *Nursing Research*, 25(5), 358–362.

Lykken, D. (1984). Polygraphic interrogation. *Nature*, 307, 681–684.

Marcer, D. (1986). *Biofeedback and Related Therapies in Clinical Practice*. Croom Helm, London.

Marks, G., Richardson, J., Graham, J. and Levine, A. (1986). Role of health locus of control beliefs and expectations of treatment efficacy in adjustment to cancer. *Journal of Personality and Social Psychology*, 51, 443–450.

Marsh, K. L. and Weary, G. (1989). Depression and attributional complexity. *Personality and Social Psychology Bulletin*, 15, 325–336.

Martin, P. (1987). Psychology and the immune system. *New Scientist*, 9 April, 46–50.

Matarazzo, J. D. (1982). Behavioural health's challenge to academic, scientific and professional psychology. *American Psychologist*, 37, 1–14.

Miller, S. and Green, M. (1984). Coping with stress and frustration; origins, nature and development. In Lewis, M. and Saarni, C. (eds) *Origins of Behaviour*, Vol. 5. Plenum Press, New York.

Miller, W. R. and Seligman, M. E. P. (1975). Depression in humans, *Journal of Abnormal Psychology*, 84, 228–238. Moores, B. and Thompson, A. G. H. (1986). What 1357 hospital inpatients think about aspects of their stay in British acute hospitals. *Journal of Advanced Nursing*, 11, 87–102.

Oberle, K. (1991). A decade of research in locus of control: what have we learned? *Journal of Advanced Nursing*, 16, 800–806.

Pearce, S. and Wardle, J. (eds) (1989). *The Practice of Behavioural Medicine*. Oxford University Press in association with BPS Books, London.

Pennebaker, J. W. (1982). *The Psychology of Physical Symptoms*. Springer, New York.

Peterson, C. and Stunkard, A. J. (1989). Personal control and health promotion. *Social Science and Medicine*, 28(8), 819–828.

Ridgeway, V. and Mathews, A. (1982). Psychological preparation for surgery. *British Journal of Clinical Psychology*, 21, 271–280.

Rodin, J. (1983). *Will This Hurt? Preparing Children for Hospital and Medical Procedures*. Royal College of Nursing, London.

Rodin, J. (1986). Health, control and aging. In Baltes, M. M. and Baltes, P. B. (eds) *The Psychology of Control and Aging*. Erlbaum, Hillsdale, NJ.

Rodin, J. (1987). Personal control throughout the life course. In Abeles, R. (ed.) *Life-span Perspectives and Social Psychology*. Erlbaum, Hillsdale, NJ.

Rosenstock, I. M. (1985). Understanding and enhancing patient compliance with diabetic regimens. *Diabetes Care*, 8, 610–616.

Rotter, J. B. (1966). Generalized expectancies for the internal versus external control of reinforcement. *Psychological Monographs*, 80(1, whole of number 609).

Ryden, M. R. (1984). Morale and perceived control in institutionalized elderly. *Nursing Research*, 33, 130–136.

Sarafino, E. P. (1994). *Health Psychology: Biopsychosocial Interactions*, 2nd edn. John Wiley, New York.

Schulz, R. (1976). Effects of control and predictability on the physical and psychological well-being of the institutionalized elderly. *Journal of Personality and Social Psychology*, 33(5), 563–573.

Schwartzer, R. and Leppin, A. (1989). Social support and health: a meta-analysis. *Health Psychology*, 3, 1–15.

Schwarz, G. (1982) Testing the biopsychosocial model: the ultimate challenge facing behavioural medicine, *Journal of Consulting and Clinical Psychology*, 50, 1040–1053.

Seligman, M. E. (1975). *Helplessness: On Depression, Development and Death*. Freeman, San Francisco.

Skilbeck, C. E., Tulip, J. G. and Ley, P. (1977) Effects of fear arousal, fear exposure and sidedness on compliance with dietary instruction. *European Journal of Social Psychology*, 7, 221–249.

Skinner, B. F. (1938). *The Behaviour of Organisms*. Appleton-Century-Crofts, New York.

Sklar, L. S. and Anisman, H. (1979). Stress and coping factors influence tumour growth. *Science*, 205, pp. 513–515.

Slenker, S. E., Price, J. H., and O'Connell, J. K. (1985). Health locus of control of joggers and nonexercisers. *Perceptual Motor Skills*, 61(1), 323–328.

Sutton, S. R. (1982). Fear-arousing communications: a critical examination of research and theory. In Eiser, J. R. (ed.) *Social Psychology and Behavioral Medicine.* John Wiley, New York.

Szasz, T. (1987). *Insanity: The Idea and Its Consequences.* John Wiley, New York.

Taylor, R., Lam, D., Roppel, C. and Barter, J. (1984) Friends can be good medicine: excursion into mental health promotion. *Community Mental Health Journal,* 20, 294–303.

Temoshok, L. and Heller, B. W. (1984). On comparing apples, oranges and fruit salad: a methodological overview of medical outcome studies in psychosocial oncology. In Cooper, C. L. (ed.) *Psychosocial Stress and Cancer.* John Wiley.

Thompson, S. (1981). Will it hurt less if I can control it? A complex answer to a simple question. *Psychological Bulletin,* 90, 89–101.

Vaughan, B. and Taylor, K. (1988). Homeward bound. *Nursing Times,* 84(15), 28–31.

Wallace, L. M. (1986). Communication variables in the design of pre-surgical preparatory information. *British Journal of Clinical Psychology,* 25, 111–118.

Wallston, K. A. and Wallston, B. S. (1981). Health locus of control scales. In Lefcourt, H. M. (ed.) *Research with the Locus of Control Construct.* Academic Press, New York.

Wallston, K. A., Wallston, B. S., Kaplan, G. D. and Maides, S. A. (1976). Development and validation of the health locus of control (HLC) scale. *Journal of Consulting and Clinical Psychology,* 44, 580–585.

Wallston, K. A., Wallston, B. S. and Devillis, R. F. (1978). Development of the multidimensional health locus of control (MHLC) scales. *Health Education Monographs,* 6, 161–170.

Weary, G., Elbin, S. and Hill, M. G. (1987). Attributional and social comparison processes in depression. *Journal of Personality and Social Psychology,* 52, 605–610.

Wessler, R. (1984). Cognitive-social psychological theories and social skills. In Trower, P. (ed.) *Radical Approaches to Social Skills Training.* Croom Helm, London.

Wills, T. A. (1984). Supportive functions of interpersonal relationships. In Cohen, S. and Syme, L. (eds) *Social Support and Health.* Academic Press, New York.

Wilson-Barnett, J. (1979). *Stress in Hospital.* Churchill Livingstone, Edinburgh.

Wilson-Barnett, J. (ed.) (1983). *Patient Teaching.* Churchill Livingstone, Edinburgh.

Wilson-Barnett, J. (1989a). Distressing hospital procedures. In Byrne, T. and Lacey, H. (eds) *Psychological Management of the Physically Ill.* Churchill Livingstone, Edinburgh.

Wilson-Barnett, J. (1989b). Limited autonomy and partnership: professional relationships in health care. *Journal of Medical Ethics,* 15(1), 12–16.

Wilson-Barnett, J. (1991). Providing relevant information for patients and families. In Corney R. (ed.) (1991) *Developing Communication and Counselling Skills in Medicine.* Tavistock/Routledge, London.

Further reading

Broome, A. (ed.) (1989). *Health Psychology: Processes and Applications.* Chapman & Hall, London. This edited text is divided into two parts. Part 1 looks at psychological processes (such as stress and existing health beliefs) relevant to the prevention, alleviation and management of illness and to health-care delivery. Part 2 focuses on the application of psychological insights and skills in a range of specialties including diabetes mellitus, cardiac disorders, chronic pain, paediatrics and childhood cancer.

Corney R. (ed.) (1991). *Developing Communication and Counselling Skills in Medicine.* Tavistock/Routledge, London. This excellent collection of short papers provides a valuable practical guide on how to communicate effectively with patients and clients. Contributors include Jenifer Wilson-Barnett, Peter Maguire and Anthony Clare.

Ley, P. (1988). *Communicating with Patients: Improving Communication, Satisfaction and Compliance.* Croom Helm, London. This text provides a systematic review of numerous research papers concerned with patient satisfaction, patients' understanding of and memory for medical information, patient compliance, the use of written information for patients and the content of communications with patients, and the benefits of improved communication. Highly recommended.

Niven, N. (1989). *Health Psychology: An Introduction for Nurses and other Health Care Professionals.* Churchill Livingstone, Edinburgh.

Pearce, S. and Wardle, J. (eds) (1989). *The Practice of Behavioural Medicine.* Oxford University Press in association with BPS Books, London. A useful collection of current perspectives on a range of health issues, including diabetes mellitus, heart disease, cancer, HIV and AIDS and head injury.

Watson, M. (1991). *Cancer Patient Care: Psychosocial Treatment Methods.* BPS Books/Cambridge University Press, Cambridge. An edited text of 14 chapters which examines a range of psychological issues in cancer care and treatment in adults, children and the families of sufferers. It covers various types of cancer as well as examining different psychosocial approaches. Each chapter provides a review of the relevant literature as well as valuable clinical insights.

4

NURSING: CURRENT ISSUES AND THE PATIENT'S PERSPECTIVE

Jane Schober

Introduction

Society's need for efficient health care is recognised as one of the most topical and politically sensitive issues facing those who manage and deliver the service. With nurses making up the major part of the health-care workforce in the United Kingdom, pressure on them to provide quality care is of significant professional and managerial importance. Over the years, particularly since the advent of the National Health Service (NHS) in 1948, nurses have found themselves reacting to what appears to have been constant change, usually from developments in health policy, changes in the organisation of health or nursing care and educational and professional initiatives. More recently, since 1990, a range of documents have been published which highlight legal developments, e.g. *NHS Community Care Act* (HMSO, 1990), and policy and practice initiatives, e.g. *The Health of the Nation*, [Department of Health (DoH), 1992], *The Patient's Charter* (DoH, 1991) and *The Named Nurse, Midwife and Health Visitor* (DoH, 1993a). These are examples of initiatives designed to have an impact on the delivery of care, to improve the quality of the service and the well-being of those requiring care. As such they have an impact on the way nurses plan and deliver care.

In addition, the annual report from the Chief Medical Officer to the Secretary of State for Health (DoH, 1993b) highlights six long-term strategic aims for health care as follows:

- to promote efforts to ensure health for all
- to achieve the targets in the Strategy for Health
- to involve patients and the public in choices and decision making
- to establish an effective intelligence system for public health and clinical practice
- to ensure a health service based on an assessment of health needs, quality of care and effectiveness of outcome
- to provide a highly professional team of staff with strong educational research and ethical standards

(Calman, 1994, p. 35).

These aims exemplify many of the features evident in professional nursing objectives, in particular the emphasis on quality, health promotion, patient-centred decision making and sound professional preparation and practice. All these elements are monitored through auditing aspects of health care which highlight both how the Strategy for Health (DoH, 1992) is being achieved and any new health concerns requiring further research and monitoring. Calman (1994) also highlights current health issues commanding particular attention and those which have required action as follows.

Health of black and ethnic minority groups

The NHS Executive has established an Ethnic Health Unit.

Clinical audit and outcomes of health care

Clinical audit has become an integral part of the monitoring of the service both in hospitals and with general practitioners in the community.

Medical education and manpower

Developments relating to continuing medical education are under way leading on from those made to undergraduate medical education.

Men's health

Initiatives continue to be taken locally both to highlight the particular health needs of men and to encourage as 'well-men' clinics.

Mentally disordered offenders

Initiatives begun in 1993 to continue give priority to providing care for mentally disordered offenders. This includes capital funding for the Medium Secure Unit Building programme to continue the transfer of patients from prisons to in-patient care and regional training initiatives (National Association for the Care and Resettlement of Offenders, 1994).

In addition Calman (1994) highlights a range of issues which are viewed as of particular concern to the state of public health and which will be reported and acted on as priority areas during 1995. These include the following:

The health of adolescents

There is concern relating to the rate of injury and poisoning in this group which accounts for 50 percent of deaths. Also, lifestyle is a central factor with such factors as cigarette smoking, physical activity, aspects of sexual activity, diet and alcohol consumption possibly setting trends which may adversely influence health in later life. There is also concern for the management and continuing care of those with chronic diseases, e.g. cancer, cystic fibrosis and asthma.

Genetic factors and disease

The rate at which the understanding of molecular genetics is developing has a range of implications, e.g. for screening and treatment along with associated ethical issues.

Changing patterns of infectious diseases

Communicable diseases continue to prevail with verocytotoxin-producing *Escherichia coli* (VTEC) and human immunodeficiency syndrome (HIV) along with influenza, tuberculosis, malaria and drug-resistant bacteria causing particular concern. Emphasis continues on sophisticated surveillance systems involving the Public Health Laboratory Service, District Directors of Public Health, Consultants in Communicable Disease Control and Environmental Health Officers. Locally, infection control nurses, health visitors, district nurses and general practitioners continue to provide an essential service involving screening, health promotion, the monitoring and use of treatments and prevention activities (e.g. immunisation programmes) and advice relating to travelling abroad.

Asthma

The increase in those with asthma since 1984 has led to intensive research programmes which are placing particular emphasis on treatments and the effects of air pollution.

(Adapted from Calman, 1994, p. 36.)

Nurses are adept in working in a wide range of health care and social settings, and as such need to be aware of current health issues and such aims as these in order to respond appropriately to strategic policies and local initiatives. The complexity of nursing as a service and the wide ranging demands on nurses make it necessary for them to acquire the necessary abilities to practice in accordance with professional, ethical, contractual, legal and educational requirements. With the access nurses have to patients, they have unique and privileged opportunities to contribute to and manage individual health-care needs.

It is from this background of recognising the demands on nurses from those purchasing and requiring care and the expectation that nurses will respond to policy and practice-related innovations, that this chapter will develop. Thus it is the concern for the quality of nursing practice and its influence on those requiring care which forms the focus of the chapter. It seeks to highlight, challenge and discuss issues which militate for and against nurses being able to provide and execute optimum care for those in need. A major cause for concern is the notion that nursing may not be reaching its potential for those who require care. There are factors which could enhance the contribution of nurses to the overall quality of the service, e.g. care planning could adopt a multidisciplinary approach which nurses may coordinate in a range of settings where currently this is not custom and practice. Secondly, educational opportunities for nurses need to maintain and develop the strongest possible link with clinical practice and research and be regarded as integral to the ways in which academic and educational policy decisions are executed.

Further, it is suggested that nursing is, in itself, a paradox, whereby the very motivation and commitment to care which inspires those who enter nursing is often compromised by the nature of the so-called care they witness and experience. Therefore exploration of the needs of 'patients' will serve to set the scene for the chapter and how developments contributing to the strengthening of nursing as a profession have served to meet this end.

Additionally, this chapter seeks to explore issues pertinent to the practice of nursing as a caring art and science which, in general, is well recognised (Watson, 1988) and a curing art which, perhaps is not. To this end, the following themes will be discussed:

- the health needs of those requiring nursing services
- the professionalisation of nursing and the influence on practice
- principles of good practice and nursing as a caring and curing art.

This chapter begins by exploring aspects of nursing and health care from the patient's viewpoint. It is not intended to discuss whether recipients of health and nursing care are 'patients' or 'clients' but to use the term 'patient' as a generic term, acknowledging that the degree to which people actively participate in and contribute to their health care may play a part in their potential status as a client. In addition, despite initiatives which focus on health maintenance and its promotion, it remains that the majority of nursing work focuses on the needs of those experiencing states of ill-health, and this will be the starting point here.

Psychological reactions and the illness experience

For most of us, the thought of being ill, disabled, dependent on others (be they professional carers or family members and partners), is an alien and rather horrifying one. Though contact with the health service is inevitable for many reasons (e.g. pre- and post-natal care, immunisations, and health screening), the fear that can be generated and experienced, for example, because of the uncertainty of diagnosis and prognosis, the impact of acute and traumatic experiences and the long-term effects of chronic illness, incapacity dependency and degeneration, are far reaching both for the individual affected and for those who intend (or are expected) to support them.

It is not the intention to reiterate the debate about the nature of health and thus, what constitutes ill-health as this is fully explored in Chapter 1. However it is important to emphasise how the intricate reactions which result from changes in health and experiences of illness may affect the individual particularly at a time when socio-economic inequalities in health appear to be increasing particularly in relation to young men from deprived areas, family and child poverty (Davey *et al.*, 1994) and elderly people.

The knowledge, and even the suspicion, that illness is present has the potential to cause a range of reactions. Many of these will be affected by and dependant on such factors as age and stage of maturation, the presence of mental illness, learning disability and behavioural problems. Illness is often regarded as 'the person's subjective experience of ill-health' (Field, 1993, p. 100). Cornwall (1984) found a range of perceptions of illness which were categorised as:

- normal – those that may be expected, e.g. chicken pox
- real – those which result in disabling and life-threatening diseases
- health problems – natural processes such as childbirth and ageing.

Illness tends to be regarded as a change in an individual's physical state, it is alien and undesired and disrupts usual social activities. When caused by a recognised disease, the illness may be perceived as acceptable. Conversely, a range of diseases carry with them stereotypical responses which may influence the response to the individuals concerned, e.g. mental illness still carries with it stigma and labels which may alienate those suffering the symptoms from mainstream society. Goffman (1990) identified three sources of stigma, namely:

- 'abominations of the body', e.g. facial scarring, physical disability
- 'blemishes of individual character', e.g. homosexuality, mental illness
- 'the tribal stigma of race nation and religion', e.g. language and dress differences.

Illness as a source of stress for the individual is recognised as a significant life event (Holmes and Rahe, 1967). The response to illness is complex in as much as it may be a direct consequence of a stressor on the body, resulting in, for example physiological effects of stress such as increased blood glucose levels, increased corticosteroid activity, increases in blood pressure and heart rate, as well as general health-related responses, for example headaches, dizziness, diarrhoea, insomnia and sweating. The emphasis on physiological response described by Selye (1957) and the corresponding defence reactions which he refers to as the general adaptation syndrome (GAS), while contributing to an understanding of how stress and illness influence the body, do not provide necessary insight into how the psychological reactions to stress link with the physiological and thus affect the individual.

Behavioural and cognitive responses to stress are well recognised (Cox, 1978) and include excessive eating, drinking, smoking, trembling, hesitancy, nervous laughter, restlessness, crying and lack of eye contact.

Stress affects individuals in different ways and illness is no exception. The transactional model of stress described by Lazarus (1966, 1978) provides valuable insight into the importance of assessing how individuals perceive their situation. Individuals have the capacity of acting on and responding to the environment rather than being passive responders. Thus it is advocated that individuals are encouraged to extrapolate their experiences, recognising that their insights and awareness may be affected by coping mechanisms such as denial and disbelief. Those faced with changes in health, particularly those which necessitate care and support, react in a wide range of ways which may include the adoption of a number of the following, cognitive, emotional and behavioural strategies such as:

- shock
- disbelief
- confusion
- denial
- anger
- acceptance
- assuming a sick role
- learned helplessness.

Key aspects of these will now be explored.

Loss and coping

There are marked similarities here with reactions to loss, death and bereavement, in as much as shock, disbelief, denial, anger and grief, and ultimately, acceptance, are clearly recognised as psychological and emotional responses (Murray Parkes, 1975; Saunders, 1990). There is a need to come to terms with the inner turmoil which is central to the experience of losing control over one's destiny. The grieving, sense of insecurity and potential isolation come from the threat to mortality and highlight, by way of introduction, links with the need for spiritual well-being.

Learned helplessness

Originally, the theory of learned helplessness was suggested as a model for understanding depression (Seligman, 1992). Seligman suggested, from animal experiments, that without a warning or predictor of danger or pain, the resulting continual stress may result in the development of ulcers. He went on to observe that among soldiers tortured in Vietnam, those who were able to maintain a degree of hope survived while others became ill and often died. The factor which appears to be crucial in this example of extreme and life-threatening onslaught is the element of control which individuals perceived they had over their situation. Feeling and being in control at times when there is a need or desire to adapt and cope depends on a wide range of factors including the understanding of the situation, a factor which will be seen later to be central to patients' satisfaction with their care.

Reactions to illness and disease may also be influenced by attitudes and values associated with our understanding of the mind, body and spirit. Kidel (1986) suggests that the body is seen as 'inferior to the mind and spirit' and may thus influence how messages about the functioning of the body are interpreted. Our sense of self-consciousness inhibits our body and, as Kidel (1986) discusses, denial is a form of defensiveness, making coping with illness and disease harder to bear. The dualism associated with the traditional medical model in which the functions of the body are seen as separate from the mind and psychological responses has been a far-reaching influence on how both the providers of health-care services, particularly nurses and doctors, and recipients have perceived their roles. The price has been the suppression of the emotional impact of the illness experience while prioritising the physical, treatment-related components. The challenge is for us to take responsibility for our bodies, to listen to them and to take steps to understand the emotional impact of the illness experience and thus to draw on our individual reserves as a means of coping.

Of our reaction to disease and illness Kidel suggested that:

> Insecurity lies at the heart of our reaction to disease: when illness strikes, we feel as if under attack. The defences which have enabled us to ignore our potential for frailty and vulnerability are suddenly removed. We are no longer able to fulfil the social roles which provide us with a sense of identity. Business cannot be 'as usual' and instead of being busy, we are slowed down or immobilized and forced to break routines, go to bed, seek help and take stock. We no longer 'feel ourselves', as we are confronted with the full force of the unknown and the unpredictable (p. 19)

and

> At the heart of our feelings about illness lies a universal fear of death, and associated anxieties about aging, decay and change.

Also he states:

> It seems to me essential that we should come to terms with the unpredictability of our diseases and syndromes. We can never be certain of improvement, recovery, recurrence or deterioration. Our reconciliation with illness requires before all else a surrender to uncertainty and an acceptance of mortality (p. 20).

This central theme of uncertainty and unpredictability reaches to the core of our perceptions of our own mortality and the avoidance of the inevitability of death. The fear generated by experiences of ill-health is also part of this process of recognising the personal impact of illness for ourselves and how, as practitioners, we recognise the impact in those needing care. For nurses to work with and on such challenges which are before them in the experiences of patients, requires a commitment to the development of the well-being of vulnerable individuals and goes beyond the need simply to meet the health needs and deficiencies being presented.

The sick role

The characteristics of the sick role as originally described by Parsons (1951) are:

- the individual is exempt from the usual social responsibilities
- it is recognised that the individual is not to blame for her or his illness
- the individual perceives that the sick role is undesirable and intends to get well
- the individual is obliged to get well.

The assumptions proposed by Parsons appear to have had far-reaching influence. While it can be acknowledged that not all patients fit this mould, the expectations which have been assigned patients usually by clinical staff, have had powerful consequences. The notion of 'good' patients refers to those, who, for example, conform, comply with instructions, appear passive (Leigh and Reiser, 1980) and present with 'popular' personalities and conditions (Stockwell, 1972). This may have played a significant part in the approach to patients, which have implied lower status, and resulted in poor information-giving and lack of involvement in decision making.

The experience of being a patient

In a detailed study by Morrison (1994), an attempt has been made to understand patients further. Ten patients in a general hospital setting were interviewed to discuss:

- what the nurses did and how they did their work
- the type of relationship that developed between the nurses and the patients
- how patients perceived caring acts or caring individuals, and
- what, if anything, the patients gave to the nurses
(Morrison, 1994, p. 23).

An existential phenomenological approach was used to facilitate interviews which, on analysis, revealed a number of themes described as follows (Morrison, 1994, p. 25):

- patients experienced crushing vulnerability
- patients adopted a particular mode of self-presentation
- patients evaluated the service provided in hospital
- patients' personal concerns assumed great importance

As this is a recent study some of the detail associated with each of these themes will be highlighted here, not least because there are a range of findings which are positive and which reinforce many principles of effective care, but also there are many which highlight deficiencies in care which have been exposed before in a range of other studies.

Crushing vulnerability

The theme of crushing vulnerability appears as a major theme in this study. For some of the patients this experience is associated with a range of issues which include:

The uncertainties

- the uncertainty of how to behave and what to do in a strange hospital environment
- trying to make sense of a situation and trying to analyse the behaviour of staff when diagnosis is unknown
- lack of control over the situation
- 'the shattering impact of cancer'

                                       (Morrison, 1994, p. 56).

The feelings

- feelings of being in hospital under duress
- feelings of fear about being in hospital
- feelings of being 'treated like an object' and needing some contact with trained staff
- being aware of the impersonal approach taken by staff
- feeling forgotten about
- feeling ignored during handovers
- needing to cope with major changes in body image
- needing to know the truth
- feeling let down when an operation was cancelled at the last minute.

The embarrassments

- the lack of privacy
- feeling like 'a smelly mess compared with the nurses' (the effects of faecal incontinence)
- being talked about in front of other patients
- being dependent and needing help to use the toilet
- coping with a stoma.

The positive experiences

- feeling valued as a person which contributed to feelings of well-being
- being called by their first name (acknowledging the detrimental affects of over-familiarity)
- the respect of personal wishes
- feeling hopeful despite the uncertainties of diagnosis and prognosis
- supportive nurses and doctors
- nurses who judged and responded to improving independence.

Reflective point

In the light of the experiences relating to crushing vulnerability, suggest ways that nurses may co-ordinate care in a way to reduce the negative experiences and promote the positive ones.

In Morrison's (1994) study, only one patient felt particularly critical of the care received. However, the experience of feeling like an object resulted from the lack of involvement in the care process and highlights the need for nurses to be sensitive to the situation that patients find themselves in. This is particularly important at times when crushing vulnerability may be experienced, for example, when there are uncertainties relating to diagnosis, when frightened and feeling isolated.

The mode of self-presentation

It is suggested that patients cope with aspects of the hospital experience by presenting themselves in a particular way (Morrison, 1994). The strategies adopted by patients in the study included:

- becoming obedient and compliant
- conforming to ward rituals and routines
- putting on a brave face and becoming outwardly cheerful

- being honest and open with personal information
- supporting each other
- being reluctant to ask questions despite wanting answers
- needing to be up-to-date with information
- preferring to distance themselves from staff
- feeling that nursing staff 'were not interested in, or supposed to get closer to, patients in hospital' (p. 75)
- trying not be a nuisance
- feeling they provided positive feedback to the staff
- showing gratitude to staff
- admiring the dedication of nursing staff.

The evaluation of hospital services

Perhaps the most significant findings here relate to an overriding reluctance by patients to criticise staff. A range of reasons for this are suggested by Morrison (1994) including lack of status, reluctance to complain about care to those giving care, and lack of influence over decision making. While there appears to be general satisfaction with care, Morrison (1994) states

> The level of contact between professional carers and the patients did appear very limited (p. 87).

There are no clear data given in the study on what proportion of nurses' time is given to interacting with patients. However, patients did disclose that contact with registered nurses was limited to such occasions as the administration of medicines rather than nurse-initiated interaction. On the other hand patients appeared to conclude that despite many examples of positive care, sympathetic student nurses and approachable medical staff,

> Several important criticisms also emerged that highlighted the need for staff to listen carefully to what patients have to say in order to evaluate nursing and medical care from the patients' perspective (Morrison, 1994, p. 97).

This theme is developed in the final part of the study which highlights the way the 'patients' personal concerns assumed great importance'. It is interesting to note that many of the concerns patients had were discussed with the researcher and not with the nurses on the ward. The patient's priority, in general, was on having the treatment, getting better and leaving the hospital.

This very understandable priority highlights again that, for those requiring care, there is a central need to be healed, and to return to their 'normality'. With this in mind, the notion of patients' rights will now be examined.

Patients' rights

In exploring the nature of patients rights, it is important to consider them in the context of the rights of citizens, the fact that, in the United Kingdom, there is no Bill of Rights, and that the reference to patients having rights has been shaped by legislation, ethical and professional codes of practice, and more recently the Citizen's Charter and *The Patient's Charter* (DoH, 1991). Dimond (1993) suggests that the concern with patients' rights has developed from the rise in expectations associated with increased living standards, advances in treatments and accessibility to health care as well as a concern to protect people from the potential harm caused by medical intervention. This includes iatrogenic illness, and the use of medical intervention, e.g. drugs.

Dimond (1993) suggests four main areas of rights (see Fig. 4.1); and each will be explored in turn.

A right to medical assistance and health care

At a time when there is regular reference to the finite resources of the NHS (DoH, 1994a) it is pertinent to be reminded that the right to medical assistance is not absolute. The National Health Service Act (1977) highlights the statutory duties of the Secretary of State (see Fig. 4.2) but the actions to enforce these duties may only come into effect in the case of the availability of emergency services,

Patients' rights
• A right to medical assistance and health care
• A right to a reasonable standard of care
• A right to consent
• A right of access to health records
from Dimond (1993, p. 4)

Fig. 4.1. *Patients' rights.*

e.g. the ambulance service, accident and emergency services and general practitioner (GP) services.

A key factor in the debate about rights to medical assistance is associated with the availability and accessibility of health-care services and resources. Dimond (1993) suggests that the demand for health care is tempered by waiting lists, the number of intensive-care beds and inadequate staffing, either because of the lack of specialist preparation or inappropriate staffing levels. In addition, new technologies, techniques and shifting patterns of health care need make demands on a range of resources.

The publication of *The Patient's Charter* (DOH, 1991) highlights for all citizens their NHS rights, three new rights and local charter standards which came into effect in April 1992, together with nine national charter standards of service. These are summarised in Fig. 4.3.

Despite reactions to *The Patient's Charter* which welcome these initiatives, particularly in respect of standard setting (Hogg, 1986), information-giving (Turner, 1991; NHSME, 1992) waiting times (Turner, 1991), and the handling of complaints, (Winkler and Ford, 1992), it remains that the nine national charter standards are stated as aims and, as such, are difficult to enforce. Though there has

been a pronouncement of further detailed standards in the revised *Patient's Charter* (DoH, 1995), many of the aims remain broad. They include the following:

- a three- to four-hour national limit for 'trolley waits'
- the current 18-month limit on waiting times for hip, knee and cataract surgery will now apply to all operations
- one-year limit for a coronary artery bypass operation (from the time of investigation)
- community nurses are expected to arrange convenient visit times and to arrive within two hours of that time
- patients for elective surgery will be warned if they are or are not to be admitted to a single-sex ward
- ward bathroom facilities will be single sexed
- community psychiatric nurses to see clients with a mental illness within four hours if the case is urgent and within two working days, if not.

Just from these examples, it is clear where some criticisms may lie. For example, despite the range of public and professional concerns about mixed-sex wards, they remain. Also, community psychi-

---

Section 1(1)
It is the Secretary of State's duty to continue the promotion in England and Wales of a comprehensive health service designed to secure improvement

  (a) in the physical and mental health of the people of those countries, and
  (b) in the prevention, diagnosis and treatment of illness, and for the purpose to provide or secure the effective provision of services in accordance with this act.

Section 3(1)
It is the Secretary of State's duty to provide throughout England and Wales, to such extent as he considers necessary to meet all reasonable requirements:

  (a) hospital accommodation
  (b) other accommodation for the purpose of any service provided under this act
  (c) medical, dental, nursing and ambulance services
  (d) such other facilities for the care of expectant and nursing mothers and young children as he considers are appropriate as part of the health service
  (e) such facilities for the prevention of illness, the care of persons suffering from illness and the after-care of persons who have suffered from illness as he considers are appropriate as part of the health service
  (f) such other services as are required for the diagnosis and treatment of illness.

The Defendants (R v. Secretary of State for Social Services, ex parte Hincks, 1979) in Dimond (1993, p. 8).

Fig. 4.2. Statutory duties of the Secretary of State.

Every citizen already has the following National Health Service rights:

- to receive health care on the basis of clinical need, regardless of ability to pay
- to be registered with a GP
- to receive emergency medical care at any time, through your GP or the emergency departments
- to be referred to a consultant, acceptable to you, when your GP thinks it necessary and to be referred for a second opinion if you and your GP agree this is desirable
- to be given a clear explanation of any treatment proposed, including any risks and any alternatives, before you decide whether you will agree to the treatment
- to have access to your health records, and to know that those working for the NHS will, by law, keep their content confidential
- to choose whether or not you wish to take part in medical research or medical student training.

Three new rights

From 1 April 1992, you will have three important new rights:

- to be given detailed information on local health services, including quality standards and maximum waiting times. You will be able to get this information from your health authority, GP or Community Health Council
- to be guaranteed admission for virtually all treatments by a specific date no later than two years from the day when your consultant places you on a waiting list. Most patients will be admitted before this date. Currently, 90 percent are admitted within a year
- to have any complaint about NHS services – whoever provides them – investigated, and to receive a full and prompt written reply from the chief executive of your health authority or general manager of your hospital. If you are still unhappy, you will be able to take the case up with the Health Service Commissioner.

National charter standards

There are nine standards of service which the NHS will be aiming to provide for you:

- respect for privacy, dignity and religious and cultural beliefs
- arrangements to ensure everyone, including people with special needs, can use the services
- information to relatives and friends about the progress of your treatment, subject, of course, to your wishes
- an emergency ambulance should arrive within 14 minutes in an urban area, 19 minutes in a rural area
- when attending an accident and emergency department, you will be seen immediately and your need for treatment assessed
- when you go to an outpatient clinic, you will be given a specific appointment time and will be seen within 30 minutes of it.
- your operation should not be cancelled on the day you are due to arrive in hospital. If, exceptionally, your operation has to be postponed twice you will be admitted to hospital within one month of the second cancelled operation
- a named qualified nurse, midwife or health visitor responsible for your nursing or midwifery care
- a decision should be made about any continuing health or social health or social care need you may have, before you are discharged from hospital.

Local charter standards will include information about:

- first outpatients appointments
- waiting times in accident and emergency departments, after initial assessment
- waiting times for taking you home after treatment, where your doctor says you have a medical need for NHS transport
- enabling you and your visitors to find your way around hospitals, through enquiry points and better signposting
- ensuring that the staff you meet face to face wear name badges

From Department of Health, *The Patient's Charter* (1991).

Fig. 4.3. The Patient's Charter – *a summary of rights.*

atric nurses may well be concerned about the implementation of their standard as it appears to undermine the existing strategies of referral and the roles of other members of the multidisciplinary team working with the mentally ill. This could delay aspects of formal assessment.

These standard statements attract more criticism when their interpretation and implementation may appear not to give priority to the interests of patients as the first priority. Mixed-sex wards are a case in point where for many units, the return to single-sex wards is implicated by the number of beds within the directorate, skilled nursing staff may not be available to more than the designated ward/s and it may be regarded as 'inefficient' to segregate patients by gender, for example, rather than by their diagnostic and treatment needs.

Reflective point

Consider all the details contained here in The Patient's Charter, *in relation to your area of practice. What are the implications for nurses of* The Named Nurse, Midwife and Health Visitor *initiative?*

Wright (1993) suggests that every aspect of *The Patient's Charter* has implications for nurses, midwives and health visitors. However, there are a range of interpretations as to what constitutes the 'named nurse, midwife and health visitor' from issues relating to the allocation of these staff members to patients and therefore the organisational features [often likened to the characteristics of primary nursing (Hancock, 1992)], to local initiatives which identify the nurse responsible for care. Wright summarises key aspects of this by suggesting factors which make the named nurse known to patients:

- nurses identify themselves to the patient on first contact and make their responsibilities clear
- in some places, nurses have adapted a 'business card' system to give to patients/other carers
- clear readable name badges are worn
- the nurse's name may be included on the bed notice, on medical and surgical records/in literature such as information books and letters about the ward service
- the nurse may make copies of the duty rota

available to patients, where appropriate, or details of these can be displayed clearly on notice boards
- notice boards can be used to display names/photographs of nurses and the groups of nurses they are responsible for
- nurses clearly explain to patients who is caring for them, for example, at reporting and change-over times, and ensure that time is planned in care for conversation and problem solving and so on.

(Wright, 1993, p. 16).

This initiative does much to communicate to the public the fact that they can expect to have an identified nurse, midwife or health visitor responsible for their care and that they will have direct access to that staff member. To some extent, this mimics the situation characterised by the 'named' consultant or GP, having responsibility for a caseload of patients and the corresponding medical management.

There is no doubt that the coordination and continuity of care are the keys to the benefits to patients of this initiative. Where there are existing organisational systems of nursing care which promote, for example, primary nursing or the caseload method of delivery, the benefits to patients may in turn lead to increased patient satisfaction.

A right to a reasonable standard of care

Patients have rights to reasonable (that is, adequate) care from health-care professionals, who have a corresponding duty of care. Judgements about whether care has been of a reasonable standard, or not, emerge when actions are brought in law and other professionals with appropriate expertise contribute to the case to establish whether there has been an act of negligence which has caused harm. This process, and procedure, for bringing complaints about care, should be readily available to patients regardless of the location of their care. However, despite the more open approach encouraged, for example, by *The Patient's Charter* (DoH, 1991), it remains that patients are reluctant to complain about their care. This phenomenon is well recognised in nursing (Morrison, 1994). Recurrent problems in the quality of communication, particularly between nurses and patients and doctors and patients, continue to be a significant cause for complaint (Audit Commission, 1993; Health Service Commissioner, 1993).

Patients face a range of significant uncertainties here. Though the overall number of complaints have risen in recent years (Audit Commission, 1993), unless the cause for complaint is obviously severe, for example a patient remaining unconscious following minor surgery, patients may not understand what constitutes an inappropriate professional act or standard which is either an act of negligence or omission. Thus, they may not realise that an unreasonable standard of care has occurred, e.g. the quality of discharge procedures, teaching about the self-administration of medicines and the frequency of home visits by a nurse member of the primary health-care team. Proving fault is just one of the difficulties here. In addition, access to and understanding of the principles of, in the case of these examples, good nursing practice are not usually available to the general public.

The work of the Health Service Commissioner

By way of illustration, some recent examples of cases brought before the Health Service Commissioner (1993) are given here because they are of particular concern to nurses and serve to illustrate key issues relating to standards of communication, and the nature of problems ultimately being considered by him. The Health Service Commissioner (W. K. Reid) states:

> My purpose in publishing selected investigations is three-fold. It informs Parliament and the Ministers responsible for the National Health Service of the results of my work. It enables health authorities, boards and trusts to improve their standards to service to patients. It should assist Health Service staff in monitoring the quality of their work and in avoiding the repetition of the mistakes my investigations describe. I am glad to say that I do not find every complaint to be justified.
>
> Health Service Commissioner (1993, p. iii).

These are some of the matters considered where the complaint was justified

- Removal of lymph glands without formal consent during a mastectomy – unreassuring response to complainant.
- Failure of hospital staff to give timely advice to relatives about assistance with funeral arrangements.
- Transfer arrangements – patient's state of dress for and method of transport – response to complaint.

- Communication to relatives about a patient's condition – lack of nursing care – a ward sister's attitude – lack of support to relative when the patient died.
- Care of a disturbed elderly patient – inadequate supervision resulting in a fall – movement and treatment of a patient – health authority's response to complaint.
- Delay in seeing a patient after a diagnosis of breast cancer and further delay in telling her of her diagnosis.

There follows two of the cases as described in the epitomes of cases (full details are given in the report).

Case 1. Failure in communications before surgery

Matters considered

Removal of lymph glands without formal consent during a mastectomy – unreassuring response to complainant.

Summary of case

Before undergoing a mastectomy, a woman signed a consent form believing that only her breast would be removed. During her recovery she discovered that some lymph glands had been removed also. She maintained that she had not been told before the operation about the removal of glands, nor had she consented to that. The health authority's reply to her complaint had been less than reassuring that mistakes made in her case would not recur.

Findings

I found that the woman would normally have seen the consultant to discuss the operation in detail, but he had been absent and she had learnt of the need for surgery during a brief consultation with a registrar. He had made a note in her medical records for the consultant to see and decide what course to follow, but there was no evidence that any action had been taken. The woman would normally have been offered an opportunity to see the breast-care nurse, but she was absent also. The first real opportunity to discuss her concerns had arisen a few days before the operation when a house officer saw her to obtain formal consent. I was unable to ascertain whether the removal of the lymph glands had been discussed then, but I upheld the complaint to the extent that the arrangements for counselling before the operation had been inadequate. I also found that a business manager had not investigated the complaint with sufficient vigour, and the vague and brief reply to the woman's letter of complaint had quite understandably led her to conclude that her complaint had not been taken seriously.

Remedy

The health authority agreed to ensure that adequate alternative arrangements would be made for the counselling of patients when key personnel were not available. Apologies were offered for the shortcomings found (Health Service Commissioner, 1993, p. 2).

Case 2. Deficiencies in nursing care and attitudes

Communications to relatives about a patient's condition – lack of nursing care – a ward sister's attitude – lack of support to relative when the patient died.

Summary of case

An elderly man, who had had several heart attacks, was admitted to hospital for observation. At the insistence of a ward nurse, his wife gave her daughter's name, address and telephone number, as well as her own, for contact in a emergency. The next morning the daughter was telephoned about her father's deteriorating condition, and she and her mother went to the hospital. They were told that he was very poorly and that the next 24 hours would be critical. He died the next day. The man's wife complained that the ward staff should have telephoned her about his condition, and not her daughter who did not know about his admission, and that during her husband's stay he had received minimal nursing care, food and drink had not been offered, nurses had not helped to lift him, and a commode had been provided too late on two occasions. She felt that the ward sister had been unsympathetic and unhelpful and when her husband was dying, she had had to ask twice for a doctor. After her husband's death, she had been left on her own.

Findings

The hospital's policy was to obtain a second telephone number of a younger relative who could be called in preference to alarming an elderly next-of-kin, but the nurses had not explained that and the man's wife, who expected him to be discharged the next day, had not seen any need to tell her daughter or to insist on being contacted herself. I found that the relatives and the medical and nursing staff had very different perceptions both about the gravity of the man's condition and about what nursing care and nourishment would be provided and by whom.

The ward was very busy and the nurses were working under great pressure. They had not been able to respond to the man's needs promptly enough to prevent distressing accidents and when he died, neither they nor the doctor on duty had provided the necessary help and support. While the ward sister had not intended to be unsympathetic, I found her manner and expression to have been seen in that way.

Remedy

The health authority apologised for the hospital's shortcomings and assured me that the NHS Trust which now manages the hospital would implement my recommendations. These were that the arrangements and procedures for notifying relatives when a patient's condition deteriorates should be reviewed; that the extent of relatives' involvement in providing care should be agreed with them and recorded in the care plan; and that nursing cover for busy periods should be reviewed to ensure adequate standards of care.

(Health Service Commissioner, 1993, p. 5).

> **Reflective point**
> Clearly there are a range of issues and dilemmas raised by these two scenarios. Carefully consider them, and identify existing sources of support and guidance which, when appropriately applied, go a long way towards preventing such incidents.

These examples highlight some of the negative realities of care and remind us of the vulnerability of patients despite the existence of professional codes, policies and procedures and an ever-developing body of research evidence which can guide education and practice. Dimond (1993) recognises that ultimately there may be an issue of liability and states:

Crucial to the issue of liability will therefore be the question of what standards were followed and which should have been followed (Dimond, 1993, p. 27).

She goes on to suggest the following guidelines in relation to standards in the case of liability. The nurse, midwife and health visitor should:

1. inform herself of the guidelines for any given situation
2. monitor the extent to which these are followed
3. follow the advice of the United Kingdom

Central Council (UKCC) in its Code of Professional Conduct

4. if conflicts exist between the Code and the instructions of management, ensure that these are taken up, preferably in writing, with senior management (Dimond, 1993, p. 27).

It could be suggested that all nurses, midwives and health visitors have a professional responsibility to comply with these guidelines (despite concerns raised in relation to whistle blowing), not least because of the jeopardy placed on patients when systems of effective, sensitive communication and care break down.

As access to and understanding of details of nursing and health care become more accessible to the public, there are moves to improve the NHS complaints procedures further in order to make them more available to patients. *The Report of a Review Committee on NHS Complaints Procedures* (DoH, 1994) makes a wide range of recommendations for changes, which have implications for nurses and other health-service personnel. These include the following:

- we recommend that every purchaser and provider of NHS services should have simple, readily available written information about how to complain
- we recommend that complaints procedures empower NHS staff to give a rapid, often oral, response when a complaint is made about a service within their responsibility, and to initiate appropriate action as a result of the information received (informal responses)
- we recommend that training in complaints handling should be extended to all NHS practitioners and staff who are, or are likely to be, in contact with patients
- we recommend that all NHS practitioners and staff should be made aware of the support available when a complaint is made against them
- we recommend that written complaints are acknowledged within two working days
- we recommend that all stages of a complaints procedure should normally be complete within three months
- we recommend that information derived from complaints is incorporated into quality review mechanisms
- we recommend that NHS practitioners and staff in all disciplines and professions receive thorough training in communication skills. These should be incorporated at an early stage into training for

professional qualification, staff induction courses, and basic training at all levels
- we recommend that community staff should have particular training in responding to complaints because they may not have immediate access to advice from more senior managers or specialist staff, when they are visiting patients in their own homes. (DoH, 1994, pp. 72–77).

There are 67 recommendations in this report, and they cover all aspects of the complaints process. There are many similarities with existing procedures but it appears that changes may occur which improve the efficiency and streamlining of hospital and community procedures as well as improving information about the process for patients. Whether such developments result in an increasing number of complaints and whether such complaints are upheld, remains to be seen. However, the trend continues towards making patients more aware of their rights, clarifying what those rights are and encouraging greater involvement and participation by patients and those close to them, in their care.

A right to consent

The notion of consent continues the theme of rights for individuals in relation to the right to know, and avoiding patients taking action which may result in compensation being sought.

Tschudin (1992) suggests that there are four aspects of the consent process:

- who may give consent
- the competency of the individual
- who should provide the information
- the content of the information
(Tschudin, 1992, p. 21).

There is great emphasis placed on informed consent relating to the process of treatment, research, and experiments, and in law, not all consent needs to be given in writing (Dimond, 1993). Tschudin (1992) recognises that consent is 'a caring act which involves relating to one another'. Therefore nurses are faced with making judgements about what constitutes the best interests of patients, in terms of the quantity and quality of information offered in relation to patient's needs for information both in terms of their own interventions and in relation to medical treatments. The overriding right here appears to be in relation to 'being given information about significant risks of substantial harm' (Dimond, 1993).

Nurses would do well to note this advice by Lord Templeman in relation to therapeutic privilege:

An obligation to give patients all the information available to the doctor would be inconsistent with the doctor's contractual obligation to have regard to the patient's best interest. Some information might confuse, other information might alarm a particular patient, ... the doctor must decide in the light of his training and experience and in the light of his knowledge of the patient what should be said and how it should be said [Lord Templeman, p. 665 in Dimond (1993, p. 38)].

There are three types of consent, verbal, written and implied.

Reflective point
Give three or four examples of these three different types of consent in your area of practice. What evidence (other than signed written consent forms) exists in your area to establish that consent is obtained relating to nursing interventions?

Key sources which guide this process include, protocols standard statements and patient-care plans.

In general, patients' vulnerability is exacerbated by the lack or the poor quality of information. Parents of adolescents under the age of 16 have the right to give consent and professionals may be called on to act in the best interests of patients under certain circumstances, e.g. when a patient is mentally incapacitated, for children, particularly in emergency situations and, for example, for unconscious patients when there is no obligation to obtain the consent of the next of kin if the person is over 16 years of age.

A right of access to health records

The Access to Health Records Act (1990), gives patients, those with parental responsibility, individuals, e.g. solicitors, nominated by the patient and patients' representatives following their death, the right to access to written records made by health-care professionals (excluding social workers).

They have a right to:

- inspect the records
- take a copy of the records

- an explanation of details contained within them
- suggest corrections to inaccurate records (Dimond, 1994).

Though this act contains corresponding exclusion clauses in the case of information leading to deleterious effects on patients, it is a stark reminder to all personnel who keep records of patients of the need for accurate, factual and unambiguous records.

The issue of patients' rights has both ethical, moral and legal dimensions. The respect of human rights and thus patients' rights depends on the values, beliefs and decision-making potential, particularly of those who have the greater contact with patients. While nurses may not have the professional power of doctors in terms of diagnostic and treatment decisions, they may influence this process greatly. Above all, nurses, midwives and health visitors have the potential to promote the physical and mental well-being of patients (which is often given the greater priority) as well as the contextual elements namely the socio-cultural and spiritual needs to enhance the overall well-being of individuals and their satisfaction with care – it is to this theme that we now turn.

Patient satisfaction – a means to understanding the quality of care for individuals

---

Having examined issues associated with patients' experiences and rights, factors which contribute to an understanding of patient satisfaction will now be explored. It is recognised that for patients to make judgements about how satisfied they are with care, they need knowledge and understanding of what they can expect, the available choices, the standards of practice and any alternatives to these. However as Lamont (1993) points out:

there is as yet no central consumer agency that seeks to measure standards uniquely from the patients' point of view (p. 115).

Fitzpatrick (1993) suggests that there are three aspects to the study of patient satisfaction:

- local surveys of hospital, community and primary care services
- systematic research projects (usually undertaken in the USA) addressing patients' perceptions of the contrasts between fee-paying and non-fee-paying health services.
- surveys of patient satisfaction with medical care.

Overall there is a dearth of reliable data relating to the satisfaction of patients with nursing care, though there are a wide range of studies, particularly in relation to satisfaction with medical care. In addition, since the publication of the *NHS Management Enquiry* (1993, Griffiths Report), the White Paper, *Working for Patients* (HMSO, 1989) and the growing emphasis on consumerism in health care, the assessment of patient satisfaction is recognised as an important activity. However there has been a tendency for studies to be undertaken which avoid issues associated with the quality of professional intervention but focus on such elements as the quality of waiting areas, waiting times and catering services. What exists then is evidence from a range of studies over a number of years which highlights features of patient satisfaction in a range of care environments. Interestingly, many studies which appear to have a medical focus, contain explicit reference to aspects of nursing care and factors which are of direct relevance to nurses.

Indicators of patient satisfaction

There are a number of factors which contribute to the overall satisfaction that patients have with their care. Studies exploring satisfaction with medical care offer valuable insights which bear a marked resemblance to factors often highlighted and emphasised by nurses, in particular the use of effective interpersonal skills, information-giving, listening and responding to personal concerns and the need for continuity of care. Cleary and McNeil (1988) identified nine different dimensions of patient satisfaction. These are:

- the art of care
- technical quality
- accessibility
- convenience
- finance
- physical environment
- availability
- continuity
- outcome.

Similar findings are given by Hall and Dornan (1988) who have also made explicit reference to the need to attend to patients' psychosocial problems.

From these two studies some key themes emerge, namely that patients have expectations relating to how their care is organised, managed and conducted as well as the more obvious needs associated with the outcomes of care and treatment. Patients express satisfaction with doctors who offer comprehensive information (Pendleton, 1983), who facilitate the expression of personal needs and worries (Roter, 1989), and who encourage them to express personal views and insights about their problems (Stiles *et al.*, 1979). In studies undertaken among GPs, continuity of care has been found to be a significant factor (Hjortdahl and Laerum, 1989) and in a study by Williams *et al.* (1991), the general level of satisfaction with doctors was higher when satisfaction with their interpersonal skills was also high. An example of a long-term outcome of the effectiveness of interpersonal skills was found in a study by the Headache Study Group (1986) who found that the patients who were able to tell the doctor everything had the best results after one year of treatment.

More recently the King Edward Hospital Fund for London has developed the CASPE system for the continuous monitoring of patient satisfaction which can measure in-patient and out-patient satisfaction using separate questionnaires (Gritzner, 1993). This is currently being used in more than 20 health authorities. The main topics included on the questionnaires relate to ward facilities, organisational aspects of care, treatment and general (hotel) services. Patients are asked questions about what they think about the following:

- your surroundings
- noise on the ward
- the way your day is organised
- atmosphere in the ward
- visiting arrangements on the ward
- the information that is given to you about your treatment
- the clinical treatment that you receive
- the control of any pain
- nurses
- doctors

- radio, TV, day room
- food
- telephones
- bathrooms and toilets
- overall, how satisfied are you with your hospital stay (Gritzner, 1993, p. 37).

In addition, comments are encouraged along with a second batch of questions which are generated locally and which often relate to such issues and local policies, e.g. smoking and privacy. Response rates are encouraged in a number of ways including the fact that 'the core questionnaires for both in-patients and out-patients have been translated into Polish, Bengali, Chinese, Turkish, French and German' (Gritzner, 1993).

A range of outcomes have been identified from this extensive work, which include:

- the development of specific questionnaires relating to key aspects of the core question-naires, e.g. noise, food and pain control
- the development of questionnaires relating to specific services, e.g. obstetrics, ante-natal care, accident and emergency, acute psychiatry, paediatrics and intensive care
- the development of questionnaires specific to doctors and, more recently, nurses
- the dissemination of results of questionnaires to managers, clinicians, ward staff and patients
- the comparison of outcomes between health districts
- large- and small-scale improvements in services when low satisfaction outcomes are revealed, e.g. nursing staff were encouraged to wear soft-soled shoes at night to reduce noise levels, a ward day room was designated as a non-smoking area, improvements were made to consultancy and to waiting areas in a genito-urinary clinic to improve privacy (Gritzner, 1993).

It is interesting to note from these examples from the CASPE study that while findings from the survey are having an impact on the service, the nature of some of the findings highlights issues pertinent to the responsibility that nurses have for aspects of the services. From the two examples mentioned here, i.e. the noise associated with nurses' footwear and the patient day room smoking facility, it could be argued that these issues should be addressed along with local policies relating to uniform and health promotion respectively,

which may be managed appropriately at director-ate level.

Complementary to work relating to patient satis-faction surveys is a series commissioned by the NHS Management Executive asking patients what they think makes a quality service. Five specific areas are highlighted here as examples of specific services:

- maternity services of Asian women
- breast cancer services
- haemophilia services
- fracture clinics
- sickle cell anaemia.

Maternity services for Asian women (women from the Indian sub-continent)

The main concerns of this group related to the quality of information and 'making their wishes understood' (NHSME, 1993a). Pre-natal mortality is 16.4 per 1000 births among Pakistani-born mothers and is therefore of considerable concern (NHSME, 1993a). In addition, peri-natal deaths from con-genital malformation are higher (three in ten child-ren among Pakistani families compared to two in ten of UK mothers). Information relating to a wide range of ante- and post-natal aspects of care is highlighted, e.g. the need to encourage attendance at ante-natal clinics, clear accessible written and verbal information sympathetic to the range of cult-ural backgrounds. Assessments of risk factors by midwives, for example, need to include reference to poor housing, poor nutrition and ignorance of clinical care.

These are some of the comments gleaned from the women interviewed.

This midwife, she was so wonderful. She stayed two hours at my house, drawing pictures and telling my young sister-in-law to explain to me about the place of the baby, and what I would see in X-ray. So when we went to the appointment, we could ask questions.

The midwife told me to come to classes to learn about feeding and bathing. I went one time but it was in English and I couldn't understand so much. I wanted to tell her that bottle is better because the baby gets more milk and I am shy in front of all my brothers-in-law and father-in-law to feed from the breasts.

He died after five days. I think because I didn't breathe rightly. But they say nothing to me, why – only that they are sorry. Why don't they explain?

They sent me home so quickly and I was unhappy. In hospital, I didn't like the food, but I had rest and some time. At home, we have a small flat, it's crowded and so cold, but I was afraid to ask for more time and ashamed to tell them about our house (NHSME, 1993a, pp. 6–13).

These comments clearly illustrate how focused, sensitive information-giving contributes to patient confidence and well-being. Conversely the distress which results from the lack of knowledge and understanding of socio-economic factors, cultural norms and poor information-giving is clearly expressed. The challenges for purchasers are recognised in relation to service provision, consumer choice and involvement and quality of care. These are some of the questions posed.

How do you ensure that Asian women are informed and understand about the full range of services and options available to them such as:

- access to women doctors
- methods of family planning
- where they can have their baby
- types of delivery
- who can be with them when they attend clinics and during labour
- methods of pain control
- approaches to feeding
- help with post-natal depression?

Is information available through different media such as print, video, audio cassette and advocacy?

How do you address the issue of individual choice?

What arrangements are there for clients and their families to provide feedback on the service they receive both to their purchasers and to those providing the service? (NHSME, 1993a, p. 22).

What arrangements are there in place to ensure that each woman has a comprehensive care package which includes specific language, cultural and religious needs? (NHSME, 1993a, p. 23).

Reflective point
Consider the needs of a minority ethnic group who require care in your area of practice. To what extent are their individual cultural, language, dietary and religious needs acknowledged and integrated into their care plan?

It is valuable to examine local charter standards, mission statements as well as such statements as ward/unit philosophies to ascertain the extent to which the needs of minority groups are being catered for.

Breast cancer services

There are in excess of 150,000 women with breast cancer in the UK and it is the commonest cancer in women with 27,000 new cases and 15,000 deaths per annum (NHSME, 1993b). The key characteristics of an effective service relate to efficient health promotion and screening programmes as well as treatment options and support services. Despite the priority given to the detection and treatment of breast cancer and *The Health of the Nation* targets (DoH, 1992), the experiences of women facing this devastating disease remain mixed and controversial.

Comments from women in relation to diagnosis

They've always explained things down to the last detail. They told me as they were doing things exactly what was happening.

They said they wanted to draw some fluid off and they said where the needle was going and what the test was for. But if I'd known what I was going to have to go through, I would have brought someone with me.

I didn't know what was going to happen. I didn't know it was going to be a general anaesthetic. The consultant made it seem so minor. I hadn't even made arrangements to be off work the next day.

You need a private room and time to talk. You come out in floods of tears and there you are, on the street.

It wasn't until I was in the hospital that I was told I had breast cancer by the consultant. He didn't say a lot. I was so shocked, I didn't ask him any questions. There were half a dozen people round the bed when he told me. Then they walked away.

Yes, I was able to ask questions but not much came to mind at the time ... the situation of being told, half-naked, lying down ... I can't speak to a strange man easily.

In relation to treatment options

I can't speak highly enough of the doctor. He was very gentle and kind and didn't hurry even though it was a busy clinic. He let me get dressed, then he sat me down and asked what I thought was wrong. When I said 'cancer', he said that was right but I shouldn't worry too much as the lump was small. When he'd let that sink in a bit, he asked me if I knew about all the different treatments and all the pros and cons. He asked me if I'd understood and whether I had anyone outside to take me home or if there was anyone the nurse could phone for me. He told me there was no hurry and that he wanted me to go home and think about what treatment I wanted and come back next week to talk again. He gave me the number of a nurse counsellor and asked me to get in touch with her if I was worried and I hadn't understood. It might seem funny, but I went out feeling really comforted and confident.

They don't tell you a lot. They just told me I was going to have a mastectomy. No choice, no explanation. Even with the second one, it was just a lump, but I had to have a mastectomy.

Comments on admission for treatment and care

I don't know. So much happened all at once. Several people came and asked lots of questions – why couldn't one person have asked them all? I filled out a form before going to radiotherapy, but I don't remember being asked for consent.

The doctors come round and see you but they don't give you information. A lady on the ward who'd had it eight years ago told me all about how it would look when it healed up, so she set me right a lot.

The breast counsellor gave me a booklet and a leaflet. She gave me the impression that she'd got time. She brought one (a prosthesis) so that I could see what it was like and said if I wanted one later I could ring up the surgical appliance people.

I was worried about seeing the scar. They said you don't need to look while you're in hospital. The breast-care nurse took the dressing off for the first time and I looked – the tears trickled. The sister was absolutely lovely. She held my hand and talked to me. It's things like that that really make a difference (NHSME, 1993b, pp. 13–25).

So many of the experiences illustrated here reflect both the positive and the negative influences of the patient experience of illness, particularly when the threat is from cancer, and the prospect of long-term chronic illness, and changes in body image.

Kelly (1992) suggests that nurses have an important responsibility to respond to the needs of patients with a chronic illness by being technically competent, supporting patients who are faced with a range of thoughts and feelings about self-worth, their mortality, implications for their family and the effects on corresponding relationships. Finally, Kelly (1992) suggests that nurses can play a central role in helping patients make sense of the condition.

Haemophilia services

As with many chronic illnesses, haemophilia becomes very well understood by those affected and their families. The consideration of service provision by the NHSME (1993c) took into consideration those with haemophilia A, haemophilia B (Christmas disease) and von Willebrand's disease. Here are some of the patient and family experiences.

Diagnosis

David was always suffering from bruising when he was a baby and of course everyone implied we were battering him. We knew nothing about haemophilia and the first blood tests didn't find anything unusual.

My son was diagnosed at eight months and I was devastated, absolutely devastated. I just didn't know anything about haemophilia, I couldn't even spell it.

The experience of having the disease [and in one case contracting the human immunodeficiency virus (HIV)]

The damage in my teens, with the constant bleeding and lack of any real treatment, caused the joints to just get stiffer and stiffer. Nowadays my right elbow joint is totally fixed rigid, while movement in my right wrist is impaired, and movement in my left elbow and wrist is restricted. I can still walk, but getting up in the mornings is always extremely painful.

Having HIV has had a devastating effect on my family, and my own GP just doesn't know how to handle the situation. He just refers me to the haemophilia centre, but that is just in its infancy. I feel I'm in no-man's-land.

Care and treatment

I feel I am very lucky because we have an excellent haemophilia centre nearby. You need continuity of care and the sister at the centre has been there since it opened. They will listen to you and provide you with what you need.

My son has had home treatments since he was three. But if ever we go on holiday it is always to somewhere where there is a good haemophilia centre. If you have to go to any other hospital you tend not to be believed (NHSME, 1993c, pp. 7–14).

The complexity of the impact of an inherited blood disorder where men are usually affected and women are carriers (except in von Willebrand's disease) and which brings the effects of a child with chronic illness into a family can be far-reaching.

The NHSME (1993c) recommendations for service provision are based on aspects which have been found to be valued by families and include:

- home treatment programmes wherever possible to minimise trips to hospital and ensure bleeds are treated promptly
- access to a haemophilia centre and specialist staff 24 hours a day, seven days a week
- immediate treatment on arrival
- someone with some knowledge of haemophilia if no member of the haemophilia centre staff is available
- adequate supplies of blood products to meet their needs, including prophylaxis when necessary, and to cover holiday requirements
- reassurance on the safety and effectiveness of the blood products they are receiving (NHSME, 1993c, p. 17).

The principles of continuity, sensitivity, expertise and proactive care are emphasised here, reflecting the needs of individuals and families to what can be a life-threatening condition. However the illness more often results in families sharing responsibilities for care and treatment and contributing to the management of pain.

Fracture clinics

There is a huge demand for fracture clinic services. In 1990 650,000 people (3:100) attended a fracture or orthopaedic clinic (NHSME, 1993d). The key issues and problems for these patients relate to changes and deficiencies in mobility, the effects of a painful injury, frustration at the nature of the injury and, for elderly people in particular, insecurity following an accident. Patients also experienced problems relating to accessing clinics. Here are some of their experiences.

There were signposts to everything except the fracture clinic. No-one seemed to know where it was.

One of the League of Friends hostesses could see I was in trouble. She found me a wheelchair, took my crutches and pushed me to the clinic. It was much appreciated.

My appointment was for 9 a.m. and the appointment card warned that if I were late risked not being seen ... I needn't have worried. Everyone had the same appointment time and it was about four hours later that I was seen.

Every time anyone walked past my leg, which stuck out into the corridor, I was petrified.

My wheelchair would go into the toilet forwards, and come out backwards. Anything else was virtually impossible (NHSME, 1993d, pp. 9–14).

The organisation of the service, particularly in relation to access and information appears to be the key issue and reflects the priorities of the patients.

A range of questions is raised in relation to service provision, consumer choice and involvement and the quality of care (NHSME, 1993d) to meet what could be regarded as fundamental needs of patients with a disability.

Sickle cell anaemia

Finally, the experiences of those faced with another inherited blood disorder are given. There are three principal types of sickle cell disorders: sickle cell disease, haemoglobin sickle cell and sickle beta thalassaemia, affecting around 6000 people in the UK (NHSME, 1994). Patients are prone to extremes of pain and anaemia, organ damage and sickle cell crises.

Here are some of their experiences of living with the disease

Will it get worse? Will I survive? How much damage will it do to my insides?

No one likes to watch a child suffering. I can't stand it when they get the pain.

When the pain starts it hurts him a lot. I didn't realise how painful it was. Its terrible. He doesn't sleep, he doesn't eat. It's just the crying ... it scares me.

When needing admission to hospital

To me the most important thing is getting the pain under control and then you can relax and I have the drip put in. You can answer questions and you can be examined. But when they want to examine you first, put the drip in and ask all these questions, it is very difficult. You sometimes tend to lash out at them and they think you are being awkward.

Every time I come to casualty they always seem to assume I am a junkie desperate for drugs, which I find very insulting and upsetting.

Of in-patient care

As I regularly attend hospital for exchange blood transfusions I was often in the care of different doctors and nurses most of whom I have never met or been introduced to, but recently things have changed. During the time of my admission I have been introduced to a nurse who would take care of me during my stay. When that nurse's shift was over, she would introduce me to my next nurse. I have found this system helps to keep me informed of the treatment I'm being given, because 'my nurse' would be there to answer my questions and generally take away any fears I may have (NHSME, 1994).

Reflective point
Looking back over the patients' perceptions of care as illustrated in these five care areas. Why do you think it is that nurses and nursing care hardly feature?

It is notable that reference to the care offered by nurses barely features, but where it does, the reference is positive reflecting the attention to patients' needs so central to the overall satisfaction patients have with care. Despite patients clearly expressing needs for information, support, care and continuity of services, it appears their access to nurses was limited, though in many of these experiences, nurses or midwives may have been ideally placed to meet their needs.

There is evidence from a range of sources that nurses continue to struggle to meet the needs of patients highlighted here. Discussing issues pertinent to the development of the role, responsibility,

status and competence of nurses can shed some light on this apparent paradox where the commitment nurses have to individual care does not always manifest itself in practice. In tracing the development of an occupational group such as nurses, an approach is to consider how the process of professionalisation in nursing may or may not have contributed to developments in practice and indeed, may have resulted in initiatives which have supported the development of nurses but it is debatable whether the patient's voice has been heard clearly enough to shape professional prioritisation.

The professionalisation of nursing

Historically nursing as a profession, in the lay sense of the word, appears to have been socially accepted and generally accepted by other professions until the 1960s when questions arose from sources inside and outside the profession as to the nature of its professional status. There were uncertainties about nursing roles, relationships with other professional groups within the NHS, particularly the medical profession, and doubts that the education of nurses was preparing them appropriately for registration.

Owing to the broad use of the terms 'profession' and 'professional', it is necessary primarily to establish interpretations of them. Social scientists appear to have found analysis of the concept of a profession extremely difficult. The term implies respectability and status, but it has also been used to describe a job, occupation or work and, historically, has been appropriated by groups made up, almost exclusively, of men. This confusion is increased by the comparison of the terms 'professional' and amateur. However, despite the increase in occupations claiming professional status during the 1950s and 1960s (Etzioni, 1969), a defining feature is their collective orientation rather than self-orientation (Parsons, 1958). The positive social force of a profession is widely accepted and this is perhaps the feature which allowed nursing its unchallenged position from Miss Nightingale's era until the 1960s. To clarify the features of nursing as a profession still further, it is interesting to utilise the trait approach. A traditional approach to the interpretation of an occupation as a profession, it is useful as part of the review of nursing as a profession. The list of traits by Brook (1974) centres on acceptably common attributes. These are as follows:

- the ideal of altruistic service
- practice based upon a foundation of theoretical, esoteric knowledge
- a long period of education (usually five years duration)
- control of entry and standards of practice
- an organisation – probably a professional council with disciplinary powers.

Professionalism is a process by which the characteristics of a profession are acquired, where the occupational associations control recruitment and practice and where there is marketable expert skill and knowledge. There is much controversy in the nursing literature about the value of the nurse acquiring professional status (Jolley, 1989), indeed there is a range of writers who suggest that the development of professional power and activities may have a detrimental effect on those they serve (e.g. Illich, 1977; Friedson, 1983). However, Hall (1980) suggests that the

> primary responsibility of nursing, and therefore the purposes of professionalism, is to provide direct care to the patient, client, family or community; it is concerned with maintaining, promoting and protecting the sick, and providing rehabilitation. It deals with the psychosomatic and psycho-social (and spiritual) aspects of life as these affect health, illness and dying (Hall, 1980, p. 153).

Is this a definition of the outcomes of the professionalisation of nursing or a statement summarising the main purposes of nursing actions? Here is the confusion. On the one hand, nurses seem clear that their role is to provide care. However, in practice, nurses may not be able to manage and exert enough control over themselves, their resources and the organisations and environments to deliver effective care. If the assumptions suggested by Hall (1980) are tenable, and there is much nursing literature to suggest that there is agreement about nurses prioritising care (Leininger, 1981; Benner and Wrubel, 1989) health promotion (Seedhouse and Cribb, 1989) and promoting the physical, psychological, social and spiritual well-being of patients (Fawcett, 1994; UKCC, 1986), then perhaps it is the acceptance and development of the key characteristics of a profession which will facilitate this process.

Nurses appear to have come a long way towards demonstrating professional status. Firstly, nursing practice has strengthened its theoretical and scientific knowledge base from a situation where a reliance on intuition, habit, routine and tradition justified aspects of practice. The preparation of registered practitioners, who remained in an ambiguous position owing to their student/worker status until the early 1990s, has developed with the advent of pre-registration diploma courses (Project 2000, UKCC, 1986) and integration of schools or colleges of nursing with institutions of higher education. With an unreliable knowledge base, and a relatively short period of education and training, much content centred around a medical rather than nursing model. It is no wonder then that nursing was so vulnerable to criticism as a profession. Indeed, the term 'semi-profession' was used by Etzioni (1969) as a description of the professional status of nursing because of the features described. While this is not meant as a derogatory term, Etzioni (1969) highlights a feature of nursing practice which contrasts greatly with other professionals, namely the lack of autonomy and accountability of the practising nurse compared with other professionals. This subject has been the focus of much debate over the past 20 years, particularly in relation to nursing practice. Following the Nurses, Midwives and Health Visitors Act (1979) and the formation of the United Kingdom Central Council (UKCC) the subsequent development of the *Code of Professional Practice for Nurse Midwives and Health Visitors* in 1982 (UKCC, 1982) did much to rectify this situation, highlighting for both the nurse and the consumer the required standards for professional conduct and practice. The UKCC has a responsibility 'to determine circumstances in which the means by which a person may, for misconduct ... be removed from the register' (Nurses Midwives and Health Visitors Act 1979). The powers of the UKCC therefore gives the nursing profession 'the legal status of a protected monopoly' (Edgar, 1994) who goes on to suggest that:

> This may be seen as a key element in the reinforcing of the professional status of nursing. A profession will have a governing body, free of external interference, that controls admission to the profession, and may expel members from the profession. The legal protection of clients is there by devolved on to this governing body (p. 152).

The Code of Professional Conduct for Nurses Midwives and Health Visitors (now in its third edition, UKCC, 1992), provides a professional framework both to guide the behaviour and role of nurses and to contribute to the development and evaluation of the professional orientation of nursing. The code is a valuable statement of general principles about care and serves to reinforce ideals about the service ethic. However, it is generalised, open to wide interpretation, and easily ignored. It fails to encourage debate and professional development, the nurse is responsible for individualised care as a result of his or her own decision making and therefore answerable for his or her actions. Clearer guidelines relating to these general principles would guide the interpretation and application of the code and would encourage much wider debate, highlighting the moral and ethical questions which are inevitably part of nursing and health-care decision making.

Despite these developments to strengthen the framework of accountability and responsibility, nurses are often supervised and corrected by senior nurses or even doctors. One of the most significant and controversial issues which had a detrimental effect on the professional role of the nurse as an accountable being has been the ratio and function of auxiliaries or health-care assistants to nurses in clinical areas. Since the Second World War, the ratio of auxiliaries to students rose, these 'unqualified' personnel forming an average of two-thirds of the ward team. During the 1970s and 1980s, this issue was severely criticised, particularly in relation to them being delegated a whole range of clinical tasks (Armstrong-Esther, 1981). As the majority of care was given by unqualified staff, particularly in institutions, it is no wonder that the notion of accountability was jeopardised. This is a central issue regarding accountability for without appropriate preparation nurses may be unable to accept, develop or maintain the level of professional autonomy necessary to underpin wider managerial responsibilities, for example, of managing groups, clinical resources, implementing policies and monitoring quality. It wasn't until the late 1970s that the links between individualised care and the nursing process were seen as an integral part of the preparation of nurses (General Nursing Council, 1977).

The 1960s saw the rise in scientific and medical knowledge, advances in technology and the advent of para-medical specialities and also influenced professionalisation. Observations of developments and changes in nursing at that time may be interpreted as a response to the apparent threat of these advances on the status of the nursing profession. The adoption of delegated medical tasks by nurses may have been an attempt to assert a higher clinical status and the Royal College of Nursing (1979) pioneered the concept of the extended clinical role of the nurse. However, this was never meant to lose sight of the commitment to nursing care, but it appeared to encourage a rise in 'technical' commitment, rather than the intended specialist knowledge under the auspices of the Clinical Nurse Specialist. The fact that few nurses practised under this title may be because of the outcry by the medical profession at the time to this 'consultant' nurse's role, or the lack of foundation of specialist knowledge.

A further reaction to the insecurity of this period was the exodus of experienced clinical nurses into the administrative structure, resulting from the Salmon report (1966). This attempt to create a career structure for clinical nurses was shown to be detrimental to patient care, standards and morale (McFarlane, 1980), because younger, less experienced staff were left in their place particularly at ward level.

Promotion prospects further aggravated this situation as candidates were encouraged to find opportunities only in the management and educational tiers. These few examples show how the profession was struggling for status through administrative decisions and untested means. It is interesting that at a time when the most experienced clinical nurses were leaving the bedside, Henderson's (1966) description of the unique function of the nurse emerged as what is now the most widely accepted statement of the role of the nurse. It reads:

> The unique function of the nurse is to assist the individual; sick or well, in the performance of those activities contributing to health or its recovery (or to a peaceful death) that he would perform unaided if he had the recovery strength, will or knowledge. And to do this in such a way as to help him gain independence as rapidly as possible (Henderson, 1966).

It appears that the interpretation of the role of the nurse has changed little over the past 40 years, and the following statements by Frederick and Northan (1938) and King (1968) confirm this.

They suggest:

> Modern nursing is by no means limited to the giving of expert physical care to the sick, important though it is. It is more far reaching, including as it does helping the patient to unalterable situations such as personal, family and economic conditions, teaching him and others in the home and in the community to care for themselves, guiding him in the prevention of the illness through hygienic living, and helping him to use available community resources to these ends (Frederick and Northan, 1938, p. 41).

and

> Nursing is defined as a process of action, reaction, interaction and transaction whereby nurses assist individuals of any age group to meet their basic human needs in coping with their health status at some particular point in their life cycle (King, 1968, p. 28).

An observation by Bevis (1978) further complements and strengthens the clarification of the nurse's role by Henderson (1966). Bevis (1978) identified humanistic existentialism as an important influence of change in nursing. The assumptions were that as a value system, humanism placed priority on caring about people and existentialism provided the model within which humans are unique thinking beings, making choices and being accountable. (This is discussed more fully in Chapter 5.) This may be viewed as a significant contribution to strengthening the status of the profession. The profession was striving for change amidst the realisation that traditional 'knowledge' and much current practice were founded on unsupported and unresearched declarations rather than a proven body of knowledge. The Royal College of Nursing (1979) stressed that the profession has a responsibility to evaluate the quality of service and the competence of its practitioners. A way forward appeared to be emerging which would facilitate not only the redirection of nursing practice back to the central issue of individualised care (McFarlane, 1980), but also increase the scientific knowledge-base which would only enhance the status of the profession. It is suggested that the nursing process was seen as the means to this end. With a problem-solving approach to nursing practice as its baseline, the nursing process was regarded as the means to high standards of clinical practice (Royal College of Nursing, 1981). However with the adoption of this approach came a range of assumptions, particularly in relation to what constitutes individualised care and meeting individual needs. The changing status of patients during this period cannot be ignored, indeed this emerges as an enormously significant feature and demonstrates the move away from the traditional, more subordinate role of the patient, implied but not necessarily realised by task allocation and routinised care. As nurses utilised this new approach to nursing so their accountability to the patient became more exacting. Therefore, any decisions taken together should result in the nurse being able to justify her actions to the patient. The nursing process, as a problem-solving approach, provided a systematic framework for decision making but lacked a theoretical and philosophical base to guide the application, interpretation and analysis of patient need. Work by a range of nurse theorists, under the general auspices of nursing models, appears to have bridged the gap between the simple decision-making model of the nursing process and the need to be able to justify, communicate and develop approaches to nursing care which met patient needs. The application of nursing theories to practice appear to have gone some way towards providing a rationale for aspects of care planning, but there is little evidence that they have contributed to the body of knowledge relating to the further understanding of nursing interventions and outcomes of care.

McFarlane (1980) saw the striving for excellence in nursing practice in itself as a means of professionalisation. However, with this process comes the demand for a greater degree of accountability for all grades of qualified nurses, not only to the patients but also to each other and themselves.

The emphasis on the nursing process appears to have provided a catalyst for those concerned with practice, i.e. nursing policy-makers, nursing leaders, educationalists and practitioners. Here was seen a means for managing care in a systematic way (Aggleton and Chalmers, 1986). It was seen as a means for developing and improving the totality of care, having written records to reflect this, and for ensuring that the registered nurse supervises care when it is delivered by an unqualified member of the nursing team. However, the nursing process was interpreted more as a tool for monitoring care, rather than as a belief system for analysing the health and nursing needs of patients.

Assessing, creating and implementing a plan of care needs purpose, direction and reciprocity with the patient and, for example, associated members of the health-care team. Difficulties with the nursing process have stemmed from too much emphasis on the 'stages' of problem solving and not enough concern with the purpose of nursing. Assessment, for example, without a clear sense of priority, purpose, commitment and logical thinking, may result in observations, interactions and interviews which fulfil criteria synonymous with history taking. Thus there is a responsibility for the nurse to:

- prioritise the needs of the patient and the corresponding nursing interventions
- identify the purpose of nursing for this person as a patient
- demonstrate a commitment to caring by responding to the impact of the patient's health state in a sensitive, professional manner
- utilise logical thinking/decision making continually to monitor, anticipate, prioritise and evaluate care.

By exploring the nature and purpose of nursing, as required for the patient being cared for, there is a demand that nurses utilise and adapt their nursing knowledge. Thus, the purpose of nursing may be influenced and shaped in a range of ways. The main cue should be from recipients of nursing, and for nurses to respond individually, competently, professionally and morally. However, as the limitations of the nursing process became clearer, particularly in relation to difficulties with the assessment process, continuity of care, record keeping and care plan design, two major issues for practice emerged. First, how could care be organised in a way which would facilitate continuity, and how could the nursing process be developed to facilitate individualised care. The interpretation and use of nursing knowledge may be seen as central to this process.

Some developments in nursing in the UK which have done much to shape professional nursing particularly in relation to the delivery of care. These are:

- developments in nursing knowledge and research
- holism in nursing
- nursing as a therapeutic response to patients' need
- aspects of professional development in nursing.

Developments in nursing knowledge and research

Nursing may be regarded as a subject discipline in its own right. Meleis (1991) suggests that:

The discipline of nursing, therefore, includes the content and processes related to all roles that nurses play, ... A discipline also includes the theories developed to describe, explain and prescribe as well as the research findings related to the discipline's central phenomenon and the knowledge from related disciplines that is essential for informing members of a particular discipline. All disciplines are formed around a domain of knowledge (p. 97).

The 'domain of knowledge' referred to here is a range of interrelated components which are essentially theoretical and practical. The central phenomenon of the nursing domain is the interaction between nurses and patients, and how nurses respond to individual and group needs. The interaction between patients and their environments consists of nursing activities and competencies which focus on the health and nursing needs of patients.

The definition offered by Meleis (1991) offers a more 'scientific' interpretation of the nature of nursing knowledge which tends to value knowledge which is generisable, factual and verifiable. Empirical research is the approach to generating knowledge scientifically which relies on induction, i.e. methods of data collect and analysis from, for example, pure observation, clinical trials, surveys and experimentation which aim to predict, explain or describe people, events or situations.

As well as this 'scientific' or empirical approach to the generation of knowledge, Carper (1978) also offers three other types of 'knowing' (Carper, 1978) as aesthetics (the art of nursing), personal knowledge and ethical knowledge. Research into the art of nursing depends on qualitative methods which focus on such phenomena as compassion, empathy and perception. Second, personal knowledge may also utilise qualitative methods to understand such experiences as the relationships between carers and patients and models of therapeutic interaction. Finally ethical knowledge may be generated from the relationship between ethical theories and moral values (such as honesty) and clinical dilemmas relating to truth telling, for example.

That nursing knowledge needs aesthetic and empirical dimensions is not disputed (Leininger,

1981; Rogers, 1970), nor are the relationships between knowledge and theory in nursing. Indeed there are a range of nursing theories which usually offer a perspective about the interrelationship between nursing, health, man and/or the environment (the latter usually being the least well defined or explained). These theories are mainly deductive, except Orlando's theory which is inductive (Orlando, 1961). As a result, much of the nursing theory development appears to have been pursuing the 'what is nursing' question which has also been posed by a number of nurse writers, e.g. Webb (1992). Many of the nursing theorists have attempted to say something about the relationship between nurses and patients, usually emphasising that the relationship may be therapeutic (Peplau, 1982) and dependent on the application of interpersonal skills to establish and develop effective relationships with patients (Roper *et al.*, 1990; Orem, 1995). However, there is some evidence to indicate that 'close' relationships with nurses is not what patients want (Salvage, 1990; Morrison, 1994). Nurses recognise the inappropriateness of gathering data about patients, designing elaborate care plans and leading patients towards a form of dependence and relationship which, after a matter of hours or a few days, comes to a close as the patient is transferred or discharged. This situation is, of course, particularly poignant in hospital wards and units but may also feature where opportunities for the continuity of care are interrupted through irregular staff allocation, and high staff turnover.

Salvage suggests:

> Patients' desire to be treated with warmth, kindness and sensitivity does not necessarily mean they want close relationships of a quasi-psychotherapeutic kind (1990, p. 44).

Perhaps practitioners have depended too heavily on nursing theories for answers to their problems with individualised care and care planning. Here is another dimension to the paradox – nurses appear to have struggled to adapt care to established but often theoretical frameworks rather than taking their cues from patients and prioritising care on the basis of professional decision making and the patient's perspective. There are over 30 well-documented nursing theories. Of these, many remain abstract and untested in practice areas in the UK. Yet some of the more 'popular' theories, namely the works of Orem (1995), Roy (Andrews

and Roy, 1986), Peplau (1982), Neuman (1995), Rogers (1970) and King (1971) are used as a basis for ward/unit philosophies and care-plan documentation. Nurses frequently attempt to mould their assessment on patients on criteria offered by these theories.

This leads us to consider sources of nursing knowledge and the contribution of nursing research to the professionalisation of nursing.

The status of nursing research

Nurses have not traditionally given priority to nursing research. Universities have played a central role in the development and testing of knowledge, research activities being a core activity. The existence of departments of nursing studies in universities or polytechnics in the UK was rare until the 1970s, when there was also the beginning of the emergence of a national approach to post-registration education with the establishment of the Joint Board of Clinical Nursing Studies (JBCNS) in 1971. Even then, the dependence by nurses on the discipline of medicine was so great that they failed to recognise the need for nurses, midwives and health visitors to question, check or challenge the knowledge they were being asked to use in order to practice. This period saw a corresponding growth in undergraduate and post-graduate nurse education, as well as educational initiatives to inform nurses about research which the JBCNS pioneered. Subsequently the English National Board has continued this initiative with their Course 870. The Royal College of Nursing promoted and published a series of nursing research projects in the 1970s including *The Unpopular Patient* (Stockwell, 1972), the findings from which are still valued today.

In 1991, there were still only 15 nursing departments in universities in Britain, but educational reforms (UKCC, 1986) which demanded academic as well as professional validation of courses leading to entry to a part of the UKCC professional register also saw deliberate emphasis being placed on the appreciation, use, application and in the case of post-registration degrees, the generation of research.

Nursing education, in its broadest sense, could be viewed as facing an even greater challenge in the present day than it has ever had. With most nurse, midwife and health visitor education now emanating from institutions of higher education, the opportunities for nursing (and associated) research to become an integral part of educational programmes has never been greater. The culture for the generation of research is established, indeed it is an expectation that this is integral to academic function. However, for the discipline of nursing, the maintenance and development of professional perspectives are paramount. Thus, the way that nursing knowledge is interpreted, understood and prioritised in curricula for pre- and post-registration courses will have a significant impact on practice. Employers of nurses demand skilled practitioners to undertake the 'work' and that the work nurses do has many facets. Reed and Procter (1993) describe nursing work as 'dirty', 'natural', 'invisible' and 'skilled'. They describe:

- **Dirty work** as nurses having to deal with such matters as cleaning up blood, vomit, faeces, etc.
- **Natural work** as managing similar matters to dirty work, but it is recognised as natural because it is not unusual for lay carers to undertake similar work. The distinction here lies in the differences in commitment, responsibility, roles and relationships between the carer and 'patient'. However, despite the apparent 'natural' aspect to these activities, there is a body of knowledge to support them, for example, the professional carers need to be able to assess, interpret and manage the impact for an individual, of the effects of vomiting on, for example, hydration, and nutrition.
- **Invisible work** is that which only nurses and patients see and experience. Reed and Procter suggest (1993) that:

Much of nursing work is taken for granted, such as comforting gestures, or attendance to hygiene, and so has been largely ignored in research and discussion (p. 17).

They recognise that the nature of much of this 'invisible' work is of a intimate and personal nature, making access to it by researchers problematic. Perhaps this is what contributes to the notion of aspects of nursing work being undervalued by nurses, and a source of much concern to patients because of what nurses have to do. It may also be an issue of seemingly low priority for educationalists, who neither have the research evidence to promote these aspects of caring, nor the means to undertake teaching activities which would facilitate continuity of observation, supervision, facilitation and support of student nurses in practice areas. This also raises questions about whether nurses are being appropriately assessed to establish their competence in managing intimate situations.

Skilled work

There is a risk that with so much nursing activity going unnoticed, except by nurses and patients, the skills required will be unrecognised and under-valued by resource managers and nurses themselves. They may fail to recognise the potential for skilled interventions to promote focused care, interactions, on-going assessment and evaluation despite evidence indicating that qualified nurses offer more skilled and cost-effective care (Audit Commission, 1992).

It could be argued that all work that nurses do is skilled, therefore another paradox is that while registered nurses assess and plan care, the delivery of that care can be delegated to those who are untrained. This calls into question the effects on the way that outcomes of care are judged and interpreted. Patients perceive that the untrained nurse has more time, for example, to talk, and be with them. It could be significant to the well-being of patients that information gained by the inexperienced and untrained nurse may not be valued as highly as activities usually undertaken by the registered nurse, for example, technical activities, record keeping, counselling, supporting bereaved relatives and caring for high dependency patients. There are many research questions here, for example:

1. how is nursing work delegated between trained and untrained nursing staff?
2. what do patients perceive to be the role of registered nurses in practice settings?
3. how are outcomes of care judged and by whom?
4. what are patients' expectations of the role of the registered nurse?
5. how do individual patients perceive that their needs are being met by nurses?

These broad questions are offered as a means of raising awareness of significant issues requiring research and focused study, for example, in relation to (5) it would be interesting to know more about patients' expectations of nurses in relation to information-giving.

While nurses continue to rely on nursing theories, further exploration of their use and relevance in relation to care planning is vital. With individual needs of patients being so diverse, over-reliance on one theory of nursing may result in nursing priorities failing to coincide with the patient's priorities of need. The same could be said for the way that Roper *et al.*'s (1990) approach to the promotion of independence has been interpreted and applied. While the activities of living are a useful way of looking at independent function, it remains true that the theoretical underpinning of the work is vague and largely untested in practice. This is particularly so when the concepts of independence and need are examined. It would be valuable, for example, to explore the interrelationship between the pursuit of the promotion of independence and the notion of a hierarchy of need (Maslow, 1954) which the authors offer as a way of describing elements of human need. Nurses have been frustrated by assessment criteria which do not make explicit reference to needs central to the concerns of many patients, for example, information needs and the management of pain/discomfort. It may be argued that these needs can be incorporated using this approach, for example, in relation to 'communicating' and 'maintaining a safe environment' respectively. However, the rigid interpretation of the activities of living may be, in part, due to the goal of independence being too nebulous and long term for nurses to identify with. The model offers useful principles to guide certain aspects of practice, particularly the need for nurses to assess the biopsychosocial perspective of each activity of living, and as such, it may be a useful tool for guiding the application of theory from a range of subject disciplines to the needs of patients.

Overall, nursing theories offer valuable insights into the nature of and approaches to nursing. More research is needed to test and analyse the concepts central to nursing, for example, caring, compassion, commitment and comforting which represent the type of responses being sought by patients. We need to know more about the realities and experiences of patients.

Nurses and/or those researching nursing are offering more indicators and evidence of the effects of nursing actions on care, for example, the use of touch in nursing (Tutton, 1991), counselling patients following myocardial infarction (Thompson *et al.*, 1990), and therapeutic aspects of the nurse–patient relationship (Ersser, 1991).

However a concept that has found its way into the nursing parlance from debates and experiences of individualised care and nursing process is that of holism. This will now be considered in relation to nursing in general and patient need in particular.

Holism in nursing

The use of, and reference to, holism among nurses is not new. It is frequently referred to in the context of individualised care which considers the biopsychosocial, spiritual and cultural needs of people needing nursing. Many nurses claim a holistic approach to caring without the requisite evidence that the individual is regarded as a 'whole'.

The American Holistic Nurses Association (1992) defines holism as follows:

> the concept of wellness: that state of harmony between mind, body, emotions and spirit in an ever changing environment.

In considering this definition, the idea of nurses being able to promote harmony of mind, body and spirit is a significant challenge when most patients are compromised by the very nature of their health state, the environment in which care takes place and uncertainties for their future well-being. For most of us, coming to terms with our vulnerability and mortality is challenging enough, thus gaining insight into the inner-self is not a natural part of the illness or ill-health experience. Many would rather avoid such self-examination, suppress the fears and uncertainties and reach for a means of cure. Kidel (1986) views illness as inevitable and 'offering us an opportunity for deepening awareness' (p. 25). He goes on to suggest:

> As long as we chase exclusively after 'health', we shall fail to grasp the meaning of true wholeness (p. 25).

This is certainly food for thought for nurses who have, in recent years, sought to promote health education. The challenge of holism is for nurses to combine the holistic principles of nursing, with the understanding of people as 'wholes'. However, in practice, taking Kidel's (1986) views, the real challenge is to recognise and respond to the impact on the individual's state of health of his or her spiritual self.

Buckle suggests:

I believe it is possible to call orthodox nursing holistic, if this principle of caring for that spiritual part of us is incorporated into our nursing. Being spiritual does not mean being saintly, vegetarian, teetotal or believing in dogma. It simply means being whole (1993, p. 744).

She goes on to suggest that a reason for the resurgence in complementary therapies may be a reaction to the lack of spiritual awareness and support. Thus, holistic nursing may or may not utilise complementary approaches to care but it does need seriously to consider the spiritual dimension of caring (Buckle, 1993).

Narayanasamy (1991) suggests:

The influence of spirituality and religion is commonly seen in the following aspects of a person's life: relationships with others, living style and habits; required and prohibited behaviours; the general frame of reference for thinking about oneself and the world (p. 2).

Spirituality may be viewed as a way of experiencing and expressing inner beliefs, convictions, a process of finding meaning and personal growth. Narayanasamy (1991) goes on to suggest characteristics of spiritual need as follows:

the need for meaning and purpose
the need for love and harmonious relationship
the need for forgiveness
the need for a source of hope and strength
the need for trust
the need for expression of personal beliefs and values
the need for spiritual practices, expression of concept of God or Deity and creativity (p. 7).

Certain aspects of religious need may be closely aligned with aspects of cultural need (Sampson, 1982), which places particular emphasis on each of the following (some examples are given to illustrate issues particularly pertinent to holistic nursing).

Beliefs

We need to be aware of the key beliefs of major religions, the differences between religious sects, and their main religious books, for example the Koran and the Holy Bible.

Religious observations

Iincluding religious festivals, for example, the Jewish Passover and Muslim Ramadhan, and religious articles, for example rosaries, prayer shawls and crucifixes.

The body and clothing

Sensitivities to the exposure or use of parts of the body are characteristic of some religions. Hindu women, for example, may refuse to undress in front of a male doctor or nurse and prefer long, close-fitting hospital gowns, which do not risk exposure. Jewish men and women prefer to keep their heads covered and orthodox Jewish baby boys have to be circumcised on the eighth postnatal day. Sikh men wear a number of religious symbols at all times, these are white shorts, a symbolic dagger, a comb (usually worn under the turban), a steel bangle and uncut hair. Rastafarians do not cut their hair and are also reluctant to wash it or shave.

Diet, alcohol and drugs

There are many religious and cultural factors associated with such activities as fasting, abstinence and dietary observances. Vegetarianism is not uncommon among Hindus and Rastafarians; Jains are vegans. Mormons do not drink tea, coffee, cola or alcohol. Orthodox Jews eat a Kosher diet. As well as avoiding all pig products, they also will not eat seafood which does not have scales and fins, and meat and milk are not taken at the same meal. Muslims and Rastafarians may refuse or be very reluctant to take prescribed drugs.

These are just a few examples to illustrate the range of needs which health-care personnel should respond to in a sympathetic, sensitive and knowledgeable way, though one of the main barriers continues to be language and finding effective ways to communicate, when English is not the patient's first language.

These needs illustrate a complex range of concerns for nurses who have more opportunity to respond holistically than the majority of health-care personnel, not least because of the intimate nature of the physical and emotional support they offer.

It is interesting to note that in this debate about holistic nursing, few of the nursing theorists have developed insight into spiritual need. Neuman (1989) incorporates the notion of spirituality into her work but its contribution to care is not developed. Additionally, most nurse theorists have tended not to consider holism as a concept for theory development. Levine (1971) considers the concept of holistic nursing, but tends to rely on physiological aspects of caring and does not define or explain the application of the concept.

Nurses need to proceed with caution. Holism is a far-reaching concept demanding a comprehensive understanding of the nature of being human. Holistic nursing, perhaps, goes even further, as it is an approach based on responding to the experiences of people at their most vulnerable, often without understanding how that person is when well, and often at times when the opportunity for exploring such personal matters as how illness is usually coped with.

For holistic nursing to become a reality for patient care, there should be further attention given to three factors which, viewed together, may be seen as prerequisites of holistic nursing because of their potential for facilitating a creative nurse–patient relationship. Namely, therapeutic nurse–patient interaction, patient participation in care and empowerment of both nurse and patient because of their influence on the style, expectations, purpose and outcome of the caring relationship.

That nursing care has the potential to contribute to processes of healing is central to this concern for the whole person. The process of healing has strong associations with spirituality, teaching, health promotion and caring interventions. It is well recognised that nurses can have a direct influence on aspects of healing (Pearson, 1991; McMahon, 1991). Also, nurses have an active role to play in determining interventions rather than a passive role which is dependent on reacting to medical interventions. Muetzel (1988) suggests that the following characteristics shape therapeutic interventions:

- intimacy – characterised by, for example, closeness and vulnerability which encourages openness and the expression of feelings
- partnership – characterised by recognising the need for nurses and patients to share information, to encourage patient involvement in care
- reciprocity – characterised by the balance between how the nurse and patient respond to aspects of the interaction, and the way nurses utilise their presence and helping skills to meet the patients priorities for care.

Like Peplau (1982), Muetzel (1988) appears to be suggesting that the very nature of the nurse–patient relationship has the potential to heal. Pearson (1991) views therapeutic nursing as a means not only of encouraging and facilitating a holistic response to holistic needs, but also as a means for the continual development of nursing. He regards this approach as a way of liberating nursing practice, at the same time recognising the need for research to examine the therapeutic effects of nursing. Is this yet another element to the professionalisation of nursing? Certainly the concern with the dynamics of the interaction with the whole patient is very firmly in the nursing domain, but perhaps, we, as nurses, still need to look to ourselves, our beliefs, knowledge, experience and professionalism properly to assess the feasibility of such a far-reaching approach for nursing.

The professional development of nurses has been laboured, not least because of the reluctance of nurses to establish opportunities for specialist rather than generalist practice and education. The 'watering down' of professional responsibility has been exacerbated in the past by a disproportionately large, untrained nursing workforce and a generally uncoordinated post-registration education system. This appears to have led many nurses away from specialisation (and thus specialist expert practice) because of concerns with theoretical rather than clinically led education. The final section will explore some key issues for professional development.

Aspects of professional development in nursing

The professional development of the nurse commences with pre-registration education and consists of the statutory, academic practice requirements and the acceptance and adoption of attitudes, values, responsibilities and accountability, regarded as an integral part of being a professional nurse (UKCC, 1992).

In 1993, at the Heathrow debate, a group of Chief Nursing Officers and nurse leaders considered 'the Challenges for Nursing and Midwifery in the 21st Century' (DoH, 1994b).

It became apparent during this debate that there were a range of issues which would play a part in the professional development of the nurse. They identified a range of 'benchmarks' – assumptions about key aspects of health care. These are listed in Fig. 4.4.

The main assumption lies with the trend for diagnosis and treatment to be away from large hospitals with dissemination of services into, for example, primary health-care settings. There appears to be influence here from *The Health of the Nation* targets (DoH, 1992) and the inevitability of continuing the initiatives of the NHS Community Care Act (HMSO, 1990).

Eight strategic issues for nursing and midwifery were then identified to highlight how nurses may be affected. These are given in Fig. 4.5.

A key word among this list of questions is substitution. Substituting machines for staff, for example, occurred when technological advances made hospital laboratories more efficient and advanced.

In the pursuit of efficiency and effectiveness, the report recognises that substitution relates to the location of care and tasks. Changes in surgical practices, for example, day case surgery and early discharge, illustrate locational developments, though there is perhaps a need for clearer evidence of the impact of such changes for patients.

The report recognises that the reallocation of tasks between nurses and other professionals is almost inevitable. Historically, the professionalisation of nursing was hindered by nurses failing to identify and pursue their central contribution to health and patient care by either forfeiting tasks to other health-care personnel or being reluctant to take on tasks.

All patients need their health needs assessed, planned intervention and care management undertaken, and judgements made about their effectiveness. Most nurses find themselves on a continuum between supporting medical intervention and having responsibility for their own case load and managing the untrained 'nurse'/health-care assistant's role in giving delegated care.

Which way do nurses want to go? Evidence suggests that nurses continue to seek and fulfil the professional dimensions of caring, and nurse leaders, researchers, professional organisations (for example, the Royal College of Nursing) and the statutory bodies confirms this. But do resource managers, in general, view nurses in the same light? There are two further professional initiatives which nurses must turn to in order to safeguard their status and integrity and to enhance the essential contribution nurses make to health, patient well-being, standards of practice, and education and research. These are *The Scope of Professional*

Practice (UKCC, 1992) and *The UKCC's Standards for Education and Practice following Registration* (UKCC, 1994).

The scope of professional practice

The Scope of Professional Practice (UKCC, 1992) is of significance for nurses, midwives and health visitors because it challenges the 'scope' of practice and thus the potential to deliver effective care. It provides nurses with the professional opportunity to assess the needs of patients in their care, and if necessary to initiate the necessary negotiation, education and interprofessional agreements for nurses to extend and expand their role. There follow key extracts from *The Scope of Professional Practice* (UKCC, 1992, pp. 5–8) to highlight the key implications for the way that nurses function and what they do.

Section 8. Principles for adjusting the scope of practice

Although the practices of nursing, midwifery and health visiting differ widely, the same principles apply to the scope of practice in each of these professions. The following principles are based upon the Council's Code of Professional Conduct and, in particular, on the emphasis which the code places upon knowledge, skill, responsibility and accountability. The principles which should govern adjustments to the scope of professional practice are those which follow.

Section A. The registered nurse, midwife or health visitor:

9.1. must be satisfied that each aspect of practice is directed to meeting the needs and serving the interests of the patient or client

9.2. must endeavour always to achieve, maintain and develop knowledge, skill and competence to respond to those needs and interests

9.3. must honestly acknowledge any limits of personal knowledge and skill and take steps to remedy any relevant deficits in order effectively and appropriately to meet the needs of patients and clients

9.4. must ensure that any enlargement or adjustment of the scope of personal professional practice must be achieved without compromising or fragmenting existing aspects of professional practice and care and that the requirements of the Council's Code of Professional Conduct are satisfied throughout the whole area of practice

By 2002:

- health promotion targets on smoking and physical exercise are met
- for each local community there will be arrangements for pooling NHS and local authority funds to provide local access to:
  - minor surgery
  - a minor accident service
  - certain specified diagnostic services
  - therapy services
  - social work assistance.

- all mental illness and mental handicap hospitals that were open in 1985 will be closed
- everyone over 85 will have a key worker
- referrals from GPs to specialist medical services will be reduced by 30 percent
- fifteen percent of births will take place outside hospitals
- forty percent of outpatient consultations with specialist medical staff will occur in locations other than a DGH
- eighty percent of surgical interventions will be by minimal access
- sixty percent of surgery will be day-case
- hospital acute beds in DGHs will be reduced by at least 40 percent

DoH (1994, p. 6).

Figure 4.4. The benchmarks.

9.5. must recognise and honour the direct or indirect personal accountability borne for all aspects of professional practice and

9.6. must, in serving the interests of patients and clients and wider interests of society, avoid any inappropriate delegation to others which compromises those interests

10. These principles for practice should enhance trust and confidence within a health-care team and promote further the important collaborative work between medical and nursing, midwifery and health visiting practitioners upon which good practice and care depends.

11. The Council recognises that care by registered nurses, midwives and health visitors is provided in health care, social care and domestic settings. Patients and clients require skilled care from registered practitioners and support staff require direction and supervision from these same practitioners. These matters are directly concerned with standards of care. This paper, therefore, also addresses the matter of the 'identified' practitioner, practice in the personal social services and residential care sector and support for professional practice.

- What will be the context in which nurses work?
- What will be the contribution of nursing to meeting the needs of individuals?
- How will substitution impact on the role of nursing?
- How will the public react to the changed role of nursing?
- How will teamwork be developed with other carers in the health and social care spheres?
- How will professional accountability, authority and responsibility be altered?
- How will regulation impact on quality?
- What will be the implications for initial education and training, retraining and continuous training?

DoH (1994, p. 7).

Fig. 4.5. Nursing – the strategic issues.

12. The reality is that the practice of nursing, and education for that practice, will continue to be shaped by developments in care and treatment, and by other events which influence it. This equally applies to midwifery and health visiting. **In order to bring into proper focus the professional responsibility and consequent accountability of individual practitioners, it is the Council's principles for practice rather than certificates for tasks which should form the basis for adjustments to the scope of practice.**

The development of practice is central to the professionalisation of nurses but it may not be achieved in isolation. While ethico-legal factors distinguish the roles of health-care workers, the coordination and continuity of care will depend on the extent to which strategies and working practices can be coordinated to encourage multidisciplinary approaches to care, and the necessary teamwork to put this into effect. For nurses, the Scope of Professional Practice is more than an opportunity to undertake additional tasks and/or technical skills (usually activities previously undertaken by doctors). It is the opportunity to evaluate current practice, to determine how care may be managed and coordinated to provide the most holistic approach to the individual's health needs and to assess how, for example, overlapping responsibilities between roles may best be managed according to the resource requirements of units, wards, health centres, etc. Some examples include, nurse prescribing, multidisciplinary record-keeping, information-giving, undertaking diagnostic tests, managing parenteral nutrition, intravenous cannulation and associated drug administration. Also, there are aspects of out-patient assessments, management of wounds, continence and clinic work. There is also potential for nurses to play a more active role in the health education of parents caring for young children, family therapy, the promotion of nutritional awareness, sexual health and bereavement counselling. (It is acknowledged that there are already examples of these initiatives in practice.)

The future of professional practice (UKCC, 1994)

For standards of care to improve, attention has turned to standards of post-registration education and practice. The framework for this has developed from and is based upon 'the diploma programmes leading to registration as a nurse or midwife' (UKCC, 1994).

This report is the result of the Post Registration Education and Practice Project (PREPP) and makes explicit standards for practice, education and teaching. It also details features of advanced nursing and midwifery practice as well as standards for a new specialist discipline of community health-care nursing and the range of roles for nurses in the community including general practice nursing, community mental health and community children's nursing specialists.

There are four statutory requirements for maintaining an effective registration. These are:

- completion of five study days every three years
- completion of a Notification of Practice form every three years
- completion of a Return to Practice programme if there is a break in practice of five years or more and
- maintenance of details of professional development in a personal professional profile (UKCC, 1994, p. 3).

There are a range of initiatives which have significant potential for practice and they demand appropriate education and preparation. These include aspects of specialist practice. The UKCC (1994) makes clear distinctions here between nursing roles in the community, and states 'The Council will determine the range of specialist nursing for which additional preparation is required' (UKCC, 1994, p. 10).

Here again is another means for highlighting aspects of nursing and midwifery practice which require education beyond registration.

Preparation for specialist nursing practice will relate to:

- clinical nursing practice
- care and programme management
- clinical practice development
- clinical practice leadership.

These have implications for courses of preparation, and a key feature is the focus on practice which the academic and theoretical elements can support, through such initiatives as assessment methods which highlight the integration of theory within the practice setting, the accreditation of practice-based learning, and the continuous assessment of clinical practice. The identification of the range of community-based roles is in stark contrast with the hospital-based picture. This is also an historical feature compensated for, in the hospital sector, by the English National Board clinical courses and the development of clinical nurse specialists. The time may be right to extend this notion of specialist practice within the hospital sector, particularly in relation to critical care nursing, elderly care and the care of people with cancer, where specialist skills of nurses do much to coordinate and manage the care of the whole person.

Conclusions

This chapter began and will finish with the patient.

It has explored and discussed issues pertinent to the well-being and nursing of patients in the light of current health and policy initiatives and issues associated with the professionalisation of nursing. Developments in nursing education and research are providing more and more evidence of how nurses make a significant difference to the experiences of being a patient. However, the potential of the nurse in health-care practice is yet to be realised. Perhaps we are now moving nearer to a time when statutory and professional frameworks are in place to facilitate the roles nurses have striven for. The more that can be done to strengthen the status and roles of nurses as experts in their field, the more patients will benefit. If this means developing specialist practice then it should be to enhance rather than fragment the potential of holistic nursing.

References

Aggleton, P. and Chalmers, H. (1986). *Nursing Models and the Nursing Process*. Macmillan, Basingstoke.

Andrews, H. A. and Roy, C. (1986). *Essentials of the Roy Adaptation Model*. Appleton-Century-Crofts, Norwalk, CT.

American Holistic Nurses Association (1992). Manifesto document. *Journal of American Holistic Nurses Association*, September, Sage, California.

Armstrong-Esther, C. (1981). Standards of nursing care. *Nursing Times*, 77(1), 19–22.

Audit Commission (1992). *Effective Implementation of Ward Caring Systems*. HMSO, London.

Audit Commission (1993). *What Seems to be the Matter: Communication between Hospital and Patients*. HMSO, London.

Benner, P. and Wrubel, J. (1989). *The Primacy of Caring: Stress and Coping in Health and Illness*. Addison-Wesley, California.

Bevis, E. O. (1978). *Curriculum Building in Nursing: a Process*, 2nd edn. C. V. Mosby, St Louis.

Brook, D. (1974). *Education for the Professions*, Macmillan, London.

Buckle, J. (1993). When is holism not complementary? *British Journal of Nursing*, 15, 744–745.

Calman, K. (1994). On the state of public health. *Health Trends*, 26(2), 35–37.

Carper, B. A. (1978). Fundamental patterns of knowing in nursing. *Advances in Nursing Science*, 1(1), 13–23.

Cleary, P. and McNeil, B. (1988). Patient satisfaction as indicators of quality of care. *Inquiry*, 25, 25–36.

Cornwall, J. (1984). *Hard Earned Lives*. Tavistock, London.

Cox, T. (1978). *Stress*. Macmillan, London.

Davey Smith, G. and Morris, J. (1994) Increasing inequalities in the Health of the National. *British Medical Journal*, 8(1309), 1453–1454.

Department of Health (1966). Report of the Committee on Senior Nursing Staff (Salmon Report). HMSO, London.

Department of Health and Social Security (1978). *Early Discharge from Hospital for Patients with Hernia or Varicose Veins. Report of a Randomised Control Trial*. HMSO, London.

Department of Health and Social Security (1983). NHS Management Enquiry (Chairman Griffiths, R.). HMSO, London.

Department of Health (1991). *The Patient's Charter*. HMSO, London.

Department of Health (1992). *The Health of the Nation*. HMSO, London.

Department of Health (1993a). *The Named Nurse, Midwife and Health Visitor*. HMSO, London.

Department of Health (1993b). On the state of public health: the annual report of the Chief Medical Officer of the Department of Health for the year 1992. HMSO, London.

Department of Health (1994a). *Being Heard. The Report of a Review Committee on NHS Complaints Procedures*. DoH, London.

Department of Health (1994b). *Targeting Practice the Challenges for Nursing and Midwifery in the 21st Century*. DoH, London.

Department of Health (1995). *The Patient's Charter – A Summary*. HMSO, London.

Dimond, B. (1993). *Patients Rights. Responsibilities and the Nurse.* Quay.

Edgar, A. (1994). The values of codes of conduct. In Hunt, G. (ed.) *Ethical Issues in Nursing.* Routledge, London.

Ersser, S. (1991). A search for the therapeutic dimensions of nursing–patient interaction. In McMahon, R. and Pearson, A. (eds) *Nursing as Therapy.* Chapman & Hall, London.

Etzioni, A. (1969). *The Semi Professions and their Organisation.* The Free Press, New York.

Fawcett, J. (1994). *Analysis and Evaluation of Conceptual Models of Nursing.* F. A. Davis.

Field, D. (1993). Social definitions of health and illness. In Taylor, S. and Field, D. (eds) *Sociology of Health and Health Care.* Blackwell Scientific, London.

Fitzpatrick, R. (1993). Scope and measurement of patient satisfaction. In Fitzpatrick, R. and Hopkins, A. (eds) *Measurement of Patient Satisfaction with their Care.* Royal College of Physicians, London.

Frederick, J. and Northan, E. (1938). *A Textbook of Nursing Practice.* Macmillan, New York.

Friedson, E. (1983). The theory of professions: the state of the art. In Dingwall, R. and Lewis, P. (eds) *The Sociology of the Professions.* Macmillan, London.

General Nursing Council (1977). Circular 17/19. GNC, London.

Goffman, E. (1990). *Stigma.* Penguin Books, Harmondsworth.

Gritzner, C. (1993). The CASPE patient satisfaction system. In Fitzpatrick, R. and Hopkins, A. (eds) *Measurement of Patients Satisfaction with their Care.* Royal College of Physicians, London.

Hall, C. (1980). The nature of nursing and the education of the nurse. *Journal of Advanced Nursing,* 5(2), 149–159.

Hancock, C. (1992). The named nurse concept. *Nursing Standard,* 6(17), 16–18.

Health Service Commissioner (1993). *Report of the Health Service Commissioner. Selected Investigations completed October 1992–March 1993.* HMSO, London.

Henderson, V. (1966). *Nature of Nursing.* Macmillan, New York.

HMSO (1989). *Working for Patients.* HMSO, London.

HMSO (1990). *The NHS Community Care Act.* HMSO, London.

Hjortdahl, P. and Laerum, E. (1992). Continuity of care in general practice: effect on patient satisfaction. *British Medical Journal,* 304, 1287–1290.

Hogg, C. (1986) *Patient's Charter – Guidelines for Food Practice.* Association of Community Health Councils, London.

Holmes, T. H. and Rahe, R. H. (1967). The social re-adjustments and rating scale. *Journal of Psychosomatic Research,* 11, 213–218.

Illich, I. (1977) *Disabling Professions.* Marion Boyars, London.

Jolley, M. (1989) The professionalisation of nursing: the uncertain path. In Jolley, M. and Allen, P. (eds) *Current Issues in Nursing.* Chapman & Hall, London.

Kelly, M. P. (1992). *Colitis.* Tavistock/Routledge, London.

Kidel, M. (1986). The meaning of illness. *Holistic Medicine,* 1, 15–26.

King, I. M. (1968). The conceptual frame of reference for nursing. *Nursing Research,* 17, 27–31.

King, I. M. (1971). *Toward a Theory of Nursing.* John Wiley, New York.

Lamont, L. (1993). The consumer's preference. In Fitzpatrick, R. and Hopkins, A. (eds) *Measurement of Patients Satisfaction with their Care.* Royal College of Physicians, London.

Lazarus, R. (1966). *Psychological Stress and the Coping Process.* McGraw-Hill, New York.

Lazarus, R (1978). Stress related transactions between persons and environment. In Previn, L. A. and Lewis, M. (eds) *Perspectives in International Psychology.* Plenum Press, New York.

Leigh, H. and Reiser, M. E. (1980). *The Patient Biological, Psychological and Social Dimensions of Medical Practice.* Plenum Press, New York.

Leininger, M. (1981). *Caring: An Essential Human Need.* Charles B. Slack, New Jersey.

Levine, M. E. (1971). Holistic nursing. *Nursing Clinics of North America,* 6(2), 253–264.

McFarlane, J. (1980). *Accountability in Nursing.* Report RCN, London.

McMahon, R. and Pearson, A. (1991) *Nursing as Therapy.* Chapman & Hall, London.

Maslow, A. H. (1954). *Motivation and Personality.* Harper & Row, New York.

Meleis, A. I. (1991). *Theoretical Nursing. Development and Progress,* 2nd edn. J. P. Lippincott, New York.

Morrison, P. (1994). *Understanding Patients.* Baillière Tindall, London.

Muetzel, P. (1988). Therapeutic nursing. In Pearson, A. (ed.) *Primary Nursing.* Croom Helm, London.

Murray Parkes, C. (1975). *Bereavement: Studies of Grief in Adult Life.* Penguin Books, Harmondsworth.

Narayanasamy, B. (1991). *Spiritual Care. A Resource Guide.* Quay.

National Association for the Care and Resettlement of Offenders, Department of Health (1994). *Working with Mentally Disordered Offenders: A Training Pack for Social Services Staff and Others.* NACRO, London.

Neuman, B. (1995). *The Neuman Systems Model: Application to Nursing Education and Practice,* 3rd edn. Appleton-Century-Crofts, Norwalk, CT.

NHSME (1992). Empowerment through information. *NHSME News,* No. 53, 11 January.

NHSME (1993a). *Maternity Service for Asian Women.* DoH, London.

NHSME (1993b). *Breast Cancer.* DoH, London.

NHSME (1993c). *Haemophilia.* DoH, London.

NHSME (1993d). *Fracture Clinics.* DoH, London.

NHSME (1994). *Sickle Cell Anaemia*. DoH, London.

Nurses, Midwives and Health Visitors Act (1979). HMSO, London.

Orem, D. E. (1995). *Nursing Concepts of Practice*, 5th edn. McGraw-Hill, New York.

Orlando, I. J. (1961). *The Dynamic Nurse–Patient Relationship*. Putnam, New York.

Parsons, T. (1951). *The Social System*. Routledge & Kegan Paul, London.

Parsons, T. (1958). Some ingredients of a general theory of organisations. In Etzioni, A. (ed.) (1969). *The Semi Professions and their Organization*. The Free Press, New York.

Pearson, A. (1991). Taking up the challenge. In McMahon, R. and Pearson, A. (eds) *Nursing as Therapy*. Chapman & Hall, London.

Pendleton, D. (1983). Doctor–patient communication and review. In Pendleton, D. and Hadler, J. (eds) *Doctor–Patient Communication*. Academic Press, London.

Peplau, H. (1982). *Interpersonal Relations in Nursing*, 2nd edn. Macmillan.

Reed, J. and Procter, S. (1993). Nursing knowledge: a critical examination. In Reed, J. and Procter, S. (eds) *Name Education, A Reflective Approach*. Edward Arnold, London.

Rogers, M. E. (1970). *An Introduction to the Theoretical Basis of Nursing*. F. A. Davis, Philadelphia.

Roper, N. (1988). *Principles of Nursing in Process Context*, 4th edn. Churchill Livingstone, Edinburgh.

Roper, N., Logan, W. W. and Tierney, A. J. (1990). *The Elements of Nursing*, 3rd edn. Churchill Livingstone, Edinburgh.

Roter, D. (1989). Which facets of communication have strong effects on outcome: a meta-analysis. In Stewart, M. and Roter, D. (eds) *Communicating with Medical Patients*. Sage, London.

Royal College of Nursing (1979). *The Extended Clinical Role of the Nurse*. RCN, London.

Royal College of Nursing (1981). *Standards of Nursing Care*. RCN, London.

Salvage, J. (1990). The theory and practice of the 'new nursing'. *Nursing Times*, 84(4), 42–45.

Sampson, C. (1982). *The Neglected Ethic. Religious and Cultural Factors in the Care of Patients*. McGraw-Hill, Maidenhead.

Saunders, C. (1990). *Hospice and Palliative Care, An Interdisciplinary Approach*. Edward Arnold.

Seedhouse, D. and Cribb, A. (1989). *Changing Ideas in the Health Service*. John Wiley, Chichester.

Seligman, M. E. P. (1992). *Helplessness, On Depression, Development and Death*. Freeman, San Francisco.

Selye, H. (1957). *The Stress of Life*. McGraw-Hill, New York.

Stiles, W., Putnam, S., Wolf, M. and Janes, S. (1979). Interaction exchange structure and patient satisfaction with medical interviews. *Medical Care*, 17, 667–681.

Stockwell, F. (1972) *The Unpopular Patient*. RCN, London.

Thompson, D. R., Webster, R. A. and Meddis, R. (1990). In-hospital counselling for first time myocardial infarction patients and spouses; effects on satisfaction. *Journal of Advanced Nursing*, 15, 1064–1069.

Tschudin, V. (1992) *Ethics in Nursing – The Caring Relationship*, 2nd edn. Butterworth Heineman, Oxford.

Turner, T. (1991) Patients rights. *Nursing Times*, 87, 13 November, 20–21.

Tutton, E. (1991). An exploration of touch and its use in nursing. In McMahon, R. and Pearson, A. (eds) *Nursing as Therapy*. Chapman & Hall, London.

United Kingdom Central Council for Nursing, Midwifery and Health Visiting (1982). *The Code of Professional Conduct for Nurses, Midwives and Health Visitors*. UKCC, London.

United Kingdom Central Council for Nursing, Midwifery and Health Visiting (1986). *Project 2000*. UKCC, London.

United Kingdom Central Council for Nursing, Midwifery and Health Visiting (1992). *The Code of Professional Conduct for Nurses, Midwives and Health Visitors*, 3rd edn. UKCC, London

United Kingdom Central Council for Nursing, Midwifery and Health Visiting (1992). *The Scope of Professional Practice*. UKCC, London.

United Kingdom Central Council for Nursing, Midwifery and Health Visiting (1994). *The Future of Professional Practice the Council's Standards for Education and Practice Following Registration*. UKCC, London.

Watson, J. (1988). New dimensions of human caring theory. *Nursing Science Quarterly*, 9(4),175–181.

Webb, C. (1992). What is nursing? *British Journal of Nursing*, 1(11), 567–568.

Williams, S. and Calnan, M. (1991). Key determinants of consumer satisfaction with general practice. *Family Practice*, 8, 237–242.

Winkler, F. and Ford, B. (1992). Cause for complaint. The Patient's Charter and the FHSA complaints procedure. *Health Direct*, 16 February, 11.

Wright, S. (1993). The named nurse, midwife and health visitor – principles and practice. In *The Named Nurse, Midwife and Health Visitor*. DoH, London.

Further reading

Benner, P (ed.) (1994). *Interpretative Phenomenology, Embodiment, Caring and Ethics in Health and Illness*. Sage, London. This text demonstrates another important contribution to the nursing literature by Patricia

Benner and a group of authors from the United Kingdom and United States. The authors explore important theoretical issues which contribute to nursing research and practice based on interpretative phenomenology. In addition, there is a range of chapters which explore specific aspects of this approach in practice. These include teenage motherhood, parental participation in care, effects of chronic illness, ethical issues, the dying patient in critical care and effects of disasters on rescue workers.

Department of Health (1993). *The Contribution of Nurses, Midwives and Health Visitors. The Health of the Nation.* DoH, London.

The Health of the Nation (DoH, 1992) strategy has important implications for nurses, midwives and health visitors. This document provides a useful catalyst to explore these implications further as it sets out principles of good practice, gives examples of nursing, midwifery and health visiting initiatives based on the Health of the National targets and suggests key issues for the future.

Department of Health (1993). *The Named Nurse, Midwife and Health Visitor.* DoH, London. Following an introductory chapter by Steve Wright about the principles and practice of this organisational tool, there are 38 chapters giving examples of how it may be applied and developed in practice settings.

Fawcett, J. (1994). *Analysis and Evaluation of Conceptual Models of Nursing.* F. A. Davis. The discussion about the development and contribution of nursing theories and models continues. This book makes a useful contribution to that debate.

Hunt, G. and Wainwright, P. (1994). *Expanding the Role of the Nurse, the Scope of Professional Practice.* Blackwell Scientific, Oxford.

The Scope of Professional Practice (UKCC, 1992) is an important position statement for the development of practice, education and the interface between nurses, midwives and health visitors and other health-care professionals. This book does much to contribute to and alert us to the potential of the nursing, midwife and health visitor roles. It addresses such themes as nursing competence, nurse prescribing, specialist and advanced practice and issues related to specific roles of practice nurses, midwives and nurses in accident and emergency and intensive care.

Soothill, K., Henry, C. and Kendrick, K. (eds) (1992). *Themes and Perspectives in Nursing.* Chapman & Hall, London. This book succeeds in exploring a wide range of issues relating to four main themes, namely perceptions of nursing, education and curriculum development, clinical practice (which includes advocacy and stress management), and management.

5

HUMANISM: A WEAK LINK IN NURSING THEORY?

Gosia Brykczyńska

Introduction

Humanism, which has been chosen as the fundamental philosophy in health care, is manifested in
the concept of man and in the basic values adopted
in health care (Sarvimaki and Stenbock-Hult, 1992,
p. 31).

Nursing practice is based on humanistic values,
such as respect for patients and promotion of
human dignity. Few critics would choose to disagree with this fairly obvious statement, however,
even fewer nursing commentators have concerned
themselves sufficiently to analyse what is actually
meant when they talk about 'humanistic nursing'
or claim that **humanism** underlies much of nursing
practice.

For most nurses and health-care workers,
'humanism' represents a collection of positive,
person-centred, altruistic, humanitarian and en-
nobling, that is, humanising, values. Rarely do
nurses consider that it may also represent a
specific philosophical tradition that, if one considers Renaissance humanism as its starting date, is
now fast approaching its fifth century of existence.
Philosophical movements that have been around,
albeit in varying forms, for 500 years, are not to be
dismissed out of hand. If humanism really does
underpin nursing practice, then it is worth even a
quick overview.

Certainly, many a contemporary nursing textbook refers to humanism, but few spend as much

time *describing* the movement as Sarvimaki and
Stenbock-Hult (1992). For nurses, understanding
the philosophical implications of humanism
should be of paramount importance since as
Sarvimaki and Stenbock-Hult (1992) note, 'the
humanistic concepts of man apply not only to the
patient but also to the care provider and human
beings in general'.

This chapter will therefore attempt to analyse
the philosophical movements known as 'humanism' and consider how these may be relevant to
modern nursing theory and practice. The chapter
is broken down into three main sections; first a
look at Renaissance humanism and the life of
Thomas More. Second, a look at modern
existentialism–humanism and the ideas of Jean-
Paul Sartre and Martin Heidegger; and in the third
section we will look at how nurses use the ideas of
humanism and existentialism in their development
of nursing theories.

Renaissance humanism

Solidly grounded culture is only marginally vulnerable
to material change (Carroll, 1993, p .135).

The 15th century was to become a period in European history, unsurpassed in its far-reaching effects
on the course of subsequent social, religious, and
cultural ideas. Effectively renamed 'the Renaissance', it has come to symbolise new birth and

vigour; a dawning of a new age. The word 'renaissance' comes from the Latin, via French and literally means 're-birth', re-birth of a previous ideal, a recycling – or regenerating of a previous movement. The ideal, thought or intellectual and cultural movement which the 15th century scholars and artists were harping back to and referring to, was the pagan classical scholarship of ancient Greece and Rome.

This new approach to scholarship, in contrast to the immediately preceding intellectual movement of medieval scholasticism, that stressed man's place in a hierarchical universe, structured and functioning for the greater glory of God, appeared to the scholars and artists of the day, like a breath of fresh air. The utterly secular significance and exuberant joy of Boticielli's 'The Birth of Venus', is frequently quoted as a pictorial example of the prevailing mood and atmosphere of the early years of 'the Renaissance'.

The Renaissance is a period in European cultural and social history, when a break was finally made with the old traditional approaches of scholastic-ism to learning and feudal governmental control, to the lack of adventure mindedness of man. Creative man, who was always versatile, was now additionally free of artificial controls; he could paint, write poetry and even re-arrange the world according to his needs and whims. Neither Church nor King was going to stop him.

Renaissance scholars, who had grown up on what Schiller (1912) refers to as the 'sterilising pedantry' of medieval scholasticism, now turned their interests even further back, to the writings and arts of classical Greece and Rome. Medieval scholasticism was thought of as 'sterilising pedantry', because it became so inward looking and self-absorbed, that it no longer was a creative force of learning. It represented a trivialising approach to major philosophical questions, imposing undue restraints on scholarship and inquiry. Not only was Renaissance man interested therefore in what the ancient pagan philosophers had to say about the human condition generally, they were anxious themselves to portray man as the centre and rationale for the functioning universe. This centrality of man was not however literal; they were quite prepared to shift the planets, to accommodate new celestial theories and they still saw themselves as deeply religious. Renaissance man, a child of scholasticism and the harbinger of secular humanism, was a complex

cultural phenomenon that unleashed a force, far greater than anything dreamt possible at the time (Carroll, 1993).

It was a quote attributed to the Roman philosopher/poet Terence, 'I am a man, nothing human is strange to me', that became the leading motif for the Renaissance scholars. It is, perhaps paradoxical that the Renaissance scholars and artists looked back in time for inspiration, in order to move forward beyond the ever-tightening grip of classical scholastic scholarship which was best exemplified by the writings of Duns Scotus, Thomas Aquinas or William of Occam.

The looking back of Renaissance scholars took at least two main forms, one was linguistic and one was artistic. The linguistic pre-occupation was with classical Greek, Latin and old Hebrew. The Renaissance men felt that in a re-analysis and a rediscovery of the old traditional languages, they could achieve a better understanding of their own 'contemporary' Latin, not to mention vernacular speech. Renaissance man wanted to study Greek and Latin for its own intrinsic value and not just in order to be able to converse with clerics. Renaissance men pursued the love of ancient literature and what it could offer by way of enlightenment. It is interesting to note that all subsequent major philosophical movements will also have something to say about the nature of language and its role in shaping our thought processes. For the enlightened Renaissance man, although he may have started to write in his own native tongue, e.g. Dante in Italian, Chaucer in English or Rey in Polish, they all were exceedingly well versed in Greek and Latin. For them, writing in their native tongue was a form of experimentation and liberation from the hitherto uniform approach of *church Latin*.

Writing in the vernacular, that is, a non-Latin language of the populace also implied writing potentially for a larger readership, or if not initially a larger readership, then certainly, writing for non-church-related purposes. Writing in Italian about heaven and hell and on morality, as Dante did in his epic poem, 'Inferno', liberated Dante from writing *exclusively* with a church readership in mind. He now could write on human subjects (not just clerical or religious subjects) free of the traditional stylistic and thematic constraints of scholasticism. He still wrote however as a fervent Christian, believing in God and as a faithful son of the Catholic Church.

The Renaissance artists meanwhile portrayed man in the full splendour of his youth and vigour; powerful, beautiful and above all, totally engaged with being 'human', e.g. Michelangelo's sculpture of David in Florence. Even religious pictures and statues of this period, often portrayed their subjects engaged in secular activities, e.g. eating, reading or walking and are full of human emotions, such as joy or anguish, e.g. the pieta's, such as Michelangelo's Pieta now housed in St Peter's Basilica in Rome. Renaissance artists often portrayed their subjects in a similar way to medieval artists, only now it was precisely the human aspect of the saint or religious subject that captivated the imagination of the artist. It was the humanity of man that was being celebrated, and thus increasingly secular man, without any Christian or religious connotations. Increasingly, Renaissance artists portrayed classical subjects amidst ancient Roman or Greek ruins, or even contemporary subjects with a 'classical' backdrop. From architecture to music the Renaissance spirit prevailed in European culture and rejoiced in the discovery of its human potential.

The human potential was displayed not only in the explosion of the arts and literature but also in the entrepreneurial spirit of scientific and scholarly workers, rediscovering mathematical formulas, navigating uncharted waters, exploring unknown lands and justifying new boundaries for the 'new' man. The scientific discoveries and inventions of the age, such as the printing press by Gutenberg, not only revolutionised the art of book-making, it also ensured that Renaissance writers, such as Dante, eventually had a wider audience for his epic poem and that the biblical scholars of earlier times, such as William Tynedale, had a potentially wider readership for their translated Bible.

The characteristic virtue of the Renaissance was a proud proclamation that man was special and worthy of honour, even if, at the time, it meant learned and cultured man; or was limited to the artist's impression of the 'perfect man'. The Renaissance period, however, has also been considered as the nursery of humanism; the precursor of the secular state and the bridge between medieval feudalism and capitalism. Heller (1967) considers that 'the Renaissance was the dawn of capitalism', and that it was capitalism that 'destroyed the natural relationship between individual and community', and certainly by the time that the euphoria of the Renaissance gives way to the soberness of the

reformation, individual and community are at odds. Thus, the humanism of the Renaissance period was predominantly a celebration of the achievements and potentials of the human spirit – but the very celebration of individualism that the movement required, forewarned of the 'protracted process of transition from feudalism to capitalism' (Heller, 1967) that lay ahead. Humanism, a word derived from 'studia humaniora' or liberal arts, in contrast to 'studia divina' of the traditional church scholarship, in time became synonymous with the all-round scholarship of the 'Renaissance man'. Humanism, at least in its original version, was an approach to philosophy based in the liberal arts and thus philosophers of this period can say that the 'Renaissance current of thought which is customarily called "humanism" is actually no more than one (or several) of the ideological reflexes of the Renaissance in ethical and scholarly form' (Heller, 1967).

Humanism was born as an off-shoot, or consequence, of Renaissance thinking and all the great humanists of the reformation, were also great Renaissance men. Rey (1983), refers to that 'magnificent old word "humanist"' and notes that in its 'broadest and most general sense, humanism denotes a greater preoccupation with the welfare of man than the glory of God', a point noted in the lives of great humanists, until their faith was profoundly challenged, e.g. by Thomas More. For as Rey subsequently adds, 'in Europe, all great humanistic movements had theosophical origins', even if our contemporary understanding of humanism is 'polar to theology and sacerdotalism' (Rey, 1983). The humanism of Erasmus of Rotterdam, Thomas More or William Tynedale, was a humanism that comfortably bridged classical ancient scholarship and a profound Christian religion.

The humanists of the reformation period take their intellectual lessons from their Renaissance mentors, who increasingly emphasised the role of freewill and human potential. As Carroll (1993) explains, the humanist fathers of the 15th century formulated an axiom that permeated all of their thinking, namely: 'Man is all-powerful, if his will is strong enough'. However, if man is all powerful, he is also creator, and yet how can the created be at one and the same time, the creator? Increasingly, as Renaissance man flexed his muscles and attempted to assert his latent creativity and secular scholarship in the spirit of unbridled liberty, he did so at the expense of a traditional understanding of self in the universe and of religion. Nothing hemmed in the pre-Renaissance man so effectively as the myriad of academic restrictions imposed by scholasticism and the practical interpretation of the Church's teaching and pastoral function.

Seeing man as all-powerful in his humanness was a novel approach to the question of existence; an approach, as Carroll (1993) brilliantly argues, which undermined the very dominance of God as creator and primal motivator. Now man himself stood firm in the centre of his own world, and although the foremost humanists of the 16th century fervently believed in God, it was a belief increasingly more personal and private – albeit nonetheless fervent and uncompromising. The 16th century God-fearing humanist only partially foresaw the potential dangers inherent in the proposition that man can be his own celebration. As Carroll (1993) points out, potential problems in humanism as a coherent philosophical approach to the question of being, was seen by Luther and other north European scholars and activists and splendidly portrayed in the quandaries and deliberations of Shakespeare's *Hamlet* – but, at least initially, humanism was seen by humanists as a breath of fresh air and its chief exponents manifested in their very lives, the embodiment of the slogan, I am – and I am my own author (Carroll, 1993).

Reflective point

The Renaissance was a period of artistic exuberance and joy. Think of a secular painting, executed between 1400 and 1550, and state why the painting may be considered to be portraying exuberance or joy.

Thomas More: the humanist

Of all the 16th century humanists of this period few capture the imagination as much as the personalities of Erasmus and More. Since Thomas More (1478–1535) is an example of such a prominent English-speaking Renaissance man who ultimately died at the very dawning of the Reformation because he admitted and saw through the central flaw in unfettered humanism, we shall use him as an exemplar of this enigmatic movement.

Thomas More, arguably the greatest humanist of his time, barring Erasmus, was a man of letters, and of the arts; a competent, honest professional and civil servant, a man of enormous courage and conviction, and therefore his life is useful for modern nurses to study and to analyse. Nurses claim to base their theories and models of nursing on humanistic writings and 'humanism'; therefore a closer look at Thomas More should yield some interesting information.

Thomas More, if anything, was a fascinating and, at least for some, when superficially understood, a complex, and even contradictory figure; so much so that in modern times the playwright referred to him as 'the man for all seasons', perhaps an ironic epitaph for a man who was neither a weather vane nor appeasing.

According to the philosopher Kenny, Thomas More has a guaranteed place in the intellectual history of Europe for three reasons (Kenny, 1983). The first reason, is that he was the author of the immensely popular and thought-provoking classic story in Latin *Utopia*; secondly, that he was a pre-eminent scholar and incorruptible judge, and thirdly, as a prolific and excellent writer of and in the English language. It is curious therefore that his brilliant life, has been so foreshadowed by his 'ignoble' and premature death. Not only is he now remembered more in his death than in his living, but even the very reason for his death is obscured with the passage of time and the convenience of a jaded conscience. Yet Thomas More was and remains the archetypical humanist. To study the *life* and *death* of More, is to understand 16th century humanism and its unsuccessful fight against the all-persuasive influence of secularism.

More lived at the very height of the flowering of Renaissance ideas. He lived in times very similar in their concerns, fears, excitements and joys, to our own. It was a time of transition and massive social changes. It was in his youth that the English dynasty of Tudors was consolidated; he grew up in the ecclesiastical court of John Morton, Archbishop of Canterbury at Lambeth Palace, and was educated at Oxford. The year he went up to Oxford, Christopher Columbus discovered America. Seven years later, in 1499, More met the most famous scholar of his time, the Dutch cleric, Desiderius Erasmus, and a friendship was formed between them, that spanned the rest of their lives. Erasmus and his close scholarly friends were called 'humanists', in recognition that they believed in the educational value of 'humane letters' or Greek and Latin classical texts, not only in the value of divine scriptures (Kenny, 1983). As noted earlier, with the revival of the classical texts, came a revival of secular culture and the arts, and the 'humanist' More was as much interested in classical writings as in cultivating the visual and other sensory arts.

More, during his public career was varyingly a lawyer and judge, a member of parliament, Under-sheriff of the City of London, diplomatic envoy to the court of King Henry VIII, King's Councillor and Royal Secretary, High Steward of the University of Oxford, Speaker of the House of Commons and finally Lord Chancellor. It is therefore all the more spectacular, that this extraordinarily busy professional, could find the space to cultivate in his own time, his love of the arts, music and last but not least, his love of classical literature. And yet, More the public servant is not the main focus of his own lasting fame. More is best remembered for his 'Renaissance personality' and for his humanistic scholarship – both cultured and supported by the prevailing intellectual and artistic movement of the day. More was very much a product of his time, any earlier and he may well have had difficulties reading and enjoying classical texts, and a few decades later, and his wit and charm would have been dampened by Reformation fervour.

More was probably one of the first English-speaking writers deliberately to use humour and wit to engage his readership and to challenge the status quo. More's *Utopia*, written in Latin when he was still fairly young, as a satire on the very society he was living in and working for, reads as marvellously sharp and insightful today, as when it was first written. In today's idiom it should have been awarded the Nobel prize for literature.

It is some testimony to More's English scholarship and penmanship however, that such differing critics in temporal and personality terms as Ben Johnson and C. S. Lewis, both thought that More's literary English style represented perfect English prose and was in need of admiration and emulation (Kenny, 1993). The most popular work of More's however, in his day was not his *Utopia* or religious tracts against Luther, or even satires and parodies in English, but a piece of Greek which he translated with his friend Erasmus into Latin. Together with Erasmus he translated the works of

the Greek satirist Lucian in 1506 and these became instant best-sellers. In today's publishing jargon, we would say that it went into thirteen reprints! (Kenny, 1993). It is indicative of the unique scholastic and cultural climate at the time, that so many people wanted to read (and were capable of reading) these translations and were prepared to pay for them. Such an open climate to culture and learning was not to repeat itself for several centuries. What is so characteristic of this period and of the scholarship of Thomas More, is the insistence on going back to primary sources, especially as far as understanding and commenting on the bible is concerned. More and his fellow humanists felt that only by understanding original texts, in the original Latin, Greek or Hebrew, could one be adequately prepared for the scholarly work of meaningful commentary on the theology contained in the text. This cardinal humanist principle will find interesting echoes down through the centuries, and certainly in our own century has been re-articulated by the existentialist–humanist philosopher Martin Heidegger (Steiner, 1992) who, according to some critics, made more of a legitimate academic impact on German psycholinguistics, semantics and semiotics than on philosophy!

More was not charged with treason and sent to his death for being a model judge (although that annoyed Henry VIII and Cardinal Wolsey considerably), or for writing and/or translating Greek poems, even if they were satires and sometimes bawdy, but because, as a son of a united Christendom and a lawyer by primary profession, he could not see a moral, logical or legal way in which the request of his sovereign could be granted. More was perfectly happy to 'grant to Caesar what was Caesar's', and his circumspect comments in the form of letters from the Tower of London in the summer of 1535 to his captors and friends bear witness to this. He was not prepared however, to share with Caesar what he saw as intrinsically not Caesar's, but God's by right. According to More, Henry VIII could not set himself up as head of the Catholic Church and thereby as arbiter of morality and things divine, as it was something outside of his sphere of possibilities and competencies. It was taking on powers, beyond his legitimate sphere of influence. Powers, that according to More and the Catholic Church, he simply did not have. Man, for More, was not creator of his world, but a creature within his world, a basic difference in philosophical approach. The fight between More and

Henry VIII, was not over marital propriety and injudiciousness or whim. A quick reading of his *Utopia* should dispel any doubts about his alleged prudery or 'conservatism'. The conflict was a pitting of two differing ideas concerning the powers of man and the permanent break-up of the humanistic ideology as understood in Christian northern Europe (Carroll, 1993).

More, the quintessential humanist, ultimately died, because he disagreed with the secular humanistic conclusions reached by the King concerning man's place and role in the universe (Carroll, 1993). More saw the issue primarily as one of *his* conscience and *personal* conviction and he *personally* could not see a way forward from the faulty premises of his sovereign. Ironically, like Luther, his theological opponent and rival, he had to take a stand and be prepared to take the consequences of his beliefs.

Finally, More the saint, was no sugary sanctimonious parody of virtue, rather a firm and yet witty opponent of an unyielding, obstinate, and aberrant King, who asked for service to be rendered in an area where this could not be accomplished. It was so self-evident to More that he could not grant the King's request, that he did not even rave or write vitriolic tracts against the King; the way he did against Luther and Lutheran 'heretics'. Rather, he quietly turned inward, to that which meant most to him – to that which shaped his loves and his life, that is, to his scholarship, his family and to his faith.

For nurses, the life of Thomas More illustrates both the glory and the danger of virtue and learning. Philosophies are not innocuous addenda to specific mind-sets, rather, philosophies and underlying philosophical trends profoundly affect the way we think and therefore behave at any one time, and will provide a rational for the very orientation and direction of our thinking. Thomas More, surely the perfect example of the self-actualised hero of Maslow's hierarchy (Maslow, 1972), whose very intellectual consistency and honesty ultimately proved his physical undoing, illustrates the enormous power that virtue and learning can have over the life of an individual. The key to the power manifested by More, is his intellectual and professional integrity. Ever open to change and new learning, he was nonetheless consistent with the truth as he saw it, prepared to take the consequences for his decisions but gentle and open minded towards the consciences and

learning of others, except in the area of faith. He was, therefore characteristically, a son of his time, and relentlessly ridiculed and lashed out at 'heretics' – that is, all those who did not tow the received message of the magisterium of the Church of Rome. He wrote biting and sarcastic tracts about Luther and his followers, just as the reformers wrote personalised attacks on More. He was a perfect example of a well-adjusted, well-educated man of his time, and saw his own death as much a *natural consequence* of the times and beliefs in which he lived, as Socrates saw the inevitable 'necessity' to die, in his day, rather than escape.

Nurses, eager to demonstrate professional integrity and wanting to increase their philosophical understanding of the world *they live in*, need to realise that with the understanding of philosophical orientations and increased learning, comes increased reasonability for knowledge and inevitable moral choice. Philosophical movements such as Renaissance humanism, was as much a way of being, and herald of contemporary ontological thinking, as it was a scholarly orientation after truth and increased understanding. It went hand-in-hand with a considered life-style that was anything but exclusive and elitist. It was a lifestyle that celebrated the achievements of an 'authentic' man.

Reflective point

If a modern satirist, were to write a contemporary novel, like Thomas More's Utopia, *what may he/she write about?*

Write a short satire lampooning the current state of affairs in the health-care service.

Humanism and existentialism

To raise the ontological problem is to raise the question of being as a whole and of oneself seen as a totality (Marcel, 1984, p. 17).

The glory and power of Renaissance humanism prepared the way for the work of reformation scholars and a humanism which was grounded in Greek and Latin scholarship but not necessarily in Italian arts. This, in the English context was largely due to the fear of popish and Italian or Spanish influences on Protestant scholarship and secular life. Obviously this avoidance of papist influences did not work entirely, and there was much cross-fertilisation of ideas and learning between England and the 'Catholic' continent, but, it could be said, that apart from several notable exceptions, the baroque and rococo styles in art and architecture, for example did not take root in England to the extent that they did on the continent. In England, and in English-speaking countries, as in the Protestant countries of northern Europe, culture, scholarship and learning went a separate way (Carroll, 1993). Renaissance humanism gave way to a humanistic approach to literature and liberal studies that, in comparison with continental Europe was sombre and premeditated. Gone was the apparent explosive cultural spontaneity of the 15th and 16th century continental Europe. In fact Rey (1983) goes as far as to say that the word 'humanism' itself was 'appropriated by very many various philosophers writing positive philosophy such as Comte; to describe scientific advances [!] to describe addiction to belle lettres ...' in fact it had become, according to Rey, a 'soiled word' (Rey, 1983, p. 93).

It was the Protestant emphasis on responsibility for personal action on one hand, and a particular interpretation of salvation theory on the other hand, that in essence put man *beyond* the capability of total self-redemption or at least an understanding of co-redemption. It put all the weighting therefore on God's unilateral grace. This essentially Protestant emphasis fundamentally reshaped the progress of northern European humanism.

The humanism however, most often referred to by *contemporary* scholars is the humanism of *our present times*. It does not mean that in the past 400 years philosophers and scholars had nothing to contribute to our understanding of humanism, humanity or even the 'humanities', but that in terms of sheer influence and visible effect, it is the humanism of post-war French philosophers that has affected us most. It is, therefore, interesting that the philosopher Mary Midgley (1978), in her memorable book on the roots of human nature, in reminding us that we are not the pinnacle of the self-made human pyramid, states 'any kind of humanism which deprives us of this, which insists on treating the universe as a mere projection screen for showing off human capacities; cripples and curtails humanity' (Midgley, 1978, p. 262). Humanism, in today's world must be seen to be

more than an excuse for praising man (or woman); it has to go deeper and probe more effectively into the very nature of humanity. Otherwise it will remain at the superficial and therefore rejectable level of self-indulgent admiration in the declared absence of another creator and other significant creatures (Midgley, 1978). Renaissance humanists exhalted in the nature of man, because man *was* so creative and powerful and beautiful. Some modern humanists would say the same, but they would add that man is actually capable of shaping his own creativity and utilising his own powers of being, not because this is somehow given to him, by a Creator who wishes to share His creative, vital powers with him, but because man, *Homo sapiens*, simply *is*, and it is in the being of man to be creative. Since man is all that he makes of himself and is his own creator, and 'shaper' of his own attributes, modern philosophy has had to explain this new twist of humanism, or as Carroll would say, extension to humanistic thoughts.

As the pragmatist philosopher, Schiller (1912), noted in the introduction to his text on 'pragmatic humanism', 'to claim that in its philosophic use Humanism may retain its old associations is not, however, to deny that it must enter also into new relations' (p. xxviii).

It is precisely the 'new relations' of humanism with the social thinking of the late 19th and 20th centuries that interests us here, and that I wish to explore further.

Jean-Paul Sartre: the humanist–existentialist

The modern humanist that most nurses and contemporary social scientists refer to as the chief exponent of secular humanism is Jean-Paul Sartre (1905–1980). Sartre, the brilliant French philosopher–novelist, re-interpreted and expanded upon the work of Søren Kierkegaard, Edmund Husserl and Martin Heidegger (who was his contemporary), and articulated the philosophy of existential–humanism. According to Sartre, man is nothing else but his own plan; and he exists only to the extent that he fulfils himself. He is nothing more or less than his own life.

Such a vision of man is both invigorating and harrowing. How does one promote the fulfilment of one's own life plan, how does one bear the burden of one's own acts, without a let-out clause; without a reference point beyond (or even) beside oneself? It is Carroll (1993) who clearly and graphically presents the inherent problem in modern humanism of how man can be the still centre of his own world and simultaneously be capable of moving it.

Carroll (1993) reminds us that modern humanism by putting man at the very centre of his *own* universe, and denying any other Being creative powers over man, forces man to a point of vigilant paralysis, to a fear of the study of the only thing left to fear, that is the fear of death. Just as in Greek mythology Medusa's image paralysed and killed the onlooker, so modern humanism confronts man in facing death, any death, with the inevitability of facing his *own* annihilation (Carroll, 1993). As the poet, Donne observed: 'ask not for whom the bell tolls, it tolls for thee.' Carroll continues with the observation that 'from the outset humanism was confronted with the metaphysical challenge of neutralising the fear of death' (p. 5), a challenge taken up most visibly by modern existentialist authors.

Sartre saw existentialism however as 'a doctrine that does render human life possible; a doctrine also, which affirms that every truth and every action imply both an environment and a human subjectivity' (Sartre, 1989, p. 24). It is the grounding of Sartre's humanism in a human context and a human environment that lends to his ideas a hint of phenomenological influencing. For Sartre, his humanism was based in existentialism, where human existence came before an awareness of actualisation of human essence. As he notes ... 'if God does not exist there is at least one being whose existence comes before its essence, a being which exists before it can be defined by any conception of it ... that being is man' (Sartre, 1989, p 28). Since Sartre sees each human responsible for shaping and defining his own humanness, he does not consider such a thing as a universal 'human nature'. As he wryly notes, 'there is no human nature because there is no God to have a conception of it. Man simply is' (Sartre, 1989, p. 28). Thus for Sartre, man defines himself, in the absence of a creator, who would have 'imaged' man according to some celestial blueprint; even if humankind were allowed, in freewill, to reshape and remould the very nature of this 'blueprint man'. For Sartre, the atheistic–existentialist, man is literally made in his own image; man simply is; thus 'man is nothing else but that which he makes himself' (Sartre, 1989, p 28). Sartre is, in fact, most emphatic that for him, existentialism represents a

forward-moving, liberating drive to the endeavours of man, for he states that 'man is, before all else, something which propels itself towards a future and is aware that it is doing so' (Sartre, 1989, p. 28).

For Sartre, the very existence of man is tied up with cognitive volitional functions of the adult sentient member of the race. Thus, the very forward directed 'becoming' of man is dependent on the acceptance that 'man is, indeed, a project which possesses a subjective life ...' (Sartre, 1989, p. 28). The importance of this forward moving, self-activated projection of self for the purposes of self-actualisation (or self-becoming) are that, without this endeavour, man really does not 'exist', to himself, and certainly not in authentic terms, for others; for according to Sartre, 'man will only attain existence when he is what he purposes to be.' (Sartre, 1989, p. 28). Thus for this philosopher 'becoming' is crucial in order to affirm one's being. He does not see another solution. Man must create for himself, his own authentic being, not a whim as he points out, but the fulfilment and actualisation of one's total potential. No-one can do this for another and no-one can blame another for unfulfilled, 'un-actualised' potential. Man makes his own decisions and choices for which he is responsible; for as the philosopher emphasises 'the first effect of existentialism is that it puts every man in possession of himself as he is, and places the entire responsibility for his existence squarely upon his own shoulders' (Sartre, 1989, p. 29).

Sartre places responsibility for choices on the shoulders of those who choose to be. Choice of course is not just in a narrow sense, solely for short-term personal gain of self-gratification, but rather, in a strange almost Kantian sense, choices are made for self, but also with others in mind, or as Sartre comments, 'in choosing for himself he chooses for all men' (Sartre, 1989, p. 29). Thus, there is a concept of co-responsibility for the image and essence of mankind, if not directly for the acts of others. The reason, according to Sartre, that one may need to be mindful of others in making choices and taking personal responsibility for choices affecting them, is that in making the best choice that one can, and surely he asks, one would not choose anything less than a perfect choice, one is making a public statement concerning the desirability of that choice and a wish that all choose and do likewise. Thus, he notes, 'in fashioning myself, I fashion man' (Sartre, 1989, p 30). The argument is attractive but the last statement is definitely contentious. Is it really possible or even desirable always to choose that which all should share and likewise desire. Such a burden of choice, which also demonstrates the obligations inherent in the choice, inevitably produces anguish, a notion well described by the proto-phenomenologist and existentialist Kirkegaard. Sartre realises that some people will attempt to opt for moral parasitism, but he clearly dismisses such options, on the well-versed classical lines of long-term social and moral incompatibility of selfishness with free choice and autonomy.

Sartre's greatest emphasis, however, is on the clear statement that man is his own maker, final arbitrator of standards and responsible for himself to mankind. Man makes his own future, a future of his own making, but that anguish so familiar to Søren Kirkegaard, the Danish philosopher, is there, and an overwhelming feeling of abandonment is present.

Sartre is aware of the implications of his theory of humanism existentialism re-affirming however, that 'we are left alone, without excuse ... condemned to be free. Condemned, because he did not create himself. Yet is nevertheless at liberty, and from the moment that he is thrown into this world he is responsible for everything he does' (Sartre, 1989, p. 34).

Sartre wrote his most comprehensive analysis of existentialism in his hefty tome *Being and Nothingness* (1990), where he explains that it is the very inherent nothingness of man that is man's greatest asset, for man can choose to make up the existential void and differences. His is basically a philosophy of action and presumed becoming. His theories left at this stage could be regarded as extremely self-centred, that is, self-regarding to the point of denying the existence and values of those around one. Sartre does see the primary need for society. The 'becoming' that man undertakes must be done by oneself, for oneself, moreover, it is the basic tenet of the philosophy that no-one can 'become' for another. This does not mean however that we cannot enable, and indeed see it as our responsibility to help others to reach their potentials. In fact he states that understanding of oneself (which is a fundamental prerequisite for self-actualisation and becoming), is impossible without the existence of others, other self-actualised and becoming individuals – thus he notes,

'The other is indispensable to my existence, and equally so to any knowledge I can have of myself' (Sartre, 1989, p 45). Not only does Sartre acknowledge that we need others truly to be ourselves, he considers it essential to act in our choices such, that all of humanity is better off by *our* becoming, provided however, that we are truly *authentic* to ourselves.

Sartre's existential philosophy is not a clearly thought-through blueprint of atheistic–humanism. His ideas in various books diverge, conflict and most significantly were continuously evolving. His little tract on existentialism that has formed the basis for this exposé of his ideas, originally written in 1946, right after the war, tones down but also makes far more 'user-friendly' his ideas found in his main expositional work *Being and Nothingness*. It is also popularly held today, that for an example of his thought in action, or for an illustration of the sort of ideas that he was trying to promote, one ought additionally to read his novels. It is in his novels that Sartre really demonstrates the potential power and awe of human action and inaction, the slothful murderous consequences of paralysing boredom and finally the sheer non-existence of the un-actualised.

It is not that Sartre in his novels, such as *Nausea*, chooses deliberately to show the darker or sadder side of life, at the expense of a more hopeful vision. Rather, that it is by these relatively inadequate exemplars of humanity, that a far more significant philosophical point could be illustrated. He himself, in his 1946 tract on humanism and existentialism, noted that it is not the intention of existential–humanism as he saw it to plunge man into despair, rather, 'it is a doctrine of action' and the burden on man, is the burden of freedom. Free men, make choices for which they are responsible, moreover, man is creator and arbitrator of his own laws. Man is free to shape himself and humanity. There is not external objectification of man's 'Being', except that which he himself creates and becomes. Why then the unease with the writings of Sartre? Why have so many authors and philosophers rejected his model of modern humanism, indeed, why did Sartre himself, abandon much of his early thinking in his later novels?

Sartre's existentialism and humanism were essentially based on two main pillars of thought, one that God does not exist – and therefore man must be his own guide and judge and creative motivator, or lose that which makes him uniquely human; and secondly, man can only become authentic to himself if he accepts the burden and responsibility of freedom. Whereas the second pillar in various guises can be seen today in modern thinking, and is even recognisable in the thinking of many previous philosophies, the first pillar is highly contentious, and moreover, there have been existentialist writers, some contemporary to Sartre, such as K. Jaspers, G. Marcel or M. Buber, who were not atheists and who managed to formulate a modern theory of humanism without the necessary logic of theistic abandonment which is so strong in the writings of Sartre. The unease that one feels for the writings of Sartre stems from his unequivocal denial of any genuine sense of human spirituality as the basis and rationale for self-motivation, self-creation. To take such a one-sided aspect of humanism though Carroll (1993) would say that this was possibly prophesied by the early humanists, is not only to impose a way of viewing the world and ourselves in it on others, but to manifest the inconsistency of our own logic.

As nurses, we claim to be open to a multivaried approach to life, living and the shaping of our place in the world. We claim to see man as a being with biopsychosocial and spiritual aspects to his personhood, and yet we claim to base these very ideas on the works of one man, who was not particularly flexible and did **not** say this. Whether Sartre would recognise his theory of humanistic–existentialism in the works of nurses' is something we will never know; what we do know, is that he saw man as a being in the process of becoming; becoming authentic. It is the aim of man to be his own true self. Nurses, especially in psychiatry and education, have seen the relevance of some of Sartre's notions that are, as Marcel points out, in his criticism of Sartre's ideas, both valid and powerful (Marcel, 1984, p. 48). Nonetheless, it is in the *premises* of Sartre's ideas that there lies the kernel of disquiet about his particular view of man. Sartre's premises are however rarely discussed by nursing users of Sartrean philosophy.

Possibly, the saddest and most enigmatic comment of Sartre's comes at the very end of his book *Being and Nothingness*, a comment subsequently echoed in the conclusion of this tract on humanism, namely, that 'Man is a useless passion' (Sartre, 1990). A spent force, whirling in the wind without direction ... a far cry from the determined self-assurance of the Renaissance humanists. The crucial question must therefore be

whether Sartre, the philosopher–novelist, really has much to offer nursing?

Macquarrie (1972), in his book on *Existentialism*, brings out the contribution that Sartre and other existentialist philosophers have made to modern thinking, culture, social sciences, education, the arts and theology. We owe much to the existentialists; but they do vary among themselves, so much so, that in order to incorporate their thinking into nursing work and practice one would need to have an idea of what they are trying to say as *individuals*, not only as a collective group of philosophers of various persuasions concerned with human freedom.

As Mary Warnock rightly pointed out, what is different about this group of humanist–philosophers, is that they not only write about human freedoms but ask man to experience personal freedom for themselves (Warnock, 1970, p. 2). It is because of this that existentialism has been considered 'a committed and practical philosophy' (Warnock, 1970, p. 2) and perhaps it is precisely because of this that it is not like any other passing philosophical phase. It challenges the reader for total re-evaluation of hitherto firmly held ideas about the nature, place and function of man in the universe, and as a philosophy is only vindicated when it has won a convert (Warnock, 1970).

Martin Heidegger: an ontological humanist

The other prominent existentialist who is much quoted by nurses, is the German philosopher, Martin Heidegger (1889–1976), who is considered by some to be the first *genuine* existentialist (as opposed to Kierkegaard who is considered a proto-phenomenologist–existentialist). Certainly Heidegger was the major influence on the acceptance and spread of Husserl's phenomenological ideas in France and the United States. Heidegger was a complex philosopher, who started his academic career as a theologian writing a dissertation on the medieval scholastic Duns Scotus, only later embracing wholeheartedly Husserl's philosophy of phenomenology. He was for a while Husserl's assistant. In time he came to reject phenomenology in favour of an exclusively self-styled ontological philosophy best explained in his unfinished treatise *On Being and Time* (Heidegger, 1962). Eventually, his writings increasingly moved towards psycholinguistics, anthropology and a Germanic mysticism-cum-mythology not easily understood by the casual reader of philosophy, not to mention literature or even nursing. As the critic George Steiner commented, in his extremely well-written and well-balanced classic introduction to the life and works of Heidegger, words failed the philosophers and 'at a pivotal stage in his life and work, he failed them. The symmetries of imminence are cruel' (Steiner, 1992, p. xxi). Heidegger is difficult to read, and therefore relatively inaccessible, not just because he had something difficult and complex to convey, for so did Sartre, who was and still is a celebrated best-selling novelist, but because he insisted on creating a new vocabulary and language to accommodate his new ideas.

Heidegger was a prolific writer, and on the subject of humanism the most *readable* material of his most probably is his *Letter on Humanism* (Heidegger, 1994), originally published in 1949, in which he rejects both Sartre's and Husserl's understanding of 'being'. This work, however. is rarely read and almost never cited by nurses. By far the most popular citation of Heidegger's is his early work published in 1927 on ontology, *Being and Time*, which although containing much of interest to the philosopher, is hardly written for the mass audience that a body of professional nurses would constitute (Heidegger, 1962). Mary Warnock in her text on existentialism notes 'his writing is not intended to be precise, and his plan is not a scientific plan ... his method is cumulative, and his actual vocabulary new and barbarous' (Warnock, 1970, p. 49). Not only is his writing very difficult to process, there probably never was an intention on the part of Heidegger, to make it particularly more understandable as Warnock (1970) concludes, 'total comprehension would be impossible, and probably not what was intended' (Warnock, 1970, p. 49). Heidegger nonetheless captured the imagination of nursing theorists and especially his epic but unfinished work *Being and Time*, which is an early exposition of his thoughts on ontology, in spite of the fact that subsequent works probably illuminate his overall thinking much better. Certainly, subsequent writings contain more precise and final thoughts on existentialism, and as such are more useful to compare with the writings of Sartre, with whom he differed on many points (Rockmore, 1994). *Being and Time* is considered however to be a specifically *existentialist* book, in that it addresses the issues of 'being as being'.

The single greatest consistency in Heidegger's writings moreover concerns his views on ontology and his vision of the place of man in the world, 'whose essence of human being lies in his existence, that is, in his authentic being. Nurses amazingly have taken to the writings of Heidegger, predominantly because of his insistence that to be fully present to oneself and to be creatively making oneself become in the world, and to be aware of one's being in the world, demands concern for and awareness not only of self but also of others, and a care for oneself and for others. Concern about the future creative well-being of oneself and others, in the authentically *present* individual can only stem from an understanding of the past and is the aim of the truly authentic being-in-the-world who is forever looking forward. In all of this, for Heidegger, man, is alone, and knows that he is alone.

Authenticity of being for Heidegger, as for Sartre, consists in being aware of this aloneness and transcending the present moment. This involves creative concern, motivating angst and care. What Heidegger started as a phenomenologist he concluded as a Germanic mystic poet, as Steiner (1992) remarks, 'For the later Heidegger, Being is presentness in the poetry, in the art we believe in' (p. xxi). Certainly with time he became more clearly preoccupied with language and poetry; with the role of communication in authentic being and the meaning of words and the significance that these play. As Macquarrie (1972) the philosopher, who wrote a most readable introductory text on existentialism comments; for Heidegger, 'the relation of language to reality [is] in terms of the making unhidden that which is talked about ...' and that it is obvious that 'language lays as much stress on the personal integrity of the users of language as on the logical strictness of the language itself' (p. 147). Thus for Heidegger, language itself was closely connected with facilitating and explaining ways of authentic being. This point he shared with Sartre, but went even further in his utilisation of and understanding of language.

Sartre and Heidegger were not the only existentialist–humanists or indeed philosophers writing at this time. It is a great pity that the nursing profession has become almost fixated on the writings of these two men, to the exclusion of other contemporary philosophers, not to mention existentialist philosophers, some of whom also had interesting comments to make about modern humanism. Jacques Maritain (1946), a French contemporary of Sartre, in a short essay entitled *The Crises of Modern Humanism* comments that 'one should take warning never to define humanism in such a way as to exclude from it all that is ordained to the supra-human and forswear all considerations of transcendence'. Maritain was Christian, specifically a Catholic theologian, and saw the need for a humanism that was not exclusively anthropocentric (a term he himself was not totally satisfied with) (Maritain, 1938). Like Carroll (1993) he saw the seeds of humanism's problems set at the Renaissance and that what was needed now was 'an open human nature' and 'an open reason'. Maritain was concerned with the rise of what he calls 'counter-humanism', which stems from a negation of the role of spirituality and God in our lives. Therefore he sees the need for a Christian–humanist position, which would 'remake anthropology'. It must discover the rehabilitation and the 'dignification' of the creature not in a species of isolation, thus enclosing the creature within itself, but in an opening up of the creature to the universe of the divine and the supra-rationale' (Maritain, 1946). Maritain was lashing out as much at Sartre as he was at Marxist philosopher–humanists. For Maritain, putting a soul and an after-life back into notions of man would provide the profundity and sense of dignity that is missing in atheistic humanism, for as he notes the former approach has meant that 'the world has pursued good things down the wrong pathways.' It would appear that perhaps nursing too, in some instances, has pursued good things down wrong pathways.

> ### Reflective point
> *We owe much in modern social and human sciences to existentialism. Choose one aspect of modern nursing practice and consider how existentialist thinking has shaped our perception of this phenomenon, act or idea.*

Humanism in nursing practice

Without the direction provided by ontological nursing knowledge, the end result of our efforts at

inquiry would be chaos ... (Kikuchi and Simmons, 1992, p. 35).

Nursing, immersed as it is in society, in keeping with other disciplines, seeks to affirm and demonstrate its interconnectedness with contemporary prevailing theories and ideas. As a profession which is practice-based, it is imperative to justify and identify its role in relation to contemporary self, patient and society. This it has been doing, with varying degrees of success almost since the dawn of its professional modern existence. In the last few decades, nursing theorists have been considering the theoretical and philosophical underpinnings of the practice of nursing and, in keeping with the prevailing philosophical orientations of the time, have looked at the ontological theories of contemporary humanism and existentialism.

Modern nursing theory found its early articulators situated along the northeast seaboard of the United States. The immediate post-war euphoria had started to wane, and nurses who still remembered their newly-gained powers following the necessities of military and war-time nursing, began to look around for opportunities to continue their professional development and to articulate a new vision of nursing, closer to the needs of post-war society. The flurry of nursing activities in the 1960s and 1970s, originating from such places as Yale School of Nursing and Teachers College, New York, resulted in the blossoming of nursing theories, intended to describe, explain and predict nursing functions, activities and nursing ideologies. The scarcity of graduate schools in nursing meant a heavy concentration of nursing theorists and activists in a few leading centres. This enforced proximity of leading nursing scholars led to interesting professional developments and a rich exchange of ideas. The young profession sought to base its theory and practice on sound philosophical ground and looked around for *contemporary* ideas to incorporate into its theoretical foundations.

Traditionally, the philosophical basis for nursing had been a Judeo-Christian theology of concerned professional idealism – an aesthetical orientation, owing much to nursing religious orders and military obedience and subservience (Jolley, 1989). This approach was thought not to be consistent with the modern lifestyle of new nursing recruits or with their post-war thinking. These young women were tasting for the first time the fruits of democracy, and the intoxication that comes from liberty and freedom of professional and personal choices. The nurse theorists, who were writing for this new generation of nurses, themselves were aware of the power that freedom of choice can bestow and looked around them to see what sociologists, philosophers and psychologists had to say. They were searching for new and appropriate ideas.

It is important to recognise that the very theoretical underpinnings of classical contemporary nursing theories, as we know them, were arrived at, not by asking what is nursing, or even, what is it that nursing does, that is, what is the domain of nursing, which would be an epistemological or possibly an ontological approach but by looking at *allied* disciplines and the fields of social science, and adopting, relatively wholesale, philosophical underpinnings of these non-nursing disciplines, in order to 'place' nursing in society and give it academic and scholarly standing among *other* professions.

The social sciences in the United States of the 1950s and 1960s were heavily influenced by German–Jewish thinkers of the 1930s and 1940s – since it was this group of European scholars who fled inter-war Germany to the United States, to escape the ravages of national socialism in the German Republic. These thinkers from various academic disciplines influenced many branches of science and philosophy, and by the conclusion of the 1950s had managed to leave a lasting impression on US scholarship. In the area of social sciences, the single biggest idea to transform social research and social philosophy, was the philosophical movement of phenomenology and psychological humanism and following from that, existentialism, especially French existentialism.

By the late 1950s to early 1960s French existentialism was influencing continental philosophy and making headway in English-speaking countries. It spoke of a philosophical orientation to modern life that was entirely different in its focus and in its conceptualisation, from anything that contemporary English philosophers were writing about at that time. In fact, some leading British philosophers of the time, such as Bertrand Russell, never really came to accept 'the continental philosophers', such as Heidegger. The US scholars seemed more open to new ideas and so in

US graduate schools, contemporary ideas concerning phenomenology and existentialism spread fast and with unforeseen consequences. The history and subsequent development of modern secular humanism in the west, reflected uncannily the speed of the spread of Renaissance humanism in 15th century Europe. Just as Renaissance humanism was a philosophical movement that affected the understanding of religion and man's place in the universe so, contemporary western secular humanism affected more than just philosophy and theology graduate students.

US nursing theorists accepted 'humanism' as a working philosophical approach to nursing; after all, it was about seeing the person as the centre of one's concern, it was about responsibilities for choices made, and finally, it was modern, contemporary and therefore had a semblance of current academic credibility. The nurses accepted modern post-war humanism in an unqualified fashion, together with the writings of other contemporaries such as de Chardin and Heidegger, making the reading of some nursing theorists' citations very amusing, if not haphazardly contradictory. Not only have nurses, on the whole, not qualified what form of humanism they had in mind when referring to 'humanism' in their theories and writings, but when they did, they invariably referred to the humanism and existentialism of Sartre and Nietzsche and the 'phenomenology' of Heidegger. They have totally ignored other possibly more acceptable 'humanist' philosophers, especially when considering the nature of nursing. Let us therefore look at some nurses' understanding of 'humanism', 'humanistic' and 'humanities' in nursing praxis, and then turn our attention to a few nursing theories that claim to be based on 'humanism'. How do contemporary nurses understand and explain 'humanism' and the 'humanities'?

Joseph (1985), in an article written in a US nursing journal, attempting to explain humanism to nurses, states that the 'central tenets of humanism are not engraved in stone ... the issues or tenets are evolving'. This is an interesting approach to the philosophical movement, since, it would appear, that it is precisely the *peripheral issues* in humanism that may vary and change through time and place. We have seen from Renaissance humanism, through to the ideological humanism of the revolutionaries in France and colonial America down to our own secular humanism of post-war France, that the central tenets of the movement do not vary much. The author continues by stating that whereas a philosophy steeped in naturalism rather than religion seems more appropriate in a modern university (and she sees humanism as a naturalistic philosophy), the nurse, or her patient, may however believe in God as 'part of the person's repertoire of experience'. It is not clear from the author's text whether nurses who profess a particular religion or hold a particular faith have a different understanding of humanism or not, certainly they are singled out for comment, as 'many of today's humanists differ in their belief about the existence of God and this difference breaks with an earlier tradition of strict adherence to naturalism'. It is difficult to judge exactly which 'tradition' of humanism this nurse–author is referring to, presumably not the Renaissance tradition of Erasmus or More. In the mid-1980s, French existentialism to which she may have been referring was a mere 40 years old! Not much of a tradition.

This particular attempt at explaining humanism has several flaws, that one can only presume that it was referring to a terribly narrow understanding of the philosophy; but then, even when giving examples of humanists and citing their works, there appears to be little understanding of the material quoted. Thus Buber and Sartre are both referred to in one breath, as having 'incorporated the concept of God into their beliefs'; but Buber was a deeply religious rabbi and educationalist and Sartre was a self-professed ex-Christian atheist; two more unlikely bedfellows are hard to find. They both professed an adherence to humanism, but not to the same 'current' of humanism. Finally, the author notes that since theoretical frameworks and theories are 'probably more specific in articulating basic assumptions' than multiple explanations, she proffers the following piece of text as an example of 'humanism' in nursing theory. 'The individual is an open system constantly changing as he/she interacts with the internal and external environment'. This statement is based on several tenets and suppositions but none of them need necessarily refer to humanism. In fact the author uses this passage to illustrate the point that, 'Naturalism or the first tenet of humanism is addressed' (Joseph, 1985). Perhaps some nursing theories do address 'true' humanism, but this particular text does not illustrate the *central* meaning of the philosophical approach, at all.

Maybe this is not surprising, however, from a nurse–author who can also state that humanism 'as a philosophy is particularly appealing because its basic tenets are not esoteric ... and it can help cushion some of the harsh beliefs about technology' (Joseph, 1985).

It is heartening to know that nurses are interested in the philosophical underpinnings of their theories and practice, but surely analysis should be carried out carefully and thoroughly, for half-baked analysis can be even more damaging than no analysis.

The next two authors refer to humanism in the context of nurse education. Philip Woodrow (1993) and Ann Byrnes (1986) both address the connection and differences between behaviourism and humanism in nurse education. Woodrow defines humanism through the prism of psychology and counselling, citing as his references the work's of Abraham Maslow and Carl Rogers. He states that humanism in psychology, 'emphasizes *intrinsic* rather than extrinsic values, seeking to achieve self-actualization of individuals' (Woodrow, 1993). This definition has within it the familiar ring of early Renaissance and reformation humanism, and traces of the determined rugged individualism of Sartre, especially as he goes on to say, 'Humanist education aims to enable learners to express their own needs and interests, building their self confidence, independence and creative energy'. It is the individual learner, who is a nurse, who needs/wants education, who needs to fulfil his or her potential; and a humanistic approach to education, emphasises the *process* of learning above the end *product* of the educational experience, and even more significantly, humanistic education would like to tap into the latent creativity that lies within us all. This interpretation of humanism as applied to nursing education is far more in keeping with the original philosophical tradition to which it refers, than some other uses of it in nursing.

It is interesting to note that according to Woodrow, who is primarily an educationalist, 'Humanist education becomes learning how to grow ...' especially through the arts (Woodrow, 1993). We will come back to this idea shortly, when looking at the humanities in nursing education, but certainly this claim of humanistic educationalists has found confirmation in generations of humanists of varying currents of persuasion. As he notes 'education becomes a life long process, not confined to classrooms' (Woodrow, 1993) a point understood by the northern European humanists, and modern existentialists.

Byrnes (1986) in an earlier article aimed specifically at nurse educationalists, defines humanism in educational theory, much as Woodrow (1993) did seven years later. Educationalists, consciously see the difference between humanism as an active philosophy in their profession and the legacy of behaviourism that may still play a role in some areas, but lacks the overall philosophical explanation and credibility for a global approach to student training. As she states, 'Humanistic education can be defined as a commitment to practice, in which all aspects of the teaching–learning process emphasise freedom, choice, value, dignity, and integrity of each individual' (Byrnes, 1986). Such a view of humanism in education is quite reflective of the original philosophy and neatly ties in with those aspects of humanism that have endured the passage of time, although it does not elaborate upon the inherent problems in this approach. This however, the author does somewhat later in the article.

Nurses have also commented on humanistic psychology as it affects particular aspects of nursing, thus Philip Burnard (1990) wrote a descriptive article for psychiatric nurses, explaining the origins of, and rationale for, humanistic psychology in psychiatric nursing. Burnard (1990) seems exclusively to refer to the work of Sartre on *Humanism and Existentialism* as the basis for the humanism of Maslow and Rogers, citing Sartre's often referred to phrase that man is 'what he makes of himself'. He does however ask the all-important question of whether 'humanistic psychology fits nursing?' and attempts to blow away some myths that have arisen around the philosophies of humanism. As he rightly notes, 'not all arguments are as sound as each other. There are faulty perceptions ...' (Burnard, 1990) dispelling rather adequately the insufficiencies of Joseph's (1985) premises in regards to her understanding of humanism. In nursing practice, as opposed to an educational approach, he notes that humanistic psychology may not always be the answer, rightly noting however that 'humanistic psychology has added an important richness to our perception of what it means to be human' (Burnard, 1990). This is the aspect of classical humanism not too many scholars disagree with.

His note of caution however, tinged as it is with sarcasm will ring as true heresy for many nurses who have adopted 'humanism' without ever truly considering what it actually entails and what it has to offer nursing, especially in its modern existentialist guise. Thus he concludes: 'Just as a previous generation of psychiatric nurses were overdosed with psychoanalytical theory, so a new generation of nurses runs the risk of being blinkered by the humanistic approach.' (Burnard, 1990).

Some nurses having tried 'humanism' like a style of painting, have rejected it as inadequate for their purposes and needs (McKinnon, 1991). The author states that she was using Paterson and Zderad's model of humanistic nursing, in the delivery of care, but found that it did not 'hold the nurse accountable for the quality of patient care ... as it has no guidelines or format to follow in administering patient-care, nor is there a means for evaluating the effectiveness of care' (McKinnon, 1991). It is not my intention here to analyse the particular model of nursing, but to note, that surely there is some misconception of both the primary philosophical movement of 'humanism' on one hand and what it has to offer and the role and function of models of nursing generally. The author is a fairly senior, graduate nurse, and yet she does not appear really to have understood either the philosophical underpinnings of her profession as it is practised today, or the primary rationale of models in nursing in clinical practice. Her observations are to some extent insightful and correct, as far as they go, but they are based on faulty logic and inaccurate premises, making her overall point rather dismissive.

Kate Beverley (1988) and Bonnie Duldt (1991) both approach humanism via the writings of Buber (1878–1965), the Jewish teacher/philosopher who has influenced quite a few social scientists and nursing theorists. Beverley (1988) uses Buber's metaphor 'I – thou' to elaborate on her 'humanistic' proposition that 'we be consciously aware of self as I, who is more than the sum total of the role of the nurse, and that similarly the patient/colleague is "thou"...' but she does not really explain what she herself means or understands by 'humanistic', or even what Buber might have meant by 'humanism'. Beverley's article like so many other pieces of professional literature assumes *a priori* understanding of the concept 'humanism', 'humanistic', or 'humanist' –

and does not address the issue of *humanistic* values as such, but rather is an elaboration on the transportation of Buber's 'I – thou' concept to nursing practice. It is a very good explanation of Buber's theory applied to nursing, but it in no way elucidates the problems and issues of humanism in nursing, which is rather a pity, as the article appears to be written with a certain amount of sensitivity and knowledge and an explanation of humanism would have been interesting.

Duldt (1991), has developed a communication's theory in nursing, which she has based on Buber's 'I – thou' proposition and communication theories, but although she manages to mention Buber once in her article, she does not however even reference any of his works, or explain why she has chosen Buber as her guide, or in any way refer to humanism as a philosophical and social movement in the social sciences, except in linguistic extensions! For Duldt, the words 'humanism' and 'humanistic' are vaguely interchangeable and synonymous with person-centred and human. Thus she talks of nursing as being 'humanistic in nature', that an aspect of interpersonal communication is to 'humanise', where she explains 'humanise' as: 'to develop and maintain contacts between people'. Duldt and Giffin (1985) develop a fairly coherent, if a bit transparent nursing communication theory which Duldt (1991) tries to review for its efficacy and appropriateness in general nursing practice. Although it is called a 'humanistic' model, it is only so, by virtue of it referring to humans and being concerned with decreasing dehumanising interpersonal transactions and increasing humanising interactions via meaningful communication. Although she based her original (1985) work on Buber's 'I – thou' theory, this 'evaluation' article as already noted, although entitled 'I – thou in nursing' barely mentions the original Buberian theory of interpersonal relationships. Neither does she explain in other than tautological phrases, why her particular theory should be considered 'humanistic'!

Lastly, there is an evergrowing body of nursing literature that looks at the use of the 'humanities' in promoting nursing. Nurse educators and theorists alike are beginning to realise that if nursing is to address the whole person, then an understanding of the whole person will be needed, and this can only be achieved by recognising the areas of spirituality and aesthetics – in addition to all the other aspects of being human; the areas of our lives otherwise covered by the catch all phrase of 'the arts'. Just as all people consist of biopsychosocial elements well recognised and accepted by nurses, so all people live within and play-out, a spiritual and artistic dimension to their lives. It is this artistic, spiritual and non-physical and essentially non-psychosocial dimension of our lives that is best addressed by an appreciation of 'the humanities' (Hagerty and Early, 1992). As Darbyshire (1994) points out, at the very beginning of his fascinating review of the utility of Frida Kahlo's paintings in promoting an understanding for nursing students of what it is to be chronically ill, 'of all nursing's clichés, 'nursing is an art and a science' is the least reflected in reality'. It is precisely in an attempt to redress this imbalance in the structure of nursing, that increasingly nurses are looking towards the humanities to learn about those aspects of human nature, not covered by the traditional teachings of the social sciences, and to become more sensitive themselves to the artism of life.

Some nurses have always incorporated an understanding of 'the humanities' into their work and this has been reflected in their writings (Dock and Stewart, 1925). For them, as for the US educationalists of the 1970s and 1980s a solid grounding in the 'liberal arts' or humanities was seen as a good preparation for professional education. They accepted as given that the arts can tell us something about human nature and as an end in and of itself, ennoble us; that is, 'make more human' or promote an increase in our sensitivities and understanding of life. This preparation for professional training was seen for the most part however as something additional to and apart from the core matter of nurse education. That is, students of diploma and university degree programmes in the United States were expected to come into nurse preparation courses, already with the required modules in the arts and sciences. Once in nurse training there was rarely a perceived need to refer back to them, not to mention incorporate them into an understanding of life; except the sciences, of course (Hagerty and Early, 1992; Peck and Jennings, 1989). Thus, the idea of placing nursing within a liberal university-based education lost out once again to the requirements of schools of 'health-care and medicine' which imposed a quantifiable, science-based curriculum. Thus, only a few exceptional nurse leaders, who usually had a university degree in the arts, or 'humanities' additional to nursing qualifications, extolled the virtues of the humanities in nurse preparation courses. Theirs was a lone voice in the wilderness. Now, more and more, nurses from various backgrounds, and including those who do not have specialised 'humanities' backgrounds, are calling for the inclusion of the humanities into the very fabric of nursing education programmes (Hagerty and Early, 1992; Peck and Jennings, 1989). For the most part, they understand humanities in the *Renaissance* context.

In 1986, Cushla Beckingham in Australia wrote a clear and precise article, based on work in her college, about how 'the study of literature develops perceptive, sensitive nurses'. She noted, as many others have, before and since, that 'students ... responded with maturity and unqualified enthusiasm to the many situations they have read in the novels and short stories', identifying with the emotions portrayed or realising for the first time the true extent to which they were unaware of certain strong feelings and perceptions. In the same year Bartol in North America noted that for many educationalists the humanities have value for a truly educated person, but that the sciences were still considered *essential* to the practice of nursing; and proceeded therefore to explain to fellow nurse educationalists, why they should use the humanities in nurse education programmes. In a lovely turn of phrase she comments that 'ideas inspire and nourish us by providing us with a kind of inner music that prompts us to stretch towards truth' (Bartol, 1986). It is this stretching towards inner truths, and an understanding of our emotions and feelings, that cannot be explained by the sciences (physical or social) that are best addressed by the humanities. We often urge students to be *more* empathetic and *more* understanding of themselves and their patients and yet without an introduction to the vocabulary and language of emotions and perceptions, how are students to achieve this laudable goal; as Bartol (1986) concludes, 'creative literature can assist us in gaining this necessary vision'.

Other nurse educationalists followed suit, urging their colleagues to consider the benefits that an inclusion of the humanities 'or liberal arts' into nurse education programmes could deliver. Pamela Reed (1987) notes that a nursing education model based on the arts can promote a form of personal and professional wisdom that is currently lacking.

Janne Dunham (1989), also from the United States, in an unusual article on nursing leadership, sees the room for an 'art of humanistic nursing' especially in the sphere of nursing administration and management. She talks of 'applying caring and humanism to the nursing staff as well as to our patients', invoking Paterson and Zderad's theory of humanistic nursing, among other theorists (Dunham, 1989). Unfortunately she does not explain what she means by humanism or humanistic and from her usage of the words appears to use the word 'humanism' as so many other nurses do, interchangeably with 'humane', or person-centred, or even 'humanity', thus she notes 'humanism and caring for people must pervade the entire nursing profession' or, 'humanism also transforms the organisation', and 'the humanistic nursing administrator redefines power' (Dunham, 1989).

Some nurse educators see the use of humanities not just in providing verbal insights into the minds of author–patients, but also in order to increase their students' sensitivities to life and life's events, through paintings, photography or even music (Davis, 1992; Erhart and Furlong: 1993; Penden and Staten, 1994; Darbyshire, 1994).

Davis (1992) saw the benefits of taking her students around an art gallery in order to promote an understanding of human life and living. She notes that artists portray humans being busy with the task of living, and that this artistic subjective approach to life through universally recognisable functions of living, enhances students and their sensitivities and perceptions. She notes that one of the objectives of the university museum to which she took her students was to show that 'every piece in the collection is a reflection of the political, social and cultural milieu in which it was created' (Davis, 1992), and therefore a beautiful example of the life of man and woman. She proceeded to structure an exercise for the students while at the museum's art gallery, focusing on aspects of health assessment! A rather novel and exciting use of 'the humanities'.

Penden and Staten (1994) applied the use of humanities to psychiatric nurse education; an area of nursing that seems most appropriate for the utilization of the arts in the promotion of caring and understanding. They utilized films, literature and theatre to look at the humanities focusing on material that addressed psychiatric issues, e.g. alcoholism, hallucinations, and violent behaviour.

Ehrhart and Furlong (1993) would like to see the total integration of the humanities into nursing philosophy and practice, especially as it pertains to community and psychiatric nursing. By encouraging students to utilise the arts, via literature, photography and music in presenting patient clinical cases to their colleagues for discussion of clinical competence they demonstrated not only the use of the arts in developing the student's sensitivities, but also how the arts themselves can be used therapeutically to help with the student's work with patients. Darbyshire in addition to his use of the artistic works of Frida Kahlo in promoting the understanding of the significance of illness in a person's life, (Darbyshire, 1994) also uses extensively photography in promoting sensitivities and understanding towards others (Darbyshire, 1993). Philip Darbyshire and Janet McCall have, also in 1994, run a summer institute in nursing humanities, at the Caledonian University in Glasgow, to try to reach an even wider group of nursing students and professionals with the message that the humanities have much to offer the discipline of nursing which is indeed an *art*, not just a science.

Reflective point

How do you think that studying the humanities can increase sensitivity and/or caring approaches to health-care work?

Finally, what have nurse theorists to say, who claim to base their theories and models of nursing on humanism? Most nurse theorists refer to humanism in their theories, usually just to say that they acknowledge a debt to humanism or that humanism in some way underpins their philosophical approach. Such theorists as Dorothea Orem, Imogen King, Callista Roy, all refer to humanism implicitly or explicitly but only in passing. By inference or by direct citation the form of humanism they have in mind, is usually contemporary humanism – existentialism as represented by the French existentialist, Sartre.

Other nurse theorists, such as Jean Watson, Martha Rogers, Rosemarie Parse, Madeleine Leininger, Josephine Paterson and Loretta Zderad state that they use humanism and theories of humanism in the very fabric of their theories and models. They claim humanism is an intrinsic aspect of their theories. Certainly Paterson and Zderad (1988) have even named their model of nursing, 'humanistic nursing theory'. Martha Rogers and Rosemarie Parse both imply an understanding of nursing that is humanistic and human-orientated, referring to a 'science of unitary human beings' and a 'theory of health as human being', respectively (Rogers, 1970, 1994; Parse, 1981). Jean Watson, talks about the role of humanism in nursing and a need for a 'humanistic–altruistic' approach to nursing practice in her book, *The Philosophy and Science of Nursing*, which effectively states her vision of nursing (Watson, 1985). She sees humanism and existential phenomenological factors in nursing as crucial to a well-balanced theory of nursing. She states in the introductory chapter of her book that since nursing is an academic subject, it should represent a balance 'between scientific knowledge and humanistic practice'. For Watson 'humanism' is the philosophical underpinning of 'humanistic practice' which however, she comfortably presents together with the behavioural sciences and the arts! Thus she gives us as an illustration of the difference between sciences and humanism, the fact that 'it is now possible to define an outcome of scientific activity (e.g. prolongation of life) without referring to its aesthetic–humanistic aspect (e.g. the quality of life and death)' (Watson, 1985). Humanism for Watson is a combination of arts and philosophy, i.e. 'the humanities' and the social sciences. She redefines the humanities as 'addressing themselves to the understanding and evaluation of human goals and experiences'; hence her blurring of ontology with the arts. She continues by claiming that the humanities ... cannot give predictable solutions to the problems of human nature. The humanities cannot provide the hard database that comprises the intellectual content of nursing ...' (Watson, 1985) and therefore one needs *both* academic traditions in order for nursing to have the ability really to be a science and an art. This could almost mean that, according to Watson, science *can* 'give predictable solutions to the problems of human nature', surely a faulty piece of deductive reasoning, given her other statements.

Few nurse theorists explain as well as Madeleine Leininger however, what nurses *actually* understand by the term 'humanism' (Leininger, 1978). Starting with a quote by Shakespeare from *Hamlet*, where the poet extols the qualities of man, she continues to connect unequivocably 'humanism' with a 'science' of humanities or what it is that makes us human. Thus, she writes about man manifesting 'humanistic expressions as *Homo Sapiens* ...' or 'humanism appears to be largely determined by one's cultural life style ...' or 'experiencing humanism and feeling human tend to vary a great deal with an individual's cognitive orientations about people' and so on. Even when she is differentiating between secular and sacred humanism she does not stray too far from the notion that humanism is a 'complex phenomenon with diverse emotional, cultural and social dimensions' and has much to do with 'human warmth, interest and compassion' (Leininger, 1978, pp. 178–179). For Leininger, humanism is 'about being human' – the philosophy and ontology that addresses the nature of humanness. Her chapter on humanism in her book on transcultural nursing wonderfully and comprehensively brings this out and confirms our impressions. There is no reason why humanism should not be understood in this way, as a primary definition of the idea *in a nursing context*, except that it is never prefaced as 'nursing' humanism or 'applied' humanism or even 'health-care' humanism. It is either not elaborated upon at all, or as Leininger has done, it is redefined in socio-cultural and nursing terms to suit the needs of practice! This however, only coincidently refers to and overlaps with the humanism that philosophers would recognize. For the majority of nurses, as for Leininger, humanism is the ideological process of justification for 'caring about people'.

It does not refer to the historical tradition of philosophical humanism at all. Occasionally it overlaps with the subject area of 'humanities'.

Both nurse theorists, Martha Rogers and Rosemarie Parse, her student and disciple, refer to humanism in their works (Rogers, 1970, 1994; Parse, 1981). They both have extremely complex and as of yet, unfinished theories, that are more akin to ideological propositions on the nature of nursing, reflecting a myriad of scholarly and also non-scholastic influences. Rogers, however does not appear to present her ideas on humanism in any different a light than Leininger (1985). It is not clear, to what extent Rogers, the theorist, represents anything more than her own rather individualistic approach to nursing practice. Only time will demonstrate the lasting influence and extent to which Roger's personal vision of nursing is shared and further developed by a significant group of nursing professionals. Certainly humanism, as a strong philosophical orientation in its own right, gets lost in Rogers' intricate theory of interpersonal nursing. Parse, who based her model of nursing on Roger's work and as such is highly influenced by her mentor, does not fare much better.

Lastly, Paterson and Zderad (1988) developed an entire nursing theory around the concepts of 'humanism' and 'humanistic' yet they too, refer to humanism in much the same vein as Leininger (1985). They however have a far more identifiable link with existentialism and the philosophical movement of phenomenology. As O'Connor (1993) states in describing their vision of nursing, it is viewed as 'an authentic dialogue involving meeting, relating, and presenting in a world of people, things, time and space' (O'Connor, 1993 p. ix). Loretta Zderad, the nurse theorist, also studied philosophy at Georgetown University, and this acquaintance with philosophical movements and philosophical linguistics comes through in her need to elaborate on the significance of humanism and inadequacy of existing language to describe experiences in her work (Paterson and Zderad, 1988).

In relation to humanism, their theory is based on the need to *experience* the worlds of nursing and its *meaning* to the needs of 'the person' and the persons' world. The person and the world of the person are heavily interpreted through the philosophical writings of existentialists, especially Sartre and the writings of the rabbi, educationalist, and phenomenologist, Buber. The nurse theorists are fairly adamant however that their theory is not just an application of existentialism to 'nursology' (Paterson and Zderad, 1988), but should be seen as a blossoming of existentialism, through, a 'complementary synthesis' (Paterson and Zderad, 1988). The theorists actually tell us why they chose the term 'humanistic' for their model of nursing, in favour over possibly more descriptively accurate nomenclature, such as 'existentialist' or 'phenomenological'. Thus they note that the term 'humanistic' is more embracing and has a more inclusive meaning than the limited significance of 'existentialism' or 'phenomenology'; an observation that is unique in nursing scholarship on humanism. Nonetheless, in describing their model and theory of nursing, one has the feeling that they too are forever skirting the basic need to define humanism in nursing, specifically in their nursing context. All the constructs and elements of their theory speak however to a humanism heavily indebted to modern post-war French existentialism as represented by Sartre with a characteristic American understanding and interpretation of Heidegger's phenomenology. The marriage and merger of the two philosophies are reflected however in other nurses' understanding of humanism, as presented by Leininger (1985) and are to be seen in their statement about the overall aim of nursing, which is to be present to a patient and to comfort. Thus they state; 'through her presence it is possible for other persons to be all they can be in crisis situations of their worlds' (Paterson and Zderad, 1988, p. 56). This represents the language of Heidegger with the understanding of nursing; which is considered 'humanistic', and is heavily indebted to modern humanism.

accept the concepts inherent in humanism. It is important to remember, nonetheless, that man needs to feel the joy of freedom and see the beauty of his powers, otherwise we are faced with contradictory messages concerning nursings' aims and objectives. The best news would be however, if nurses developed a uniquely nursing way of viewing man, something Taylor (1994) has attempted to do, looking at the nature of nursing and its aim of promoting 'humaneness' among its patients (and practitioners) through the very ordinariness of nursing. This is a rather splendid echo of Renaissance ideas totally infiltrating everyday life, even if she is predominantly still looking at modern humanists. Least Thomas More, the satirist, say to nurses what he noted about councillors, in his Utopia, namely that 'someone's liable to say the first thing that comes into his head and then start thinking up arguments to justify what he has said', let nurses take the initiative and before they start quoting various philosophies, consider first what they really represent.

Conclusion

Thomas More joined in the culture and pursuits of his time; he taught his children foreign languages and insisted they learn to play musical instruments. He wrote poetry and cultivated friendships all over Europe. Thomas More, the public servant, private family man, scholar and man of principles, lived the Renaissance humanism which he embodied. Several centuries later, neo-humanists of the 20th century will advocate another humanism extremely hard to reconcile with More's Renaissance humanism. It will appear devoid of the joys of man, yet full of the burdens of man, and full of the 'wreck of western culture' (Carroll, 1993). It is this later humanism unfortunately that has mostly captivated the thinking of modern nursing theorists, such as Watson and Paterson and Zderad, except for a group of *educationalists*, who increasingly are emphasising the need for a return to a *Renaissance* 'education' for nurses (Ehrhart and Furlong, 1993) and an appreciation of the *humanities* in nursing practice.

Humanism as a philosophical movement has offered much to our understanding of man and his place in the universe. Nurses working with frail vulnerable and broken man can do worse than

References

Bartol, G. (1986). Using the humanities in nursing education. *Nurse Educator*, 11(1), 21–23.

Beckingham, C. (1986). How the study of literature develops perceptive, sensitive nurses. *Australian Journal of Advanced Nursing*, 3(3), 15–20.

Beverley, K. (1988). Humanistic values and the ward environment. *Nursing: The Add on Journal of Clinical Nursing*, 3(27), 996–998.

Burnard, P. (1990). Staying in balance: humanistic psychology and psychiatric nursing. *Community Psychiatric Nursing Journal*, 10(1), 16–19.

Byrnes, A. K. (1986). Bridging the gap between humanism and behaviourism in nursing education. *Journal of Nursing Education*, 25(7), 304–305.

Carroll, J. (1993). *Humanism: The Wreck of Western Culture*. Fontana Press, London.

Darbyshire, P. (1993). Understanding caring through photography. In Diekelmann, N. and Rathers, M. (eds) *Transforming RN Education*, pp. 275–290. National League for Nursing, New York,

Darbyshire, P. (1994). Understanding the life of illness: learning through the art of Frida Kahlo. *Advances in Nursing Science*, 17(1), 52–60.

Davis, S. (1992). Nursing and the humanities: health assessment in the art gallery. *Journal of Nursing Education*, 31(2), 93–94.

Dock, L. and Stewart, J. (1925). *A Short History of Nursing*. Putnams, New York.

Duldt, B. (1991). 'I – thou' in nursing: research supporting Duldt's theory. *Perspectives in Psychiatric Care*, 27(3), 5–12.

Duldt, B. and Giffin, K. (1985). *Theoretical Perspectives for Nursing*. Little, Brown & Co., Boston.

Dunham, J. (1989). The art of humanistic nursing administration: expanding the horizons. *Nursing Administration Quarterly*, 13(3), 55–66.

Erhart, P. and Furlong, B. (1993). The Renaissance nurse: permeating clinical competence with the humanities. *Nurse Educator*, 18(3), 22–24.

Hagerty, B. and Early, S. (1992). The influence of liberal education on professional nursing practice: a proposed model. *Advances in Nursing Science,* 14(3), 29–38.

Heidegger, M. (1962). *Being and Time*. Blackwell, Oxford.

Heidegger, M. (1994). Letter on humanism. In Farrell Krell, D. (ed.) *Basic Writings*, pp. 213–265. Routledge, London.

Heller, A. (1967). *Renaissance Man*. Routledge & Kegan Paul, London.

Jolley, M. (1989). The professionalisation of nursing: the uncertain path. In Jolley, M. and Allan, P. (eds) *Current Issues in Nursing*. Chapman & Hall, London.

Joseph, D. (1985). Humanism: as a philosophy for nursing. *Nursing Forum*, XXII(4), 135–138.

Kenny, A. (1983). *Thomas More*. Oxford University Press, Oxford.

Kikuchi, J. and Simmons, H. (1992). *Philosophic Inquiry in Nursing*. Sage, Newbury Park.

Leininger, M. (1978). *Transcultural Nursing: Concepts, Theories and Practices*. John Wiley, New York.

Macquarrie, J. (1972). *Existentialism: An Introduction, Guide and Assessment*. Penguin Books, Harmondsworth.

Marcel, G. (1984). *The Philosophy of Existentialism*. Citadel Press BK; Carol Publishing Group, New York.

Maritain, J. (1938). *True Humanism*. The Centenary Press, Geoffrey Bles, London.

Maritain, J. (1946). *The Twilight of Civilization*. Sheed & Ward, London.

Maslow, A. (1972). *Motivation and Personality*. Harper & Row, London.

McKinnon, N. (1991). Humanistic nursing. *Nursing and Health Care*, 12(8), 414–416.

Midgley, M. (1978). *Beast and Man: The Roots of Human Nature*. Methuen, London.

O'Connor, N. (1993). *Paterson and Zderad: Humanistic Nursing Theories*. Sage, Newbury Park.

Parse, R. (1981). *Man–Living–Health: A Theory of Nursing*. John Wiley, New York.

Paterson, J. G. and Zderad, L. T. (1988). *Humanistic Nursing*. National League for Nursing, New York.

Peck, L. and Jennings, S. (1989). Student perceptions of the links between nursing and the liberal arts. *Journal of Nursing Education*, 28(9), 406–414.

Penden, A. and Staten, R. (1994). The use of the humanities in psychiatric nursing education. *Journal of Nursing Education*, 33(1), 41–42.

Reed, P. (1987). Liberal arts and professional nursing education integrating knowledge and wisdom. *Nurse Educator*, 12(4), 37–40.

Rey, M. (1983). *The Exile of the Soul*. Prometheus Books, Buffalo, NY.

Rockmore, G. (1994). *Heidegger and French Philosophy: Humanism, Antihumanism and Being*. Routledge, London.

Rogers, M. E. (1970). *An Introduction to the Theoretical Basis of Nursing*. F. A. Davis, Philadelphia.

Rogers, M. E. (1994). The science of unitary human beings: current perspectives. *Nursing Science Quarterly*, Spring, 7(1), 33–35.

Sartre, J. P. (1989). *Existentialism and Humanism*. Methuen, London.

Sartre, J. P. (1990). *Being and Nothingness: Essay on Phenomenological Ontology*. Routledge, London.

Sarvimaki, A. and Stenbock-Hult, B. (1992). *Caring: An Introduction to Health Care from a Humanistic Perspective*. Foundation for Nursing Education, Helsinki, Finland

Schiller, F. (1912). *Humanism, Philosophical Essays*, 2nd edn. Macmillan, London.

Steiner, G. (1992). *Heidegger*, 2nd edn. Fontana Press, London.

Taylor, Beverley J. (1994). *Being Human: Ordinariness in Nursing*. Churchill Livingstone, Edinburgh.

Warnock, M. (1970). *Existentialism*. Oxford University Press, Oxford.

Watson, J. (1985). *Nursing: The Philosophy and Science of Caring*. Colorado Association University Press, Boulder, CO.

Woodrow, P. (1993). A case for humanism in nurse education. *Senior Nurse*, 13(5), 46–50

Suggested further reading

Danto, Arthur C. (1985). *Sartre*, 2nd edn. Fontana Modern Masters, Fontana Press, London. This is a small, readable biography of Sartre, written by a writer/philosopher. A lovely introductory text, explaining the life and times of this French existentialist.

Magee, Bryan (1978). *Men of Ideas: Some Creators of Contemporary Philosophy*. Oxford University Press, Oxford. This is a collection of interviews by the philospher Magee with famous living philosophers, who explain their ideas and approach to philosophy.

Marriner-Tomey, A. (1994). *Nursing Theorists and Their Work*, 3rd edn. C. V. Mosby, St Louis, MO. This is a classic textbook describing the work of nursing theorists. A lovely introduction to nursing theories and nursing models.

More, Thomas (1965). *Utopia*. Penguin Classics, Penguin, Harmondsworth. A classic parody (satire) of life and society at the time of Sir Thomas More. A nice introduction to political and social philosophy. A good example of literature telling a serious story.

6

INTERACTION AS A THERAPEUTIC RESPONSE TO THE HEALTH OF THE INDIVIDUAL

Judith Reece

Introduction

This chapter is about an essential part of nursing, namely the art of communication. It does not profess to offer a new method of dynamic communication or add to work of other scholars such as Burnard, for example (see the Further Reading section at the end of the chapter). It aims to address the importance of communication in the delivery of care within the increasingly complex structure of health-care service provision. It will explore various issues that arise from the necessity to use effective communication skills within a complex range of practice settings. In that setting, the practitioner will have needs and feelings, both towards recipients of their care and the providers of the service for whom they work.

What it attempts is to raise a selection of issues for the nurse to consider when dealing with the many clients with whom they interact on a daily basis. The chapter explores various parallel issues and uses a few examples to illustrate the value to be gained in reflecting on how we use therapeutic interactions with a variety of clients. The writer has made a conscious decision not to include clients who have problems with their mental health status as this would entail a chapter of its own.

It is addressed essentially to the nurse working outside of mental health areas where the concept of therapeutic communication may have a unique

understanding. All the same, it is hopefully a useful chapter for the student about to undertake placement in a mental health setting in the first part of a diploma course. The client reflections which follow later in the chapter are equally applicable to other placements as well.

To gain greatest benefit it is advisable to commence a diary of reflection that is small enough to be carried around whilst on duty and into which you may record reflections and scenarios concerning work with clients in your area of practice. It is important that you take time over these exercises. Remember there is not a definitive answer on all occasions, that is not the purpose. The purpose is that we all think carefully about the therapeutic nature of communication and the positive and negative effects it can have on our clients. Certain scenarios have been included for you to consider, but these are only for guidance, what is more important is the reflection on particular situations and scenarios in which you are involved as a practitioner.

The word 'client' is used in the generic sense rather than the psychotherapeutic understanding. This allows for reflection in the wide variety of settings in which nursing is practised.

Setting the scene

We all profess to know what communication is

about. We understand the basic theory of message transmission, reception and decoding, but there has to be more to the act of communication than something as mechanistic as this. We need to take time to question what we are really communicating, as opposed to what we think we are communicating. In this respect the reader is invited to examine the role of self within this process and examine how we actually communicate with the self. This is an aspect vital to the mental health of someone constantly exposed to distress and suffering.

The chapter will define communication not only for the individual but also its relevant functions for both instigator and receiver and aims to explore the wider issues of communication, rather than be a directive manual. It is hoped that a sense of personal reflection on the subject will be gained. This assumes a basic knowledge of the principles of communication and interpersonal relating but you may like to consult a text such as Kagan and Evans (1995), especially Chapter 3.

Reflective points will be used as exercises to explore aspects of self and also to analyse aspects of practice.

The chosen examples can never hope to be definitive given the wide variety of practice settings currently in the National Health Service (NHS). In fact, many other care situations are used by clients which fall outside of these strict boundaries and their communication systems and even political ideologies may be very different both in nature and content, for example self-help and survivor groups. The survivors are perhaps survivors of traumatic incidents, or survivors of a health-care system which has not always been conducive to their recovery.

Communication is a powerful tool. It is also a potent tool for the application of ideals in practice. We need to be mindful that ideology does not become dogma which is damaging to self and client. We are constantly being made aware of the need to communicate appropriately within the NHS to allow proper channels of communication to exist between the service and its commercial partners. A failure to communicate therapeutically with recipients of care was highlighted in the Audit Commission Report (1993), which states

> The growth in consumerism, backed up by formal mechanisms such as the Patient's Charter, has made these shortcomings more obvious and is making health-care providers re-examine the ways in which they communicate with patients. Moreover,

there is a growing body of evidence to show that if providers improve communication they can in turn improve the effectiveness of care, increase the efficiency with which it is delivered, and improve their reputation locally with both patients and purchasers (p. 1).

Staff are reminded constantly of their obligation to communicate what they are doing both to the client and to each other in a systematic and meaningful manner. They have to listen to recipients of care, listen to managers' demands, listen to their NHS trust, and finally, listen to their professional bodies. All this time they are working in an environment where they are bombarded by an information revolution that almost defies description in the speed of its arrival.

Thus, communication is no longer the relatively simple matter of reading, responding to and generating written communiqués, phone calls or letters requesting information from management.

It is equally, no longer merely telling the recipients of our care what will happen to them, with little subsequent reflection on the impact of our words.

Such communications were often a feature of managerial communications as well. The result was that enormous injustices were, and still are, done to people because we do not listen to the verbal message nor the hidden inference.

In the past consumers of health-care services were at the bottom of an enormous managerial pyramid-like structure and had little access to the person at 'the top' of the structure. This possibly characterised the era that immediately followed after the Salmon structure was implemented in the 1960s. In the Salmon structure, the person at the top had little reason to communicate with the person at the bottom, and in fact may have become totally isolated from them. That has changed to a degree, both in relation to the patient and also to staff. The danger now is that staff are experiencing personal stress at a geographically closer level. The ward manager is now perceived to be more of a manager than a colleague and, as such, has perceived and actual powers over the individual. Communications to and from the ward manager possibly now have an authority that was perceived to be the function of someone higher up the structure of management, and who was therefore further away from their functioning in the system.

However what of the client? The client is now a person for whom health care is purchased from a provider and rightly, as a result, agreed standards are set. Dickson *et al.* (1993) commented that

> The past decade has witnessed a burgeoning awareness of the indispensability of effective levels of interpersonal communication to acceptable standards of practice in many professional circles (p. 4).

It is within this revolution that nurses function as one of the groups which has communication at its heart. What is more, communication is **assumed** to be therapeutic when involving care delivered to a client at all times. However, is it possible to question whether such standards of communication are possible, when as a profession, we are not accustomed or comfortable with questioning whether we **are** indeed always therapeutic. Most of all, do we know what we mean by **therapeutic**? The writer contends that any communication which is either restorative or educative in nature, or which guides a client to a more productive state (either physically or emotionally) is a therapeutic communication. This assumes that the recipient of our communication finds it to be so. Dickson *et al.* (1993) seem to allude to this in suggesting that communication is an act of rewarding.

We not only gain a personal reward, but also reward the attempts of others who communicate with us by actually listening **with** them and **to** them. We do not listen just to elicit information, but hopefully to bring about closer, more insightful relationships and to lessen the impact of professional power. We surely need to remember that though patients may have better knowledge because of greater media coverage of medical issues, they have not necessarily attained a personal insight yet into what that particular illness means to them. The use of defence mechanisms by clients who face an uncertain future can include failing to make the link between a study of survival rates in HIV infection for example and its particular progress for them. The same client on being admitted yet again for an HIV-related illness may 'check out' a nurse by making verbal approaches indicating a growing awareness of what is happening to them. This is not just taking a history it is making real efforts to come alongside and listen as well as reward their attempts to verbalise their personal and not just theoretical fears. By using true empathetic listening skills we can change the unequal relationship between us and become

more equal in a two-way communication. Johnson and Webb (1995) comment that professionals use their power to maintain distance and ultimately to label patients as popular or unpopular.

The use of communication is a very central part to this process. The question is, how well do we use communication skills to reward effort rather than label responses? Dickson (1993) reminds us that communication is behaviourally rewarding in nature. We not only gain a reward but by listening in depth to people we reward the attempts of people who communicate with us by listening **with** them and **to** them.

This failure to listen is not a problem unique to nursing. Often in the media we hear reference to 'What the majority of people want'. But are not most of us, in fact, a silent majority? When were you last asked what you wanted by the very politicians whom we berate for not giving us what we want?

Recently a commentator on a television programme said that as a nation, we were disillusioned with politicians because they do not relate to us, they do not know what we want. The politicians have simply stopped listening to us. Likewise with nursing. It is not unusual to hear nurses and other health workers commenting that managers do not listen and so they feel impotent.

Despite mission statements assuring us that our NHS trust is committed to quality and that we are a part of that quality process of feedback and standard setting, many are feeling almost alien to the process, alien because, as with the television commentator, we feel that we are not being listened to.

Perhaps the problem is not with the actual message of raising standards but with how the message is delivered. For example messages that imply a threat, either emotional or physical, may produce a sense of panic or being out of control, a sense of being disempowered.

On reflection within the setting of the internal market, has the decline in power of the medical profession brought with it the changes in equality of communication and professional respect that we all wanted? Nurses may have felt unlistened to by certain consultant colleagues. However maybe now the focus of non-listening has changed. Both groups are now stating that they are not listened to. Both groups are expressing concerns about decreased staffing levels and increased work pressures.

It is similar with nurse–client communication. Sometimes the words we use are at fault and sometimes it is the way the words are used that convey a sense that we are more powerful than the patient we are working with. This was, and still is, a situation that is common in psychiatric practice even today. Psychiatric patients still report that they very often feel 'talked about' and not 'talked to'. Their distress was, and is still, often unheeded (Reece, 1995).

This chapter will, in subsequent sections, differentiate between communicating, using counselling skills and counselling. These are often seen to be the three main dimensions of interaction within health-care practice and delivery. It will then explore further the use of communication skills with certain groups of clients. Finally it will address briefly the process of ending interactions, before considering the value of supervision, essential to the practice of interaction, and a vital part of personal and professional development.

Although within the chapter there are reflective points containing exercises, it would also be desirable for you to create your own diary of reflection and self-supervision. This would be a personal document in which you may record either critical incidents from practice and which you could use to complete the scenarios and exercises included here. Such exercises vary in length of time needed but many need a minimum of 15 minutes.

This type of reflection as a basis for reflecting and learning from practice situations is itself the foundation of what is later taken to be supervision. This is a subject that will be returned to later in the chapter.

The next section starts with just this type of exercise.

Defining the boundaries: three fundamental areas where good therapeutic communication is needed

With the inner self

> **Reflective point**
> *Who are you? Take 10 minutes to consider your response.*

> *In asking yourself this question what factors did you explore? Perhaps you actually dismissed it as irrelevant, or more likely became offended because you are sure that you know who you are. Do you actually know where the boundaries are between the 'you' who is personal and the 'you' who has to act in a professional manner?*

Another equally fundamental question is 'who am I in this working world that I occupy for a large part of my day?'. We have countless descriptions, definitions and understandings of nursing but who are 'you'? who am 'I' as a nurse?

It is likely that you are occupying a multitude of roles and if you are female, it is likely that you are occupying a greater number of roles than your male colleagues. Within that you are likely to be experiencing a higher degree of role conflict as well. If you are female and a nurse it is likely that the boundaries between caring at work and home are very blurred indeed. The type of communication may even be the same on occasions. In fact many carers go home to indulge in further caring, even nursing an older relative with an illness such as dementia. The dividing line between the roles may be so small that the two become inseparable, and as Unger and Crawford (1992) point out 'Chronic overload may lead to fatigue, short temper and lowered resistance to physical illness' (p. 474).

That is not to say that the male nurse is any less affected by having to balance roles, but the majority who have to occupy several caring roles are women, sometimes doing part-time 'paid' caring work and then adding unpaid 'voluntary' caring within the family (Finch and Groves, 1985).

What is the effect on you of these multiple roles for example. If this is not your personal dilemma then what issue is there that may be causing a block to more effective communication.

It is possible that this may impinge on the next category under consideration.

With colleagues

Defining the nature of communications between nurses and other colleagues has been attempted in many and various ways. Many writers, e.g. Dickson have concentrated on acquiring the skills of assertive, positive communication in group situations, taking personal responsibility for all the team failings and attempting compromise. But how do we communicate with colleagues and more importantly, how successful are we at this? Dickson (1982) writes of the need for us to learn to communicate more assertively with other colleagues, essentially with women in mind, but the message (and the training), does not need to exclude male colleagues.

Kagan and Evans (1995) speak of the constraints on effective communications with others. These can be multi-faceted, but they are classified into four contexts that may alter the effectiveness of communications.

1. Cultural, for example, the change from provider-led service to consumer-led services.
2. Environmental, for example, the physical layout of wards influence how much we can interact with particular patients and colleagues. How wards are constructed, i.e. provision of small group rooms in a psychiatric ward with good support facilities for the staff members as well.
3. Social, for example the roles that both staff and different patients can occupy can influence how we interact with both clients and colleagues [see Johnson and Webb (1995) as well].
4. Personal, for example, the provision or lack of personal professional support systems being addressed only recently for adult nurses, are more common in psychiatric and learning disabilities nursing.

In looking at the factors listed with all the variables which are likely to occur, it is almost inevitable that some communications with colleagues will, through no immediate faults of our own, be less than totally effective. This is not a matter of blame only of reflection, and on what can be done to improve them.

The levels of stress involved in communicating within a vast system such as an NHS trust, are likely to leave us tired, frayed and at times useless to that system without effective channels of communication and organisational management. Changes within the health-care delivery system are taking place at a frantic pace and we need to be aware of the cost that this may exact from our own and our colleagues' mental health.

Luft (1970) suggests

Interpersonal relationships throughout an organisation affect the general psychological climate, and the attitudes of the organisation, affect interpersonal relations: parts and wholes influence each other (p. 65).

If this is true, then it is not at all surprising that communications with colleagues need to be right if communications with clients are to be meaningful and therapeutic. If, as a result of all these minor breakdowns of communication within the system, we are stressed to breaking point, then it follows that the recipients of the service will experience this as well. If the system into which people come to be restored to health is itself not health promoting in its communication systems and is showing signs of stress, then clients will experience this as well.

Such breakdown is inevitable because over-stretching a system will firstly manifest itself in stress and if it is stressed to the point of no return it will eventually breakdown. The signs of impending breakdown were summarised by Selye (1956), for example, who originally explored the effects of increasing stress levels beyond a certain limit. The body as a system can only deal with a certain amount of stress and it deals with it in a series of steps.

1. Alarm reaction. The body gears up for the fighting response
2. Resistance. The body attempts to make adjustments and copes.
3. Exhaustion. If the stressor is not removed, then exhaustion and even death is the most likely outcome.

Could this equally be true of a system such as communication?

We are now reasonably accustomed to thinking of this model of stress in relation to patients and their health but what of its applicability to nurses?

Reflective point

Reflect on a recent situation that caused you a great deal of distress because in one way or another you were thwarted in your attempts to communicate in your workplace over a long period of time. What physical changes in your personality and physical health did you notice and how did you deal with the situation as it progressed? What lasting effects has this had on you?

Did you contemplate sickness, or did sickness come on you when you did not expect it?

How did you feel when you again had to deal with the situation?

Draw up an action plan for dealing with such a situation again that would be less stressful.

With clients

Nursing requires that practitioners communicate at all times with their consumers. Many nurses, for example in the community, now work from remote bases or even from home. Their phone number is always available, but when and how do we control the boundaries of when we may be communicated with?

Is it always therapeutic to be permanently available to all people all the time? We speak of being off duty but often we are merely working from a different base. For example, we stop seeing clients in order to update records, do some teaching, supervise a junior colleague. There is a limit to always being available both in terms of physical work and being continually pre-occupied with the concerns of our clients.

Peplau (1994) warns us to gain a balance between being, as she terms it, 'pseudo-close' and equally being unhealthily involved with a patient, to the extent that objective decision making is lost and as a result objective communications are not effected. There is, according to Peplau, a valid time for withdrawal in order to maintain an appropriate professional closeness, and she suggests:

> The extent of emotional involvement with patient after patient in a days work also requires consideration. Not only does emotional involvement of great intensity drain a nurse's energies and particularly so in situations in which the extant problems may not be immediately amenable to solutions, but such involvement may also becloud the perceptual field and distort her observations (p. 241).

We need to remember that the boundary between health and illness is as narrow for the nurse as it is for the client. What seems to be health-promoting communication which is seemingly therapeutic can easily become unhealthy for both consumer and nurse alike. So what does the writer understand by them?

Communicating and the use of counselling skills in nursing

Communicating

Communicating is a vital part of the process of nursing. It is that which is done in all acts of nursing care even when the patient is not consciously aware

that she or he is being cared for. It is such a vital part that we have long been guilty of taking its presence for granted. For the nurse it has many facets, it utilises all of the human senses and is directly or indirectly goal centred. It has the property of being constantly in a state of change and is ultimately unique. As such, it follows that all people's responses are also unique. How I communicate my distress may not only be unique to me, but also my mode of communication may also vary from one circumstance and situation to another.

Sundeen *et al.* (1989) point out that for the nurse another dimension is also essential – that is time. How and what we communicate with clients is both a part of a continuum and at the same time a unique moment in time for both them and us. The authors suggest:

> What happens now, at this moment, can never be recaptured. It is not the same as anything that has occurred previously, nor will it be repeated in the future. The individuality of the participants and the quality of the time dimension make communication a unique experience – something that cannot be duplicated (pp. 91–92).

This sums up precisely the problem in attempting to define communication, if the act itself is unique and changing it follows that the definition will also be changing continuously. The purpose of communication determines its definition. However it may safely be assumed by us, that the primary purpose of communication is to convey information by transmission usually it is at least verbal but it may only be vocal in nature.

The purpose of communicating is the establishment or maintenance of a relationship. Without communication no relationship can continue for very long.

It may be that a relationship for example a partner with an unconscious person is based purely on touch and verbal communication and is on a one-sided basis only. But all the while a partner feels the need to do this, then the relationship can continue, however much it defies rational explanation by others. Think particularly of the countless hours people spend with a person who has severe neurological injury. To suggest that a relationship and communication were not there, because they do not conform to accepted 'rules' of communication would be heartless in the extreme.

Luft (1970) defines communication in the following way.

Communication refers to what is expressed verbally and non-verbally; it applies to articulated words and thoughts, and to unvocalized feelings; it concerns the intentions of the communicator and the impressions received by the ones to whom the communication is addressed. Communication may be formal, as information conveyed in an organisation through regular channels, or informal as in the interactions among friends over coffee (p. 39).

Communication has the purpose of conveying a message, of giving an instruction, of teaching, but primarily it could be suggested that its ultimate purpose lies in unifying all aspects of what McMahon and Pearson (1991) have termed 'therapeutic activities in nursing'. They suggests the following are components of this relationship, based on the work of Muetzal (1988):

- developing partnership, intimacy and reciprocity in the nurse–patient relationship. Manipulating the environment (in which nursing is practised where possible)
- teaching
- providing comfort
- adopting complementary health practices
- utilising tested physical interventions
- McMahon (to which the writer would also add tested psychological interventions as well).

Reflective point

Sundeen et al. (1989) suggest the following criteria for evaluating the effectiveness of nurse–client communication:

1. *effectiveness: does this (particular) communication meet pre-set goals of the interaction?*
2. *appropriateness: is this communication relevant to the stated goals?*
3. *adequacy: is there sufficient communication and feedback to meet the stated goals?*
4. *efficiency: does this communication use the minimum amount of energy necessary to meet the goals?*
5. *flexibility is there an appropriate balance between control and permissiveness in the interaction? (p. 147).*

Record a communication between a newly qualified nurse and a patient as it happens and then compare this with a similar scenario handled by a more experienced colleague. The chosen scenarios should be as similar as possible.

Then spend time asking yourself how far the communications of both nurses meet Sundeen's criteria?

If they do, note where they do, if they do not analyse why not. How many of the criteria were met by both people? Were there situations were experience helped or where the opposite was true? How could you change your skills to meet these criteria, or suggest an alternative.

Counselling

To attempt a definition of counselling is nearly as difficult as trying to define the object of counselling, the client. Just as we make certain assumptions about who needs counselling equally we think we all know what counselling is. There are of course definitions, many of them, but the fact that there are such a variety underlines that we are not clear in the first place. Counselling as a term has been applied to a variety of settings within nursing. Some of these are inappropriate, and some are most definitely not counselling. Counselling as a term may be used as a euphemism for rebuking poor student 'attitudes' and problems. It has also been part of the language of professional disciplining. It has been prescribed by and to staff as a means of avoiding dismissal. The British Association of Counselling offers the following definition:

Counselling is a skilled and principled use of relationships which develops self-knowledge, emotional acceptance and growth and personal resources. The overall aim is to live more fully and satisfyingly. Counselling may be concerned with addressing and resolving specific problems, making decisions, coping with crises, working through feelings and inner conflict, or improving relationships with others (quoted in Bayne and Nicholson, 1993, p. 4).

Counselling has been used to tell patients they are facing death, how to change their lifestyle after a myocardial infarction and for others how to accept the fact that they are not to be released from a section of the Mental Health Act (1983), which may require them to accept treatment that they may not desire.

Essentially counselling is an act of enabling by one person to another. This should result in some kind of desired growth, a change in that person's perception of what is happening to them, or strengthening of purpose to deal with what is causing them to feel 'dis-eased'. Burnard (1994) helpfully suggests that 'The processes of counselling can be defined as the means by which one person helps another to clarify his or her life situation and to decide further lines of action' (p. 4).

Counselling has many dimensions and schools of thought. However the essential prerequisite of the counselling process is that we must like to be with people and more importantly have the ability to come alongside them and be involved with them in a professional way.

Take time also to decide clearly what is within the province of supportive counselling and what requires further specialist therapy, such as dealing with an unresolved bereavement or where there is clear evidence of psychiatric disturbance. As Buckman (1992) asserts, always know when to get further help and advice. The biggest danger of all is in thinking that we are personally endowed with the perfect theory and the perfect answers. We never own our clients in any way and neither for that matter should they own us.

In using counselling skills Burnard (1994) offers what the writer sees as cardinal 'rules' in the work, which we all ignore at our peril

1. the client knows what is best for him or her
2. interpretation by the counsellor is likely to be inaccurate and is best avoided
3. advice is rarely helpful
4. the client occupies a different personal world from that of the counsellor and vice versa
5. listening is the basis of the counselling relationship (p. 89).

Reflective point
This is a much longer one! Work or read through Burnard's book mentioned above and having done so ask yourself three essential questions:

1. *Do I frequently abuse the word counselling?*
2. *Do I need to do counselling for my own benefit or the client?*
3. *What type of counselling philosophy is best suited to my personal orientation and my career needs?*

Healthy interactions in practice

Having looked briefly at communication skills and touched briefly on counselling skills, various groups of clients have been selected as examples of how such principles may be applied. These examples are not intended to be exhaustive but rather are illustrative in nature and are also an attempt to utilise both the less obvious categories and reflect hopefully differently on more common scenarios. It is beyond the scope of this chapter to explore a wide range within nursing/midwifery. However, what is to be attempted here is a sample of the differing areas where health workers/nurses frequently make interventions and where health-promoting communications are an essential part of these interventions.

The 'unattractive'

There is surely no lack of research evidence which suggests that we are all influenced consciously or subconsciously by the attractiveness or otherwise of people with whom we come into contact (Johnson and Webb, 1995). It is a concept closely linked with sexual attraction and we are all very influenced by what we are lead to believe is attractive to others, usually of the opposite, but not always, gender (Unger and Crawford, 1992; Gross, 1992). Often it seems that our perceptions of others are based on schemata that we have built up by past contacts, or by mentally placing certain people into 'boxes' which are subconscious. This ensures that we will recognise the people again and be able if necessary, and when, under threat from them to defend ourselves against them (Fiske and Taylor, 1984). This should be a part of learning and recognition, but that may not always be the case. We may well have had one unfortunate encounter with a particular type of person and then subsequently judge all other similar people by that encounter.

Also, we live within a sexual context. We are likely to become a partner to someone who fulfils certain criteria of attractiveness. What however is attractiveness? Mathes (1975) noted that contrary to research that suggested that in theory we do not rank physical attractiveness as a prime criterion for personal liking, in behavioural terms we do. The only time this seems to lessen is when a permanent partner is taken.

For the nurse the greatest danger is to enter into stigmatisation (Goffman, 1963). The unattractive person, however that may be defined, becomes a person who is stigmatised. Such people are, in Goffman's understanding, marked out from the rest of society and may well not receive all of its benefits. The real problem with communication with such a variety of different groups is that we all vary so much in what we see as unattractive and this often spills over into the formation of negative or overtly positive attitudes to one client or another, e.g. the overweight, the underweight, the complaining, the silent. It is a small step from labels to stigmatisation. As Stockwell (1972) noted, we are in danger of creating the unpopular patient.

It seems that nurses have some degree of difficulty in adjusting to all the demands and needs of patients with whom they come into contact (the writer included!). Surely the essence of making a potentially health-destroying communication into a health-creating one is in recognising that we have the problem in the first place. When we are working with those we find unattractive, we need to remember that to another person they are someone who is attractive and it is perhaps the system that has made them the unattractive.

> ### Reflective point
> *What do you find attractive and unattractive about people in both professional and personal terms, Do you believe that the nurse in you has to like as well as work with all types of people?*
>
> *Are there times when you feel the duty to care and professional obligation conflicts more or less directly with what you personally feel is unattractive and even occasionally almost repulsive? How do you work out the dissonance between what ought to be present and what is actually there inside you? How could you resolve the conflict?*

The non-conforming

There may be many reasons why a patient cannot, or will not conform to what we perceive as health-promoting interventions. There are of course a number of accepted and well-documented reasons such as a power imbalance between carer and cared for (Sines, 1994). This is particularly true of psychiatric nursing. There may be poor past experiences going back to childhood encounters with hospitals. It may simply be that we are too keen to want people to be as we would like them. We still have a tendency to see outcomes of care in fairly closely defined boundaries. We expect people who are patients to behave as if they were dependant on us and our accepted wisdom. The patient who knows too much may be seen as difficult and presenting a threat to our sometimes slim knowledge base.

In the current environment of cost-driven health delivery, we are encouraged to promote health in order to reduce the cost to the unconsulted taxpayer. This presents a dilemma for the health-care professional. Notably, is health-promoting advice really for the benefit of the individual when there may be a conflict over what is the best? For example the promotion of a low-fat diet when the patient is subjected to media accounts that it is the type of rather than the amount of fat that is important.

The politics of health advice and moral admonitions to live a good life are linked with historical notions of what is seen as a moral and conforming patient particularly women (Ehrenreich and English, 1988).

In the past patients were assessed for benefit by the state as much on the basis of their morality as for their financial need. Is this the foundation for long imprinted attitudes that surface when the health-care professional meets the patient who challenges them?

What the patient may learn from messages by inference is probably stronger than that which is conveyed verbally. We can never hope to speak one language and avoid conveying a contradictory personal feeling even if we think we have it hidden in the depths of our subconscious.

We cannot ignore messages, sometimes unconscious messages, that are conveyed even in codified form to clients whether in hospitals or the community (Teasdale, 1993).

Non-conformity may result from a failure to have need assessed and understood even if that need cannot be met. Farrell (1991) found that psychiatric and general nurses were equally poor in assessing need. The writer found that 'The nurse's inability to perceive patients needs on an individual basis is consistent with other studies which suggest that nurses use stereotypes when perceiving patients needs' (p. 1062).

Dickson *et al.* (1993) address the issue of rewarding behaviour in communication. We are all dependent on rewards and these may be affected whether we do or do not attempt any further behaviours that may challenge us. The patient with whom we are trying to communicate and who does not conform may well have had her/his self-esteem so lowered in the past that they are reluctant to take the risk of being vulnerable again, even to themselves.

Dickson *et al.* note

> The sorts of images that some individuals form of themselves and the self-esteem on which results are based, are in part based on the regimes of rewards and punishments to which they have been exposed. Here self-concept can be thought to mediate the effects of reinforcement on behaviour, so that such individuals strive to act in a manner which sustains an acceptable self-image (p. 57).

Health-promoting interactions with the person facing surgery

Increasing demands are made on nurses in a system which is geared to a fast throughput of patients. It is therefore more important than ever that we are able to communicate immediately and effectively with people who are with us for increasingly short periods of time. In that time we are expected to listen, diagnose, inform and support.

How much of that talking is therapeutic and how much of it is ritual? How much is social in nature and how much of it is purpose-specific, especially when we frequently assert that we do not have time to talk. Health-promoting interaction primarily has therapeutic ends. That means it has to aid in the process of recuperation or else it is merely talk. Talk is fine and necessary, but we cannot make a convincing case that it is therapeutic. In fact sometimes it may be non-therapeutic.

It may well be that there is case to be made for periods of non-clinical non-therapeutic talking which is a vital part of human need and that this should be separated from therapeutic interaction. For example it is possible that making such a distinction would encourage us to abandon the suspicion that just sitting talking was a waste of time. Conversely all nurses are or should be trained to communicate in therapeutic ways and accept the necessary corollary of this, that they need personal supervision, which has a real therapeutic purpose. Faugier and Butterworth (1992) comment 'One of the primary reasons for all supervision is to ensure that the quality of therapeutic work with the client is of a consistently high standard in relation to the client's needs' (p. 10).

Communicating with the client undergoing planned surgery is communicating with a person facing possibly what is the greatest threat they will face to their bodily integrity. The degree of distress that they may feel is often a long way in excess of what we as professionals imagine to be acceptable. No two people ever experience the same operation in the same way. A routine hernia repair for one person can take on the level of major heart surgery for another individual. Clearly the need is to have focused communications. A degree of stress, as stated earlier, is necessary and even within surgery it has a place. Attempts at total removal or complete avoidance may well be counterproductive and reduce the body's natural abilities to deal with stress (Salmon, 1993).

In communicating with a patient undergoing planned surgery, unless it is simply surgery that will improve function or remove an annoyance, there is always an element of unpredictability. This element is now more than ever a communication for mental health promotion. The clients with whom we come into contact are now those who have access to more health and medical information than in any previous generation. They know as well as we do that a small growth can be exactly that, a non-malignant annoying cyst, *but* they also know that it could be more sinister. Striking a balance between minimising a verbal statement of anxiety about what is to happen, and ignoring the possibility that they are right is a difficult path to steer.

As people who work with the area of communications, it is worth remembering that the breaking bad news may not be reserved for just the 'traditional areas' such as cancer care, within terminal or chronic illnesses but for the patient it can also apply to many aspects of surgical intervention.

However, when the news is bad, the range of reaction is potentially enormous. The use of a reflective diary can be a useful aid both in teaching and learning about this range.

We can look back on how we reacted and ask what were our responses at the time, how we felt and how we could make it different in the future, as well as utilising research to help understand what was happening at the time. We are reasonably used to coping with the expected responses, it is always the unexpected ones that catch us out. Buckman (1992) gives excellent advice when he says

> When it comes to anticipating a patient's reaction, there is only one safe assumption – it is not safe to assume anything (p. 13).

In an excellent chapter devoted to patient reactions he lists some 20. Reactions which range from the unacceptable (which includes violence) to the accepted and almost standard responses of silence and tears.

The client (and possibly the next of kin) undergoing surgery has in reality three periods of time when communications may be either misheard or misinterpreted. There is the period before surgery when the levels of worry are high, then comes a time when messages are misunderstood or misheard because of the effects of anaesthesia or analgesia. Finally, after surgery, the effects of analgesia cause communications from doctors to be misheard or misinterpreted.

The writer well remembers experiencing major surgery and coming round trying hard to work out why all the people in the world seemed to have the writer's name, and the effort of trying to communicate the feelings in a world that was as strange as an untuned radio was confusing. Equally I was fortunate enough to have in the area of recovery a colleague who knowing the sense of humour I possessed responded to my complaint of pain with a humorous aside and an immediate promise to relieve the pain.

It was that type of person-centred communication that was memorable and personalised. To another person it would have seemed trite or even cruel but she knew my needs, knew my preoperative terror and was there with the right words at the right time.

At any time a breakdown in communication is possible and equally any one of these periods can provoke a cathartic release of feelings in client or relative. How we manage this may contribute negatively or positively to the mental and physical health of those for whom we care.

Reflective point

Consider the following scenario:

Amy French has entered a surgical ward after referral as an emergency from an out-patient clinic which she was attending having waited three weeks for an appointment. Her main complaint was that on two occasions she has passed small amounts of blood about six hours after taking food. On admission she is quiet, withdrawn and resents bitterly your request to weigh her. She complains little apart from this and answers most questions quite well. She lives at home with parents and is part way through her degree course at the local university. Her mother is with her and is quite distraught, fearing her daughter has cancer and that no one will tell her the truth. This is in spite of your attempts to calm her and tell her that laparoscopy does not mean cancer; her mother still insists that her daughter is dying.

Amy seems to take all this in her stride until she is made ready for emergency surgery when she becomes tearful and cannot say what is the matter. After surgery (during which a small nonmalignant cyst is found), Amy admits that she has been bulimic for several years and is sorry that nothing was found that might kill her: 'I have told you because you are kind and thoughtful and I think you want what is best for me' she says. 'Could you tell my mother'. Amy has no emotional father figure present for her.

Analyse this and suggest a range of possible responses and suggest what you might say to the mother about the cyst when she appears on the ward.

Ask yourself what would be your immediate personal rather than professional response to this scenario.

> *Consider what responses Amy's mother may have to the news you will choose to give her, and suggest a communication plan for this interaction.*
>
> *Had **you** considered the possibility of bulimia, rather than other organic causes for the bleeding? Had you thought that possibly she was pregnant?*
>
> *Her mother clearly has unresolved feelings with which she has not yet dealt with. All of these make for a highly charged situation for you. Finally **you** are great danger of being drawn into a disastrous family scenario, in which you do not know what is happening at all.*

The patient with acute cardiac problems

The difficulty with acute cardiac problems is that they happen in a short space of time. At 20 it is very easy to feel we are immortal, that things always happen to someone other than ourselves, yet suddenly with the attack of crushing central chest pain people know that time may be the very thing they may not have a lot of.

The communication with a client in this situation has of necessity to be confined to aspects to do with stabilising the physical condition and giving appropriate reassurance to reduce stress levels (and therefore the demand being made on potentially damaged cardiac tissue). But what of the psychological damage which has occurred to the person? There is an undoubted existential dimension to sudden cardiac problems, the potential of death seems to be much closer when in a coronary care unit.

However it seems that after initial shock and treatment regimes are finished then more long-term aspects take over. The concern moves to employment, finances (McCorkle and Quint-Benedict, 1983), although often unmentioned, the effects of illness on sexual activity may also be a potential point of need.

The patient (as a result of the cardiac insufficiency) may well experience either short-term or more permanent problems in mentally processing communications. The cardiac problems cause them to misunderstand, mishear or even provoke reactions of an untoward nature. The prevalence of psychiatric morbidity in a coronary care unit is not insignificant (Shiell and Shiell, 1991).

It is unlikely that all of this can be attributed to organic problems though the evidence that a technological environment is anxiety provoking is not really disputed nowadays. The fact that we submit patients and their relatives to a barrage of technology which seems to them to exist to preserve or at the very least monitor life, is almost certain to communicate a message that life can be preserved for ever. Or does it?

It is as if the mind receives one message from these external forces and at the same time the body, almost in a kind of Cartesian dualism, is trying to tell the mind the opposite – that you are vulnerable, that life is fragile after all.

In communicating with a person who is well enough to understand all this, we should remember that there is this kind of mixed message happening to the client. The environment requires management to make it more like the average home environment in which the person would normally cope when ill (Halm and Alpen, 1993).

The patient is also in a heightened sense of arousal and requires extra sensitivity in interpersonal relations. She or he may be hypersensitive and also, as a result of analgesia, be likely to misinterpret words and sounds as well as sight and sounds. The sense of touch is disturbed and an unexpected touch may be misinterpreted and have the potential for being transformed into at least an illusion, or at its extreme an hallucination.

At this stage of acute response there is a need for communication that may have to be explanatory in nature concerning what has happened, as well as being geared towards making potential changes in lifestyle.

Much of the communication at this time is actually lost and may need repetition later. In times of stress the impact of bad news can often not be processed and because of the hyperarousal of the human body, will almost certainly be misheard.

Listening is not always the same as hearing, is a good maxim in this situation. According to Undern *et al.* (1993) such 'information giving' had little effects on their cardiac outcomes and recovery but in follow-up later social and psychological variables were marked. They certainly had a better outlook on life after myocardial infarction than an uncounselled control group.

The older patient

Communication with the older person is communication with a vast data bank of experience and life skills that the younger person does not alway possess.

Yet why is it that when many older people are in similar situations to these are they are perceived to be childlike and infantile? That is they are under-stimulated and the routine does not always encourage creativity and individuality. The end result is that cognitive function becomes severely impaired (Gross, 1992).

Older people do not require simple baby-like language that is often used where the older person is being cared for. We can try to persuade ourselves that this type of language is only used in situations where cognitive understanding is lessened, i.e. dementia, but even there, such language cannot be justified. Somehow when we communicate with older people we seem to think that social boundaries are changed. First names are still being used without permission being sought.

I find expressions such as 'Flower, gran, sweetie' deeply insulting. Just because people do not contradict us does not mean that they do not mind.

The older person may have severe cognitive impairment but don't assume that all older people have such an impairment. What does need to be assumed is, however, that basic human functions may not be as efficient as they were in past years. The skill in communicating with older people is to take time and check that hearing and seeing are appropriate to your levels of speaking. What is important to remember is that stages of the counselling relationship as identified by Kagan and Evans (1995) have great relevance to a older person suddenly or not so suddenly facing impending illness that may be terminal.

Kagan suggests that there are three stages which should be followed:

1. exploring, which leads to warmth, rapport and focusing
2. understanding, which leads to clarification and goals
3. acting, which leads to encouragement and evaluation.

Remember that whatever skills for disguising feelings you may have, the older person has had them for many more years than you. They may be acutely aware of each and every indication that you are finding them either boring, smelly or even stupid and most important of all, that they are being a nuisance or wasting your time.

We must remember that with much more care being given within the community, the older person who comes into a hospital comes into something which has utterly changed from their perception of what hospitals were once like. Equally, they are aware that this admission could be the one that forces them to confront the fact that they may have to give up their independence and home life as they know it.

When helping an older person to talk through fears and concerns, the central skill of restating is required. This gentle checking of understanding is essential, but be careful not to make it appear that they are a child with limited abilities to function cognitively. However, it is necessary to make sure that communications are both clear and, most important of all, appropriate. Not all elderly people appreciate the numerous hugs and squeezes that they are often given without their permission (McKann and McKenna, 1993)

We are all getting older, the ageing process is relentless. But if we see it as a negative experience we, in communicating with the older person can reflect a negativism that may not be there at all. Some older people are poor and lonely and dependant, but not all are by any means. Older women, for example, may have the opportunity for new experiences and achievements long denied as a result of raising a family and caring for partners.

Not all elderly people need bereavement counselling to attain health after bereavement, for some it may provide a chance to go off and do what they have wished for all of their life. The nurse has a role sometimes in allowing the older person, especially the widow, to be themselves. Likewise, the nurse has a role in counselling the family to facilitate such freedom and not continue to repress feelings and expressions of activity.

Reflective point

Read the following abstract from a novel then reflect on it and ask whether you have experienced such sentiments in a family with an older relative. **Then** *ask yourself how you would approach the situation.*

(This occurs after the death of the husband.) 'Of course, she would not question the wisdom of any arrangements they might choose to make. Mother had no will of her own; all her life long, gracious and gentle, she had been wholly submissive – an appendage. It was assumed she had not enough brain to be assertive. ... She would be grateful to them for arranging her remaining few years' (Sackville-West, 1986, p. 24).

Feedback

Useful advice may be along the lines of encouraging the family to develop more positive views of the older person. Stereotypical views that all elderly people are stupid may need to be challenged. You may even be brave enough to suggest that the older women is now free to do all the things she really wants to do and perhaps they (the family!) could explore this with her. (For the best advice read the novel!)

When distress is more serious

The previous section has attempted to stimulate some thinking about types of communication scenarios within different nursing environments. Clearly not all can be covered. However there are situations when the distressed person may well be communicating more severe distress than demonstrated in the preceding sections. For example in people whose loss and distress has been so great as to temporarily cause a loss of insight into what is happening to them. They may be potentially suicidal or seriously psychologically disturbed. Where such a level of disturbance is evident then counsellors need to be proficient in what ever theory or philosophy of counselling they are using. The nurse needs to be aware of these and certainly when dealing with a highly distressed person then the use of confrontation should be used with great care. If the patient is to remain alive various strategies can be employed to maintain their physical integrity, but maintaining a rapidly diminishing psychological integrity is quite another skill.

Good therapeutic skills are invaluable in defusing a situation and avoiding the patient loosing control of either themselves or their power to act independently. Peplau (1994) suggests the following as being essential counselling skills that can be applied to people who are extremely distressed:

1. structure the situation so that client and nurse intentions are clear
2. behave like an expert (do not betray a sense of uncertainty)
3. show appreciation for what is happening to the patient
4. allow them time to explain what they feel is happening to them.

Ethical considerations

As a professional it is assumed that we act ethically, but is this always the case?

It also begs the question of what is considered ethical behaviour? At once we are faced with a decision about whether to explore this from a theological/academic/philosophical base or to ask what we mean by behaving in a manner which preserves the ultimate good of the recipient of our services.

Advances in technology and refinements of skills mean that as nurses we are practising skills that very few years ago were not within our province for example.

Within in the realm of counselling there has been an extension in the last 20 years or so into fields of counselling work that were previously not seen to be the domain of nursing at all. Within these areas, we need to develop confidence. The act of counselling sometimes demands that we make difficult decisions and maybe in the past we have been disempowered from doing just this. We have been forced into situations of dependence on doctors for example in deciding to tell a patient that she/he has cancer. We need, says Van Hooft (1990), to develop reflective habits on actions performed and this may help produce the definition of the caring attitude that has so long eluded nursing and which is an essential skill in the practice of counselling.

Four main areas come to mind.

Confidentiality

Confidentiality has always been seen as a right of all people with their medical practitioners. Often patients have made it more difficult for nursing to keep to the same rules without ever breaking them because of medicine's desire to be patriarchally dominant. Patients have often used this by telling nurses things which they know are taken to medical colleagues, the very people they were afraid for various reasons to talk with.

This is maybe to an extent be useful but what happens to the nurse when confidential information is given in the context of counselling. Yes we can all give straightforward immediate guidelines maybe even hide behind the law but how do we **feel**?

Reflective point
Try to think of an example of a situation where personal feeling and rules of confidentiality are superseded by the greater good.

You may have come to the same conclusion as Atkinson (1992) 'Dangerousness to others is usually taken as the major exception to the rule of confidentiality' (p. 114).

This argument has difficulties for the fact that the rules set up to protect children, for the client may break the very sense of trust that counsellors need to attain for effective therapeutic work to take place. A particularly vexing area concerns the Children's Act (1990). As a professional nurse we are obliged to divulge where potentially abusive situations may be occurring concerning children. However what if valuable work is being done with a survivor of abuse who still allows her abusing father access to what are his grandchildren. Breaking that rule of confidentiality may well lead to failure by the mother to disclose any further material and, as a result in perpetuating her serious self harming behaviour. Is there an **absolute** *moral right in that counselling situation?*

Power

Maintaining a healthy balance of power in helping relationships is essential. The abuse of power especially where gender is involved is an abuse which has been perpetuated in psychological terms since Freud and in open and blatant terms since the science of psychiatry emerged.

Women have, throughout psychiatric history, been labelled as the 'other' to men. This has been achieved by labelling, in terms of distress, analysing in terms of reinforcing male power over women's thought processes and even control when distressed women have refused to collude with what males have desired them to be.

In this respect the power imbalance between men and women in a counselling situation has not on the whole been as widely researched. But clearly the analogy of expert versus needing female consumer remains. The experts still have enormous powers over their clients because of the ability to find explanations for painful behaviours.

Power in counselling situations is, or at least should be, a totally different dimension. Counselling does not assume 'the power of the couch'

clients are not physically distanced from the one they are speaking with and to. It is a face-to-face type of situation.

Power can be asserted in a variety of other ways however. It can be used to great effect by the language the professional counsellor uses and that may not of necessity be anything at all to do with gender. The manner in which words are expressed is equally of great importance as well.

In counselling where the experience of loosing control of feelings is desired in order to promote catharsis, there is an inherent danger that the nurse will be afraid and seek to be over-controlling of expression. Power is not always sought in this situation for the sake of superiority but more often because a violent expression of feeling is not a something that we are used to dealing with, without making some effort to make it better for the person concerned and to 'control' their distress.

We can learn from feminist approaches to the expression of emotion which seem to have less difficulty in letting women just cry without always seeking to make things better and stop the flow of tears.

Truth

Reflective point
How far is essential that we know whether spoken distress is factually truthful?

The communication of distress is actually something that does not really require objective and literally truthful language. An interaction that is designed to be health promoting surely cannot be concerned with factual correctness.

What then as nurses are we asking for when we ask for details from patients? What parts of the nursing process are really needed to decide on nursing diagnosis and treatment plans or is it rather that we want to have all things factually correct for example.

Obviously where the person is alluding to incidents likely to cause harm to another, gentle probing to decide fact from fiction, words from potential action, is essential. In fact apart from physiological facts, how far do we actually know when patients are telling us the truth. Is it essential to know bowel habits in great degree of detail in all cases?

Is it essential to know the nature of relationships and the extent to which they are sexual or not? Clearly there are times when this information is essential, but then good use of questions is surely the key to the matter?

The opposite side of truth telling relates to truth taking. There can be little disputing the fact that patients now on the whole want to be made aware of the facts of their situation. It has, until recently, been the practice of doctors only to tell the truth when they felt the patient could take it. But such truth receiving maybe been selective.

We have assumed that patients may not wish to be told because of some catastrophic reaction to what is said. We were afraid to tell people they had cancer in case they gave up, however, we were pressured to tell a woman that she is needs have a hysterectomy. Clearly men felt that this was a medical problem and that the health needs (?) of the woman far outweigh the fact that her response might be a suicidal depression were not really considered.

Another dilemma of truth telling concerns the diagnosis of human immune deficiency virus (HIV) infection. Although clients may choose to undertake a test, the results of that diagnosis may not be withheld for fear that the person may transfer the disease to another. If a patient is suspected of having an HIV-related illness, we do not avoid telling them the truth.

Reflective point
How far can we defend non-disclosure of feelings in working with patients? In your notebook ask yourself how many times in the last week you have done precisely this.

Disclosing does not necessarily mean being out of control, what it does mean is being sufficiently self-aware that we can utilise the self in a therapeutic manner. Opening up to others and aiding them to be truthful in a health promoting way means opening up ourselves to ourselves in order that the truth-sharing growth can be a mutual event. Therefore also a truthful interaction (Johari Window, Luft, 1970).

Widening the arena of therapeutic communications

The National Health Service Community Care Act (1990) has opened up the arenas in which care is delivered to a remarkable degree. With this act, people, not only those with mental health problems, are being cared for within community settings and are on their own to a greater extent than ever before. We need therefore to make greater use of technology to increase communication efficiency.

It is likely that by the end of the century many of our clients will have as standard a video-telephone in the house, many will have modem and E-mail links, and trips to doctors and visits from nurses may have come a rarity.

In order to communicate with clients and to perform our roles we are having to struggle with more and more technology. Information super highways are no longer a dream but do they serve as communicators and will we have the technological imagination to use them so that communication becomes dialogue and not just diagnosis. Interaction has to be seen to be a means of delivering care efficiently and effectively.

The telephone is being used more and more to convey news to patients. However the telephone is possibly the most useful yet the most difficult means of conferring information. The problem is that it lacks human touch, a human face and human expression. We cannot get facial feedback from a phone. The message that we intended to give is lost and what is heard may not be what is said. The telephone may be used to inform relatives of major life events such as the death or dying phase of their life partner. How many times have we not been confronted by a grief stricken relative asking why did we not telephone quicker.

Suppose you have been asked to ring the local surgery for the results of a test. If the receptionist refuses to tell to tell you the result over the phone you immediately fear the worst. We cannot ever know how the person is responding on the other end of the telephone. The joy of a positive pregnancy test for one woman can be the final breaking point for another which tips her over into an attempt at suicide. We would never know.

This is, of course, in marked contrast to its use as a counselling service for times of crisis or when problems are so fearful that the impersonality of the telephone is its point of value. Helplines and Crisis Intervention are increasingly being taken up by survivors of all types of medical and social disasters and we have much to learn from the training methods of Samaritans and other telephone counselling services.

In the new world of information the whole balance of power in terms of information is shifting. The practice waiting rooms are full of booklets and helpful information about all types of prevention and information. The written word as a means of health-changing behaviour is accepted, but little time outside of psychotherapy is devoted to allowing the therapeutic release of emotion and monitoring of client performance in making changes.

We are not accustomed to clients writing in their care plans on the whole though, there are exceptions. We have little time, for example, to discuss with them their feelings that may have been written in **their** progress charts.

The written word when in journal form is an immensely powerful tool, yet it could so easily be part of the monitoring of progress that we are all so intent on recording. Why in hospitals is much written about patients and not by them?

Reflective point

What function does the telephone have in your working life, how could you utilise it to better effect in promoting interactions between you and your patients. How many times in the last month have you thought you have missed an unspoken message on the telephone because you could only listen and could not see the person's face at the other end?.

Did they later on when you were with them indicate that they were trying to tell you something? Did you feel that they had been checking you out in some way?

Endings

Nurses in whatever arena they work have to end relationships. They are so much part of the work that we do not usually think about them. Goodbyes are not only significant when they come

after a long period, or after times of crisis. The contact clients have with us may have been a matter or minutes or weeks but we may never learn what happened to them. Peplau (1988) focuses on the effects of relationships between nurses and clients ending. The termination phase of working between client and nurse is marked by reviewing what has been achieved and the effects the lack of the relationship will have on each other. This allows time for the nurse to reflect on how far she/he may have guided the client towards a goal of being more healthy than at the start of the relationship. Peplau never intended her model to be used solely within the arena of psychiatric nursing but inevitably that is its prime focus.

In a cost-centred health delivery system we have little time to sit and asses the value of what we are doing. The concept of celebrating recovery is usually left to major arenas of trauma or life threatening disease. What of the older person who recovers from a minor operation or problem which had ruined his/her life for several years? It is easy not to register the momentousness of that relief. Recovery is usually marked nowadays by a rushed exit with a prescription in one hand and the knowledge that by the time you have turned the corner of the ward another person may well be lying in your bed.

It is a mistake to equate departure with healing and health. The person leaving may only be leaving to return even if they are to all intents healthier than on arrival.

We refer on, we make sure there is another expert to help resolve the problem. Buckman (1992) guards against the defence of referral when really what we are doing is defending our anxiety about lack of progress.

If we allow ourselves to practice a little of what Peplau called getting inside the skin of a patient to see what they are thinking, without thinking as they are thinking, then alleviating anxiety may discourage the need for referral to another.

For some people referral requires a great degree of tact diplomacy and patience. We cannot escape the fact that for the patient referral to either a geriatrician or the local hospice does carry with it emotions that need to be resolved before for them the ultimate ending (death) can be faced.

For an increasing number of people referral can mean the beginning of a series of long and protracted illnesses as a result of HIV infection. In this arena we are learning more about interaction as therapy than in many other arenas. (See for example work done at the London Lighthouse.)

Ending can be sudden dramatic and painful for all concerned. The survivors of a suicide on a ward are as traumatised as partners and next of kin. Stresses to the carer are dealt with in elsewhere in this book (see Chapter 7).

> ### Reflective point
> *Who do you refer yourself to in order to maintain an optimum mental health state for yourself?*
>
> *Is it a trusted colleague outside of your sphere of work, or, does your long-suffering partner bear the brunt of it all?*

A brief reflection on supervision

At this time the provision of supervision as a personal resource for the practising nurse is seen as being an essential provision that must be seen to be part of practice and not a psychotherapeutic luxury belonging only to those who practice psychotherapy for whom supervision is vital to practice [see Faugier and Butterworth (1992)].

Menzies (1960) wrote of the defence systems that nurses used to defend themselves against their anxiety in dealing with the emotional stresses they had to face. These defensive behaviours were those which essentially kept the nurses emotionally distant from their clients. This was in part an early response to nursing's emergence as a fledgling discipline in its own right. As nursing moved on and developed it began in various ways and by various means to act more independently of doctors and other professions. As a result of this individual practitioners were faced in very personal ways with looking at themselves and beginning to question whether their emotional or professional skills were equal to the task being expected of them.

This is particularly true of the movement, towards more in-depth personal relationships with patients. Nursing moved towards individuality and nurse–patient partnership, with a large amount of influence of American theorists including Peplau.

As nursing changed so did the supervision and training of nurses. Students began to have mentors. As a result courses of training were devised which sought to prepare practitioners to supervise and teach students.

In July 1989 the ENB published a circular which concerned the 'Preparation of Teacher, Practitioners, Mentors and Supervisors in the context of Project 2000' This cardinal document introduced the concept of supervision and set about defining it in a way that previously had not been readily known outside of psychotherapy.

Supervision therefore arrived within nursing parlance and, for some, had connotations of managerialism, maintaining standards and enforcing some element of supervision. For others, as Faugier and Butterworth (1992) point out supervision has equal connotations of preventing staff burnout and recognising stress. This, they say it does, but is not the whole story by any means.

Supervision, according to these authors, is more than informal chats in tea breaks. It is a personal, structured system whereby skills are developed, expanded and the personal ethos of the practitioner is explored.

Wright (1989) in Butterworth and Faugier offer what seems to the writer to be one of the most succinct definitions. He draws together what is sometime a divide between the skill-based type of supervision that is characteristic of more practice-based branches of nursing and the more psychodynamic stance of, for example, either mental or learning disabilities nursing. He says

> Supervision is a meeting between two or more people who have a declared interest in examining a piece of work. The work is presented and they will together think about what was happening and why, what was done or said, and how it was handled – could it have been handled better or differently, and if so, how? (p. 11).

It is important to remember that supervision, whatever theory or model is used, must result in the improvement of the service delivered to the recipient of care. Alongside this there has to be the element of increasing skills and personal development. As such supervision has to have structure, purpose and a defined function in the life of both the individual and the organisation that they are a part of.

In short it must work efficiently and be seen as much a part of the nurses' clinical life as the giving of nursing to the client.

It must be business-like, structured and have rules of conduct that are an established part of any group work undertaken with clients. The nature of those sessions may well encompass personal developmental material, but equally they must also have an element of reflection and presentation of case work to supervisor and colleagues. It is from this that real learning derives.

Supervision is a life long process (Faugier and Butterworth, 1992). It allows for personal and professional development and increases the level of personal self awareness which is essential if nursing is to remain dynamic and onward moving.

The new idea of today is the straightjacket of tomorrow.

Conclusions

In the course of this chapter, various aspects of interpersonal relationships have been explored. The art of relating and communicating is at the heart of what we do. What we have attempted is to ask how much of what we take for granted as a skill that all nurses possess, actually exists? The therapeutic value of interpersonal interaction with our consumers depends on how well we know ourselves. How willing we are to engage in self-reflection and growth that can ultimately produce not only better-informed practice but also better balanced and health-aware practitioners. If we have learnt more about communicating with each other by knowing ourselves then the most basic of all nursing functions, caring, has a health function.

To care for others we have to care for the self. Caring involves reflection, learning and refining theory before using it clinically. It involves reflecting retrospectively on a difficult situation and asking how may it be handled more healthily next time.

References

Atkinson, J. (1992). Autonomy and mental health. In Barker, P. and Baldwin, S. (eds). *Ethical Issues and Mental Health.* Chapman & Hall, London.

Audit Commission Report No. 12 (1993). *What Seems to be the Matter: Communication between Hospitals and Patients.* HMSO, Bristol.

Bayne, R. and Nicholson, P. (1994). *Counselling and Psychology for Health Professionals.* Chapman & Hall, London.

Buckman, R. (1992). *How to Break Bad News.* PaperMac, London.

Burnard, P. (1994). *Counselling Skills for Health Professionals*, 2nd edn. Chapman & Hall, London.

Butterworth, T. and Faugier, J. (1992). *Clinical Supervision and Mentorship in Nursing.* Chapman & Hall, London.

Department of Health (1990). *The National Health Service and Community Care Act.* HMSO, London.

Dickson, A. (1982). *A Woman in your Own Right: Assertiveness and You.* Quartet, London.

Dickson, O., Saunders, C. and Stringer, M. (1993). *Rewarding People, The Skill of Responding Positively.* Routledge, London.

Ehrenreich, B. and English, D. (1988). *For Her Own Good. 150 Years of the Experts' Advice to Women.* Pluto Press, England.

Farrell, G. (1991). How accurately do nurses perceive patients' needs? A comparison of general and psychiatric settings. *Journal of Advanced Nursing,* 16, 1062–1070.

Faugier, J. and Butterworth, T. (1992). Clinical supervision. A position paper. University of Manchester.

Finch, J. and Groves, D. (1985). Community care and the family: a case for equal opportunities. In Ungerson, C. (ed.) *Women and Social Policy – A Reader.* Macmillan Press, London.

Fiske, S. T. and Taylor, S. E. (1984). *Social Cognition.* Random House, New York.

Goffman, E. (1963). *Stigma, Notes on the Management of a Spoiled Identity.* Prentice-Hall, Englewood Cliffs, NJ.

Gross, R. D. (1992). *Psychology. The Science of Mind and Behaviour.* Hodder & Stoughton, London.

Halman, M. A. and Alpen, M. A. (1993). The impact of technology on patients and families. *Nursing Clinics of North America,* 28 June, 2, 443–457.

Johnson, M. and Webb, C. (1995). Rediscovering unpopular patients: the impact of social judgement. *Journal of Advanced Nursing,* 21, 466–475.

Kagan, C. and Evans, J. (1995). *Professional Interpersonal Skills for Nurses.* Chapman & Hall, London.

Luft, J. (1970). *Group Processes – An Introduction to Group Dynamics.* Mayfield.

McCann, K. and McKenna. H. P. (1993). An examination of touch between nurses and elderly patients in a continuing care setting in Northern Ireland. *Journal of Advanced Nursing,* May 18(5), 838–846.

McCorkle, R. and Quint-Benedict, J. (1983). Symptom distress, current concerns and mood disturbance after diagnosis of life threatening disease. *Social Science and Medicine,* 17(7), 431–438.

McMahon, R. and Pearson, A. (1991). *Nursing as Therapy.* Chapman & Hall, London.

Mathes, E. (1975). The effects of physical attractions and anxiety on heterosexual attraction over a series of 5 encounters. *Journal of Marriage and Family*, 37, 769–773.

Menzies, I. (1960). *The Functioning of Social Systems as a Defence against Anxiety; A Report on a Study of the Nursing Service of a General Hospital.* Tavistock Publications, London.

Muetzel, P. (1988). Therapeutic nursing. In Pearson, A. (ed.) *Primary Nursing: Nursing in the Burford and Oxford Nursing Development Units.* Croom Helm, London

Peplau, H. (1988). *Interpersonal Relations in Nursing*, 2nd edn. Macmillan, London.

Peplau, H. (1994). *Interpersonal Theory in Nursing*. In O'Toole, A. W. and Welt, S. R. (eds) (1994). *Hildegard Peplau. Selected Works.* Macmillan, London.

Reece, J. (1995). Patriarchy and power in mental health services. Unpublished MA dissertation, University of Loughborough.

Sackville-West, V. (1986). *All Passion Spent*. Virago Press, London (first published 1931).

Salmon, P. (1993). The reduction of anxiety in surgical patients, an important nursing task or the medicalization of preparatory worry. *International Journal of Nursing Studies*, 30 August, 4, 323–360.

Selye, H. (1956). *The Stresses of Life*. McGraw-Hill, New York.

Shiell, J. and Shiell, A. (1991). The prevalence of psychiatric morbidity on a coronary care ward. *Journal of Advanced Nursing*, 16(9), 1071–1077.

Sines, D. (1994). The arrogance of power: a reflection on contemporary mental health nursing practice. *Journal of Advanced Nursing*, 20, 894–903.

Stockwell, F. (1972). *The Unpopular Patient*. RCN Publications, London, reprinted Croom Helm (1984).

Sundeen, S. J., Stuart, G. W., Rankin, E. A. and Cohen, S. A. (1989). *Nurse–Client Interaction. Implementing the Nursing Process.* C. V. Mosby, St Louis.

Teasdale, K. (1993). Information and anxiety: a critical appraisal. *Journal of Advanced Nursing Journal*, 18(7), 1125–1132.

Undern *et al.* (1993). Positive effects of increased nurse support for male patients after acute myocardial infarction. *Quality Life Research*, 2 April, 2, 121–127.

Unger, R. and Crawford, M. (1992). *Women and Gender. A Feminist Psychology*. McGraw-Hill, New York.

Van Hooft, S. (1990). Moral education for nursing decisions. *Journal of Advanced Nursing*, 15, 210–215.

Wright, H. (1989). *Groupwork: perspectives and practice*. Scutari Press, Oxford.

Further reading

The following are a selection of works that you may find useful in further developing both skill in interaction and gaining more confidence in looking into various aspects of the self.

They are essentially a personal selection but they all have a good contribution to make to our development of interpersonal skills.

Backer, S. L. (1994). *To Listen, To Comfort, To Care.* Delmar Publications. A new introduction to the subject.

Buckman, R. (1995). *How to Break Bad News.* PaperMac, London. Excellent, sometimes witty but a clear way of dealing with the subject, even though it is orientated towards doctors.

Burnard, P. (1994). *Counselling Skills for Health Professionals.* Chapman & Hall, London. This text is frequently referred to in the book in both direct and indirect ways. It is an essential text. It expands on areas covered here and is full of reflective exercises and comment. Succinctly gives the reader a theoretical basis to the practice of counselling.

Burton, G. and Dimbleby, D. (1991). *Between Ourselves.* Edward Arnold. This text is concerned with perception. How do we converse and how we present ourselves to others? The style is good and clear.

Ernst, S. and Goodison, L. (1986). *In Our Own Hands. A Book of Self Help Therapy.* The Women's Press. This is an excellent text to have because it is fun. It is of particular relevance to women. It also gives practical advice in the setting up of a self-help group. A topic becoming far more a part of our work.

Faugier, J. and Butterworth, T. (1992). *Clinical Supervision. A Position Paper.* University of Manchester. A highly readable report, the contents of which will make you ask why are not all nurses having supervision. It is not just for psychiatric nurses.

Kagan, C. and Evans, J. (1995). *Professional Interpersonal Skills for Nurses.* Chapman & Hall, London. This has been referred to a great deal and is an excellent handbook to work through, either individually or as a part of a learning package.

Luft, J. (1970). *Group Processes – An Introduction to Group Dynamics.* Mayfield. This text is a classic which explores dynamics fundamental to all group work. This includes teaching group work and training groups and communication in various types of group. The resolving of conflict in groups is also covered.

Margie, O., Saunders, C. and Dickson, D. (1994). *Social Skills in Interpersonal Counselling*. Guide to the basics in the counselling relationship, with a useful chapter on rewards

O'Toole, A. W. and Welt, S. R. (1994). *Hildegard Peplau. Selected Works*. Macmillan, London. Some of Peplau's best contributions to nursing theory. The developing relationship between nurse and patient and their stages re-visited in very thought-provoking ways. Essential reading for any psychiatric nurse!

Patterson, C. H. (1986). *Theories of Counselling and Psychotherapy*. Harper Collins, New York. An easily readable text. Whilst in some ways specialist, it gives a fairly comprehensive summary of Carl Rogers in particular (Chapter 14).

Rowan, J. (1988). *Ordinary Ecstasy*. Routledge. An introduction to humanistic psychology and self-awareness.

Some useful organisations which may help you with training

Remember advertisements which appear in the general press may not be right for you and may not be accredited in any way. Contact:

British Association of Counselling
1 Regent Place, Rugby, Warwickshire CV1 2PJ.

Your local branch of Cruse.

Your local university may run courses in counselling and psychotherapy, but they may well require you to be a graduate.

The local Relate branch often runs training for counselling, but may assume that you will do some work for them as well.

7

UNDERSTANDING STRESS AND ITS IMPLICATIONS FOR HEALTH-CARE PROFESSIONALS

Lynette Rentoul, Veronica Thomas and Robert Rentoul

Introduction

The aim of this chapter is to explore the nature of stress, its determinants and its repercussions. Special attention will be paid to the relationship between stress, health and illness, and the factors which mediate between stress and ill-health. The growing literature on the stress of caring and consequent need for coping strategies and support among nurses will be explored. In this way nurses will gain an enhanced understanding of their client groups, themselves as professional carers and the impact of the organisation in which they work.

The concept of stress, although generating a considerable degree of discussion and research, remains somewhat elusive. Selye (1976), one of the founding fathers of stress research, suggests that it suffers 'from the mixed blessing of being too well known and too little understood'. As Cox (1978) points out, 'it is a concept which is familiar to both layman and professional alike; it is understood by all when used in a general context but by very few when a more precise account is required, and this seems to be the central problem'. When you hear people say that they are under stress you understand what they mean, and because of the pervasiveness and commonality of these experiences it seems logical to assume that precise definition and conceptualisation would

not pose problems. This however is not the case. Despite a huge volume of research and interest in the subject, stress remains an elusive phenomenon. Nonetheless, the development of the concept of stress has contributed significantly to a current understanding of health and illness and is a central concept in the growing discipline of health psychology. The relationship between stress and illness has been the focus of much interest in health psychology; this includes consideration of both illness as stressor and the role that stress plays in the development of disease. Understanding health also demands a consideration of factors that have grown out of stress research such as work on coping, personal resilience and hardiness.

For all these reasons it is important that nurses should have a good understanding of stress. Health promotion, taking positive action to prevent unnecessary stress and implementing health strategies to minimise the impact of long-term stress, demands a good working knowledge of healthy coping strategies and the determinants of hardiness. If nurses lack such understanding they may be less able to manage their own lives effectively, less able to work efficiently, they may unwittingly increase their clients' experience of stress or miss opportunities to promote healthy coping strategies.

Stress tends to be thought of in negative terms. It is important to recognise that stress does not always need to be seen in this way. Indeed as Selye pointed out, some stress may act as a great spur to achievement, especially among performers and in the field of competitive sports. For most people, life has to be challenging enough, that is, interesting enough for us not to become bored and suffer from the consequences of lack of stimulation or repetitive stimulation. In this sense some stress can be seen in terms of challenge and excitement and is viewed as a good thing. However, in the field of occupational stress among health-care professionals there is increased recognition that even medium levels of stress, especially in the long term, are not conducive to well-being and effectiveness in the workplace.

Theoretical approaches to the study of stress

Stress has been conceptualised in three ways. One approach focuses upon the environment, describing stress as a stimulus. This would be the case, for example, if one describes going to the dentist as stressful or as having a job which is stressful. Events or circumstances that we perceive as threatening or harmful and which produce feelings of tension are called **stressors**. Researchers (e.g. Holmes and Rahe, 1967) who follow this approach are like to study a wide range of stressors, such as major life events or difficulties in the workplace.

The second approach considers stress as a response. In this case people refer to stress as the reaction that they feel in themselves, or the sense of tension they feel in response to threatening external events. People may, for example, refer to feeling a lot of stress when facing difficult situations, such as breaking bad news to patients or clients. The person's psychological and physiological response to a stressor is referred to as **strain**.

The third approach describes stress as a process that includes stressors and strains, but in addition adds the dimension of the relationship between the person and the environment (Cox, 1978; Lazarus and Launier, 1978; Lazarus and Folkman, 1984a, b). The emphasis of this work is upon the continuous interactions and adjustments, called transactions, between the person and the environment with each affecting and being affected by the other. According to this view stress is neither a stimulus nor a response but a process in which the way that the person thinks about and responds to the events is a crucial factor in understanding the stress experience. For example, a group of people might be in the same situation, such as a traffic jam, but their response to this may be quite different. Some people might become irate and shout and honk the horn, whilst others might sit back, turn on the radio and listen to music. In a medical setting people can respond quite differently too; some nurses might find observing an operation distressing, whilst others might be intensely interested in the clinical procedure and not at all disturbed by it.

The elaboration of this work has been referred to as the cognitive phenomenological transactional (CPT) view of stress and coping (see Bailey and Clark, 1989, p. 21). The model is cognitive because it contains the assumption that thinking, memory, and the meaning and significance of events to the individual experiencing them, are central mediators in determining levels of stress and coping. It is phenomenological because it concerns itself with the highly individual meaning of events, and finally it is transactional because it emphasises the interaction between the appraisals made by individuals and the settings in which they find themselves. For the nurse and the patient the context of these appraisals will be the environment of the hospital. In addition to the appraisal of the situation is the appraisal by the individual of his or her capacity to cope with the threat. Lazarus (1966) conceptualised three types of appraisal: **primary appraisal** is when the individual assesses the challenges of demands made by the situation; **secondary appraisal** is the individual's estimate of his or her ability to cope, that is, the 'counter-harm' resources; **reappraisal** entails a check on the relative effectiveness of any coping behaviour adopted by the individual to reduce or remove the source of threat. The similarity between this process and the nursing process has been pointed out by Bailey and Clark (1989), that is, the assessment of problems, planning to cope with problems, carrying out the plan, and reassessment of the strategies. When this view of stress and coping is presented, its application and elegance as a practical model for nurses to guide them in dealing with both their own and the patient's stress becomes evident.

Sources of stress

When we think of the sources of stress in our lives, what do we think of? Is it a longish list of what the literature refers to as the 'daily hassles of life', problems with our work colleagues, the difficulties of getting to work in long traffic jams, the problems of juggling child-care arrangements with demands of work and trying to get work done with tight deadlines or limited resources? Or do we think of more significant events, such as dealing with the death of a loved one, dealing with sudden traumatic events in hospital, facing the aftermath of divorce or living with severely disabling chronic illness? The literature on stress includes all these areas, though the emphasis is not upon the events themselves but on the way in which those events are experienced.

Daily hassles of life

Some of the stress we experience comes from lesser events, such as misplacing keys or public speaking. Some people experience more of these kinds of daily hassle than others. Lazarus and colleagues (Kanner *et al.*, 1981) have developed a scale to measure daily hassles that lists 117 items that range from mild annoyances such as silly practical mistakes to major ones like not having enough money for food. Subjects list the number of events and indicate whether they have been somewhat, moderately or extremely severe. The half-dozen most frequent hassles reported were:

- concerns about weight
- health of a family member
- rising prices of common goods
- home maintenance
- too many things to do
- misplacing or losing things.

This scale has been found to be useful and practical.

Life events

One approach to stress which emphasised external pressure was Holmes and Rahe's (1967) work on life events. Although it is not possible to list events that are stressful in the same way for all people, the life events research sought to quantify major life changes in an attempt to gauge accurately their

impact. A list of life events (major happenings in a person's life that require some degree of psychological adjustment) is developed into a scale with each event assigned a value that reflects the degree of stressfulness. The most widely used scale is the Social Readjustment Rating Scale (SRRS) developed by Holmes and Rahe (1967) (see Table 7.1). It includes a fairly wide range of events that people are likely to find stressful. The values assigned to the events were carefully determined from a large sample. One of the main uses of the SRRS has been to relate stress and illness. Many studies have adopted a retrospective approach, asking people to recall stressful events and illness over the past year or more. Other approaches have combined retrospective and prospective methods, for example, by having patients report recent life events and then following their medical record over the coming months. Studies using this approach have generally found that illness and accident rates were related to an increase in life events (Holmes and Masuda, 1974; Johnson, 1986; Rahe, 1987). However, a number of problems have arisen in interpreting the relationship between life events and illness. One problem is that there is little scope for considering the different individual meanings of particular events. Another reason is that the SRRS has items that are vague or ambiguous. No place was given in this work to the appraisal of different events and to the different views that individuals have of their own abilities to deal with events. The emphasis of work now has shifted away from categorising and attempting to quantify life events towards considering appraisal of events and their individual meanings.

In an attempt to build upon some of the advantages of the life events work and to minimise the shortcomings, other researchers have attempted to devise more precise scales. For example, Lewinsohn *et al.* (1985) developed the Unpleasant Events Schedule (UES). In this scale the items are divided into a number of categories such as sexual, marital, friendship and achievement, academic and job. Subjects are asked to rate each item on a three-point scale twice, for frequency and for unpleasantness. These ratings are multiplied, and a total score is summed for the entire schedule.

Post-traumatic stress syndrome

One area where events are seen to be stressful for the majority of people is the area of sudden

Table 7.1. *The Social Readjustment Rating Scale (Holmes and Rahe, 1967)*

Rank	Life event	Mean value
1	Death of spouse	100
2	Divorce	73
3	Marital separation	65
4	Jail term	63
5	Death of close family member	63
6	Personal injury or illness	53
7	Marriage	50
8	Fired at work	47
9	Marital reconciliation	45
10	Retirement	45
11	Change in health of family member	44
12	Pregnancy	40
13	Sex difficulties	39
14	Gain of new family member	39
15	Business readjustment	39
16	Change in financial state	38
17	Death of close friend	37
18	Change to different line of work	36
19	Change in number of arguments with spouse	35
20	Mortgage over $10,000*	31
21	Foreclosure of mortgage or loan	30
22	Change in responsibilites at work	29
23	Son or daughter leaving home	29
24	Trouble with in-laws	29
25	Outstanding personal achievement	28
26	Wife begins to stop work	26
27	Begin or end school	26
28	Change in living conditions	25
29	Revision of personal habits	24
30	Trouble with boss	23
31	Change in work hours or conditions	20
32	Change in residence	20
33	Change in schools	20
34	Change in recreation	19
35	Change in church activities	19
36	Change in social activities	18
37	Mortgage or loan less than $10,000*	17
38	Change in sleeping habits	16
39	Change in number of family get-togethers	15
40	Change in eating habits	15
41	Vacation	13
42	Christmas	12
43	Minor violations in the law	11

Interpretation of total score:
• a score of up to 149 describes no life crisis
• a score between 150 and 199 describes a mild life crisis
• a score between 200 and 299 describes a moderate life crisis
• a score over 300 desribes a major life crisis.
If your score is high you might like to consider whether it is possible to postpone any events requiring further adjustments in your life over which you may have some control, such as moving house, to prevent your score from rising still further.

*Note that in 1967, $10,000 constituted a substantial financial burden. This figure would need to be considerably increased to match today's equivalent.

traumatic events and disaster. The research which has grown out of a number of naturally occurring disasters during the late 1980s, such as the sinking of the ferry *The Spirit of Free Enterprise*, the fire at King's Cross station, the train crash at Clapham Junction and the Lockerbie air crash has developed a number of principles and themes with regard to the aftermath of disasters. The majority of people are disturbed in the short term, but a significant minority of people go on to develop what is referred to as post-traumatic stress disorder (PTSD). The main symptoms include a pervasive sense of numbness and estrangement, phobias, nightmares reliving the trauma, and anxiety which may show itself as sleep disturbance and difficulty in concentrating (Figley, 1986).

Stress of hospitalisation

For those working in the hospital environment it is important not to lose sight of how stressful it can be for patients and their families. There is now considerable evidence that hospitalisation is a stressful experience (see, for example, Franklin, 1974; Wilson-Barnett, 1986). A number of studies in the past 20 years have identified specific stressors, measured stress responses and evaluated attempts to alleviate stress (e.g. Langer *et al.*, 1975; Wilson-Barnett and Carrigy, 1978; Johnson, 1983; Wilson-Barnett, 1984). It is clearly essential for health-care professionals to be aware of the sources of stress for individual patients, so that they can prevent or reduce the impact of the stressful features of being in hospital and receiving nursing and medical care. Many patients feel that they lack information, or are provided with conflicting information, and do not have adequate opportunity to discuss the concerns that they might have. Greater insight might be gained by using the Hospital Stress Rating Scale which was created by Volicer and Bonhannon (1975) to assess the degree of stress associated with different aspects of care.

Work-related stress

Much work has been carried out on stress in the workplace, for example Hingley and Cooper (1986) provide an excellent review. They cite a range of factors that are intrinsic to particular jobs, including working conditions, work load and shift-work. They consider, too, the individual's role *vis-à-vis* the overall work organisation. This includes the degree of role ambiguity, of role conflict, and of responsibility for other people. Another area of potential stress is relationships at work; this includes relationships with colleagues of equal status, relationships with superiors and subordinates as well as with other professional groups and clients. Factors outside the working environment, such as home life, may also effect one's capacity to work productively. Stresses encountered by nurses in their place of work will be considered in more detail in a later section.

Biological responses to stress

Anyone who has experienced a very frightening event, such as near accident or other emergency, knows that there are physiological reactions to stress, for instance heartbeat and breathing rates increase, skeletal muscles may tremble, we may be aware of a sick feeling in the stomach. The body is aroused and is prepared for action. In the early part of this century, the French physiologist Claude Bernard (1927) demonstrated that a basic feature of all multicellular organisms is their ability to maintain the physical and chemical composition of the immediate fluid environment of their cells within a specific range that ensures optimal cellular functioning. Organisms are able to do this despite wide fluctuations in the external environment. Following on from this work Cannon (1932) recognised that the internal composition of the cells are repeatedly disturbed by the metabolic activities of the organism, and in the face of this, attempt to maintain relative constancy of the internal environment. This process he called homoeostasis. This refers to the tendency of the internal fluid environment to return to a steady state after each fluctuation. There are a huge number of homoeostatic mechanisms which maintain life and health, and the function of these continues to be of great interest to physiologists. In addition to his work on homoeostatic mechanisms, Cannon (1929) provided a basic description of how the body reacts to emergencies. The reaction has been called the 'fight or flight' response, because it prepares the organism to attack the threat or to escape from it.

General adaptation syndrome

What happens when the body is exposed to long periods of stress? Hans Selye a well-known researcher in this field, studied animals and people exposed to stress over extensive periods of time (Selye, 1956, 1976, 1985). Through his researches he found that the fight or flight response is only the first in a series of reactions the body makes when it is exposed to extensive stress. Selye called this series of physiological reactions the general adaptation syndrome (GAS), which it is composed of three main stages.

Alarm reaction

The first stage of the GAS is like the 'fight or flight' response to an emergency, and its function is to mobilise the body's resources. At the very beginning of the alarm reaction, arousal (as measured by blood pressure, for example) drops below normal for a moment, but then quickly rises to above normal. This fast increasing arousal results from the release of hormones by the endocrine system; the pituitary gland secretes adrenocorticotrophic hormone (ACTH), which causes a heightened release of adrenaline, noradrenaline and cortisol by the adrenal glands into the bloodstream. By the end of this stage of the GAS, the body is fully mobilised to resist the stressor strongly, but the body cannot maintain the intense arousal of the alarm reaction for very long. If the stress is extremely intense and unavoidable, and the alarm reaction continues unabated the organism may die within hours or days.

Stage of resistance

If a strong stressor continues but is not strong enough to cause death, the physiological reaction enters the stage of resistance. In this stage, the body tries to adapt to the stressor. Physiological arousal declines somewhat but remains higher than normal, and the body replenishes the hormones released by the adrenal glands. Despite this continuous physiological arousal, the organism may show few outward signs of stress, but the ability to resist new stressors is impaired. According to Selye, one outcome of this impairment is that the organism becomes increasingly vulnerable to health problems, which he referred to as 'diseases of adaptation'. These health problems include ulcers, high blood pressure, asthma, and illnesses that result from impaired immune function. They will be discussed in detail in a later section.

Stage of exhaustion

Prolonged physiological arousal produced by severe, long-term or repeated stress is costly. It depletes the body's energy reserves until the physical ability to resist is very limited. At this point, the stage of exhaustion begins. If the stress continues, disease and physiological damage becomes increasingly likely and death may occur.

Selye called the GAS 'general' because it was produced only by agents which he described as having a general effect on the body; he called it 'adaptive' because it produced a state of habituation and stimulated defence or resistance and survival in response to demand. His broad concept of stress has been very influential in understanding responses to stressful stimuli, but his ideas have been updated in response to increased knowledge drawn from both physiology and psychology.

Selye believed that the GAS is non-specific with regard to the type of stressor. That is, the series of physiological reactions described in the GAS will occur regardless of the source of the stress. However the notion of non-specificity fails to take important psychosocial variables into account. There are two reasons why this is a problem. One reason is that some stressors elicit a stronger emotional response than others. Selye (1975) pointed out that 'emotional stimuli rank very high among the most potent and prevalent natural stimuli capable of increasing pituitary–adrenal cortical activity'. In other words, stressors are most likely to trigger the release of large amounts of cortisol, adrenaline and noradrenaline if the individual's response includes a strong element of emotion.

The second reason is that cognitive appraisal appears to play an important role in people's physiological reactions to stress. A study by Tennes and Kreye (1985) assessed cortisol levels in urine samples of children taken on regular school-days and on days when school examinations were given. The expected increase in cortisol on examination days was found, but not for all children: their intelligence was an important variable. Cortisol levels increased only for children with above-average intelligence; this was not the case for children with average and below-average intel-ligence. The influence of intelligence suggests that the brighter children were more concerned about academic achievement and, as a result, appraised the tests as more threatening than other children.

The stress response

The stress response has both physiological and psychological components. Both represent attempts at coping with, reducing or removing, the source of threat. Physiological responses to stress occur at a reflexive level, although they are influenced by cog-nitive factors (Mason, 1971; Frankenhauser, 1975). In contrast, psychological coping strategies are largely based upon learning and are therefore influenced by social and cultural factors. The stress response can be functional and adaptive, in that it leads to physiological, mental and behavioural adjustments which enable the individual to cope. If coping is successful when dealing with immediate problems, then it is likely that the capacity to deal with future threats will be enhanced. However, if coping is ineffective then stress increases, and this may have long-term negative consequences on health. There may be structural and functional damage, resulting in ill-health, exhaustion and in extreme cases death.

Physiological responses to stress

Contemporary physiological studies of responses to stress concentrate on the neural and endocrino-logical mechanisms that mediate stress. Using the notion of homoeostasis or biological equilibrium, Cannon combined physiological and psycho-logical concepts in his analysis of fight or flight reactions, mediated by the sympatho-adrenal system, in particular the adrenal medulla, and the hormones adrenaline and noradrenaline. Both physical and emotional challenges to homoeostasis triggered this response, and there was a critical level of stress when such homoeostatic mechan-isms fail. The main effects of the catecholamines (adrenaline and noradrenaline) are listed in Table 7.2

Selye introduced the concept of the GAS as an attempt to identify the non-specific response to any disease or demand. This shifted attention to the adrenal cortex and the glucocorticoid hor-mone, and linked the three stages of the alarm response already described to specific physio-

Table 7.2. *Main actions of adrenaline and noradrenaline (catecholamines)*

Organ/system	Effect
Heart	Increased cardiac output
Blood vessels	Dilation of arterioles supplying skeletal muscle, constriction of arterioles supplying gut and skin
Respiratory system	Increased respiratory rate Bronchodilation
Nervous system	Increased arousal
Eyes	Pupil dilation
Metabolic effects	Glycogen breakdown to form glucose for energy production fat breakdown to release fatty acids for energy production

logical responses. The initial alarm reaction was linked with immediate activation of the sympatho-adrenomedullary system; the stage of resistance linked with the activation of the hypothalamus–pituitary–adrenal (HPA) axis; the general adapta-tion to this, in stage three of the reaction to stress, is characterised by adrenal hypertrophy, gastro-intestinal ulceration, and thymic and lymphoid shrinkage; and finally there is exhaustion and in extreme cases, death. The main effects of the glucocorticoids are listed in Table 7.3 and the symptoms of the general stress response are given in Table 7.4.

Contemporary approaches to unravelling the physiological responses to stress are concerned with the elucidation of the mechanisms underlying an integrated and interactive system which prod-uces the behavioural, physiological, and biochemi-cal changes in an attempt to return to homoeostasis. A stressor in this model is something which disrupts homoeostasis; it may be physical from the internal environment, such as anoxia or hypoglycaemia; external, such as heat or cold, noxious stimuli, or physical strain; or mixed, such as exercise or injury. Psychological stressors are conceived of as stimuli that affect emotion, generating fear, anxiety, and frustration, and are very potent activators of the HPA axis.

Bernard's notion of 'adaptation', developed at the end of the last century, described the stabilising of the internal environment in the face of external changes. It has been revised and developed to

Table 7.3. *Main actions of the glucocorticoids*

Function	Effect
Carbohydrate and fat metabolism	Inhibits glucose intake at tissues, except for brain and heart, thus increasing blood glucose levels Stimulates glucose production from stored glycogen, proteins and fats
Protein	Breaks down protein molecules
Metabolism	Depresses protein synthesis (including immunoglobulins) Deaminates; increases urea production
Immune system	Decreases mass of all lymphatic tissues
Inflammatory response	Reduces inflammation
Other functions	May enhance learning Enhances urinary excretion Promotes gastric secretion and development of peptic ulcers

Note: the effect of the glucocorticoids is slower and longer-lasting than that of the catecholamines.

Table 7.4. *List of symptoms associated with stress*

- General irritability
- Pounding of the heart
- Dryness of the throat and mouth
- Impulsive behaviour
- Urge to cry, run, or hide
- Poor concentration
- Feelings of weakness and/or dizziness
- Becoming easily fatigued
- Free-floating anxiety
- Hypervigilance; being 'keyed up' and easily startled
- Trembling, nervous twitching
- Giggling, nervous laughter
- Stuttering or other speech defects
- Teeth grinding
- Disturbed sleep/insomnia
- Feeling fidgety
- Unusually frequent urination
- Diarrhoea, nausea, vomiting
- Migraine headaches
- Lower back or neck pain
- Loss of appetite
- Increased smoking
- Increased alcohol comsumption
- Other drug use
- Nightmares
- Accident proneness

encompass the notion of behavioural adaptation. This is conceived of as the facilitation of adaptive (and the inhibition of non-adaptive) neural pathways to cope with stress, and may involve altered cognitive and sensory thresholds, increased alertness, selective enhancement of memory, stress-induced analgesia, and the suppression of feeding and reproduction. Exposure to chronic stressors is destructive and pathogenic, and is presumed to involve more catabolic activation; there may be further secondary (consequential) changes such as myopathy, fatigue, changes in glycaemia, and hypertensive cardiovascular alterations.

The response of the organism involves neural, endocrinological, autonomic, and behavioural components; neural and endocrine responses are shown in Fig. 7.1 and neural control mechanisms are displayed in Fig. 7.2. Research has focused on the role of the hypothalamus, the amygdala, the locus ceruleus, and their associated biochemistry, neural extensions, and control of the sympathetic nervous system and adrenals. Closed feedback loops tend to limit the response by reducing the release of those factors such as ACTH and corticotrophin-releasing hormone (CRH) which are involved in the endocrinological mobilisation of the reaction. This endocrinological response is organised in the central nervous system, and recent findings indicate that the activation of the locus ceruleus (LC) stimulates the general release of noradrenaline in many brain centres, producing increases in arousal, vigilance, and anxiety. Findings indicate that chronic stress produces ageing, suppresses reproductive function, produces spontaneous abortion and increased infant mortality, and retards growth. This has been described as 'abuse dwarfism' with delayed physical maturation, retardation of intellectual development and delayed psychosexual maturation (Money, 1977).

Psychological responses to stress

The work of Selye laid the foundation for our understanding of human responses to stress. How-

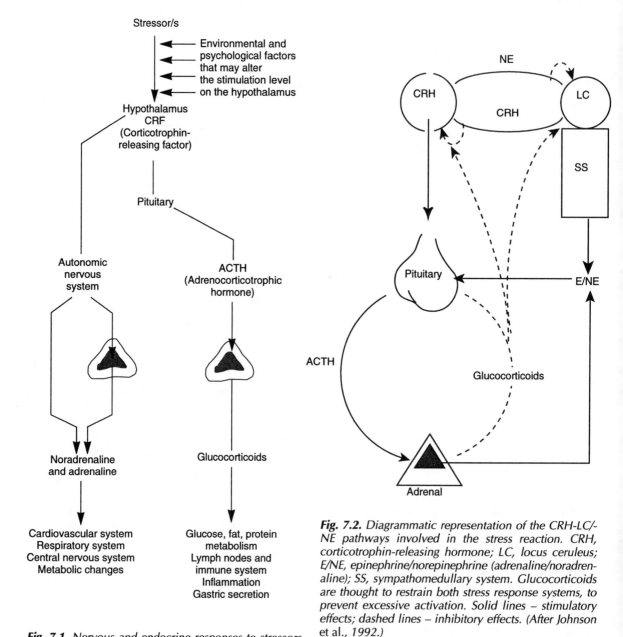

Fig. 7.1. *Nervous and endocrine responses to stressors. (After Snowley, 1992.)*

Fig. 7.2. *Diagrammatic representation of the CRH-LC/-NE pathways involved in the stress reaction. CRH, corticotrophin-releasing hormone; LC, locus ceruleus; E/NE, epinephrine/norepinephrine (adrenaline/noradrenaline); SS, sympathomedullary system. Glucocorticoids are thought to restrain both stress response systems, to prevent excessive activation. Solid lines – stimulatory effects; dashed lines – inhibitory effects. (After Johnson et al., 1992.)*

ever, because of the shortcomings of the model, research shifted towards approaches which placed greater emphasis upon the role of psychological factors, in particular the role of cognitive appraisal in assessing the significance of events. It is now generally accepted that the views individuals have about the nature and meaning of threats and potential threats as well as the views they have about their capacity to deal with events are important factors in accounting for individual variation in response to stress.

Challenges in life, including truly difficult challenges, may be viewed positively if the individual feels able to mobilise resources to deal with those challenges. Indeed many people feel enriched by stressful life events in retrospect, because they handled them positively and in the process learnt much about themselves, their support systems, and their capacity to deal with difficulties. Examples of this might include people who have responded positively to the challenge of serious ill-health; stress in the work place or even the death of a loved one.

However, the experience is quite different if the individual feels lacking in the resources to deal with problems. Negative emotions associated with the consequences of feeling constantly under great stress can be all too familiar. They include anxiety, fear, irritability, worthlessness, despair, hopelessness, anger, frustration and apathy. Lazarus refers to these emotions as 'stress emotions'. In addition to the experience of these strong emotions, there may be a sense of increasing difficulty in thinking and concentrating. At high levels of stress emotions there is some degree of cognitive impairment (see Table 7.5) as well as increased emotional lability (see Table 7.6).

The stress emotions are likely to serve as an impetus to do something about the problem. They can be seen in a positive light as a spur to action. It is in this area that Lazarus in the United States and Cox in Britain have made such a valuable contribution. The recent emphasis on stress has been to consider ways in which the negative emotions associated with stress serve to mobilise a range of actions to deal effectively with the situation. These include attempts to minimise, to reduce or to eliminate altogether the perceived sources of stress. The many ways that all of us attempt to reduce our perceived stress emotions are referred to under the umbrella term of 'coping'. Lazarus (1966) stated that coping refers to 'strategies for dealing with

Table 7.5. *Cognitive effects of too much stress*

Concentration and attention span decrease	The mind finds it hard to remain focused. Powers of observation diminish
Distractibility increases	The thread of what is being said is frequently lost
Short-term memory and long-term memory deteriorate	Memory span reduces. Recall and recognition of familiar material decline
Response speed becomes impaired, error rates increase	Actual responses reduce. Increase in errors in manipulative and cognitive tasks. Decision making suspect
Powers of organisation and long-term planning affected	The mind cannot accurately assess existing or forecast consequences
Delusion and thought disorder increase	Reality testing becomes less efficient objectivity and critical powers are reduced. Thought patterns, irrational and confused

Table 7.6. *Emotional effects*

Physical and psychological tensions	The ability to relax, muscle tone to feel good, to switch off worries and anxieties reduce
Hypochondria increases	Imagined complaints are added to real stress illnesses
Changes take place in personality traits	Neat and careful people – untidy. Caring people – indifferent. Democratic people – authoritarian
Existing personality problems increase	Existing oversensitivity, defensiveness and hostility all worsen
Moral and emotional constraints weaken	Codes of behaviour and self-control either weaken or become extremely rigid
Depression and helplessness appear	Spirits sink lower and sense of powerlessness is experienced
Self-esteem falls	Feelings of incompetence and worthlessness develop

threat'. Cox (1978) suggests that the concept of coping holds the key to understanding the complex, interactive quality of the experience of stress, and in understanding the psychological responses to it.

Coping

A person experiencing stress will remain troubled unless something can be done to remove the source of the problem or reduce the distress. According to Cohen and Lazarus (1979) the person must deal with the elements that contribute to the stress producing discrepancy between the situational demands and the internal resources. Cohen and Lazarus (1979) define coping as 'efforts, both action-oriented and intrapsychic, to reduce or minimize the conflicts of environmental and internal demands'. Therefore what a person does to manage the situation is called coping. For example, a person may choose to avoid a situation, confront it or use self-deceptive action. Coping may therefore involve both cognitive and behavioural strategies. It involves either changing the situation or adjusting to it (i.e. changing the way the situation is viewed).

Functions of coping

According to Lazarus and Folkman (1984a) coping may serve two functions: problem-solving or emotion regulation.

Problem-focused coping
This is aimed at reducing the demands of the situation or expanding the resources to deal with it; examples include studying for an exam or confronting a noisy neighbour. People tend to use problem-focused coping when they believe their resources or the demands of the situation are changeable, usually when a positive outcome is expected. For example, a 55-year-old firefighter who has a heart attack may take early retirement and change his level of aspiration. Other problem-focused approaches include learning or acquiring information. For example, a 32-year-old woman newly diagnosed with multiple sclerosis may search the library for information to facilitate an understanding of her initially vague symptoms.

Emotion-focused coping
This is aimed at controlling the emotional response

to the stress by the use of cognitive or behavioural means. Examples of behavioural means include using alcohol, drugs, seeking social support from friends or relatives and engaging in activities that distract attention. Emotion-focused coping is used when the outcome of the stressful event is thought to be unfavourable. Cognitive approaches might involve denial or changing the meaning of the situation. For example, a man who has to change his job because of a heart condition, may change the meaning by deciding that he was bored with the job anyway. He might perceive the task of changing jobs as an opportunity to do something more stimulating. Folkman *et al.* (1987) found that middle-aged men and women tend to use more problem-focused forms of coping, whilst elderly subjects use more emotion-focused approaches. Part of the explanation for these differences is concerned with the situations that people have to cope with as they age. Middle-aged people tend to report more work-related and family stresses. Direct action and confrontation tend to be more appropriate for these kinds of stress. Elderly people on the other hand have many more health-related changes, which, because of degenerative processes, may be perceived as difficult to change.

Methods of coping

There are six main modes of coping, which are: direct action, information-seeking, turning to others, resigned acceptance, emotional discharge and intrapsychic processes.

Direct action
This involves doing something specifically and directly to cope with the stressor and includes problem-focused coping strategies.

Information-seeking
This involves acquiring information about the stressful situation. For example, in the preoperative situation patients use information as a means of gaining control about unknown and stressful aspects. This informational control significantly helps to reduce anxiety and pain experience following an operation (Hayward, 1975; Johnson *et al.*,1978).

Turning to others
In this instance the person seeks help, reassurance and comfort from family and friends.

Resigned acceptance

In this case the person accepts or comes to terms with the problem. This method is especially suitable in emotion-focused coping, when the basic stressful circumstances cannot be changed, such as when a person loses a loved one.

Emotional discharge

This involves expressing feelings when under stress, such as crying or using humour to reduce tensions. Sarafino (1990) gives an example of humour when a man called himself 'semicolon' following hemi-colectomy for cancer.

Intrapsychic processes

These refer to cognitive strategies such as re-definition. Other strategies involve the use of defence mechanisms which involve distorting reality in some way. For instance, when a situation is too painful to face a person may deny its existence. Some patients faced with a terminal diagnosis frequently utilise denial and refuse to believe they are ill or that their illness may be fatal. Another defence mechanism is intellectualisation, which involves confronting the stressor on an abstract level in an attempt to keep at bay the emotional significance, which may be hard to bear. Suppression is a deliberate effort to put the stressful event out of one's mind.

The methods people use for coping can be seen as either increasing attention to the problem (approach) or minimising attention, by avoidance. Both ways can be beneficial depending on the circumstances. For example, Heim (1991) suggests that denial in the face of a diagnosis of cancer often provides a limited peace of mind.

The process of coping is dynamic; that is, at different stages of the process different strategies will be employed. The utility of a coping strategy is a function of the type of stressful encounter, the personality of the individual stressed, and the outcome measure adopted, whether subjective well-being, social functioning or health. It is likely that effective coping is the key to understanding not only the ways in which the impact of stress can be contained and harnessed, but also to distinguishing between those individuals who succumb to the deleterious effects of stress by becoming ill and those who do not.

Stress, health and illness

The relationship between stress, health and illness has been studied from a variety of different perspectives. One important area of research has focused upon the way in which life stresses are lead to problems of both physical and mental health. A further focus of study considers illness as a stressor and looks at the variety of ways in which individuals respond to this. Of particular interest in this field are the studies on the long-term impact of chronic conditions. Researchers have also looked at potentially life-threatening diseases, such as cancer and chronic heart disease, in an attempt to unravel the way in which different psychological coping strategies enhance survival.

This section will consider the first of the above questions, namely, what is it about the experience of stress that leads to illness? Much has been written about the relationship between stress and illness, though many questions remain unanswered. The causal link between stress and illness can involve either (a) a direct route or (b) an indirect route affecting health through the person's behaviour. The direct route will be considered first.

Stress, physiology and illness: the direct route

The work in this area is based upon three systems; the neuroendocrine system, the autonomic nervous system and the immunological system.

Neuroendocrine system

The pituitary–adrenocortical axis was defined by Selye as the main neuroendocrine component of the stress response. Activation of the hypothalamus leads to stimulation of the pituitary gland, which in turn is responsible for secreting adrenocorti-cotrophic hormone which stimulates the release of corticosteroids. These have a variety of effects including glucogenesis in the liver, water balance, vascular reactivity and immune function. Removal of the adrenal gland in animals has been shown to have a profound effect in reducing the animals' ability to tolerate painful stimuli (Munck *et al.*, 1984). Similarly in humans the outlook for patients with Addison's disease (adrenal insufficiency) was bleak until the use of cortisone therapeutically

(Dunlop, 1963). Selye argued that glucocorticoids are crucial in the adaptation to stressful conditions, but after prolonged stimulation diseases occurred because high levels of circulating steroids have damaging effects. Thus, the clearest connection between stress and illness involves the release of hormones, particularly catecholamines and corticosteroids by the endocrine system during arousal. One way in which these hormones can cause illness is due to their effects on the cardiovascular system. Extremely high levels of these hormones can cause the heart to beat erratically and may lead to death. In addition, chronically high levels of catecholamines and corticosteroids appear to increase the growth of fatty plaques in the arteries (McKinney *et al.*, 1984) which increase the likelihood of heart disease, cerebral vascular accidents, renal damage and disturbance of blood sugar level, possibly resulting in diabetes.

The autonomic nervous system

The sympathetic branch of the autonomic nervous system (ANS) is stimulated by psychological stress. The responses take place in the cardiovascular system and include increases in the heart rate and myocardial contractility, vasodilation in the skeletal muscles, constriction of vessels in the gut, and increases in blood pressure. In addition to this, renal function and insulin secretion are also affected. Many of these responses are potentially damaging if sustained. For example, research has shown that the electrical stability is threatened by cardiac sympathetic stimulation in conjunction with high levels of circulating catecholamines (DeSilva, 1986).

The immunological system

The release of these hormones may also impair the functioning of the immune system (Jemmot and Locke, 1984; Schleifer *et al.*, 1986). For example, research has shown that increases in adrenaline and cortisol are associated with a reduced activity of the T- and B-cells against antigens. This decrease in lymphocyte activity was found by Levy (1985) to be influential in the development of cancer. Research from psychoneuroimmunology has shown that stress-related emotions such as anxiety and depression play a critical role in the balance of immune functions. Zautra *et al.* (1989) and Willis *et al.* (1987) have shown that major

stressful events and their accompanying emotional states suppress immune processes over time.

According to Steptoe (1990) new developments in research have grown from the recognition that immunological processes are sensitive to psychological stress. Most of the work has focused on cell-mediated immunity, and it has been found that under a variety of acute and chronic stressful conditions lymphocyte proliferation is suppressed (Ader and Cohen, 1984) and immunoglobins are reduced . Experimental studies of animals indicate that tumour rejection may be reduced with an increase in the proliferation of tumour cells under stressful conditions (Anisman and Sklar, 1984). Ulcers and inflammatory bowel disease, asthma, chronic migraine, skin disorders (hives, eczema and psoriasis) are also thought to be stress induced.

The extent to which these physiological reactions are activated when a person is confronted by a potentially stressful situation is dependent on a number of factors that modify the intensity. Steptoe (1990) has identified the following variables, which have been shown to moderate the intensity of the physiological stress reaction: stimulus intensity, duration of stimulation, novelty and predictability of the stimulus.

Stimulus intensity

The magnitude of autonomic and endocrine responses is dependent on the intensity of the stressor. For example, corticosteroid responses are larger and more prolonged in major surgery as opposed to minor. Vogele and Steptoe (1986) found that ANS responses were elevated for significantly more days after major orthopaedic surgery as compared to minor surgery. Research on life events also indicates that severe illness elicits more autonomic and neuroendocrine responses.

Duration of stimulation

Steptoe (1990) has argued that no simple conclusion can be drawn by looking at duration, because it is well known that adverse consequences may result from both repeated short exposures and also occur from continuous exposure. Thus it is possible to induce hypertension and arteriosclerosis in animals who have sustained short, repeated exposure to stress. Similarly, depression (characteristically seen in patients with chronic pain) is the result of long-term painful stimulation. However, adaptation can occur either through habituation or through the development of coping resources.

Difficulty also arises when trying to draw firm distinctions between acute and chronic stressors. This is because many acute stressors such as a bereavement may have long-term consequences (exposure to new living and social environments) (Kasl, 1984), whilst acute stressful events (such as surgery) may be anticipated uneasily for weeks or months. Steptoe (1990) suggests that certain types of chronic stressors, particularly those involving constant threat (such as living near a nuclear powerplant) or those that involve constant high-level demands are especially likely to be associated with psychobiological responses.

Novelty

When we are confronted with new forms of environmental stressors, stress responses tend to be more intense. Studies of parachuting and other potentially dangerous activities indicate that intense corticosteroid, catecholamine and ANS activity are elicited on the first occasion, with effects diminishing on repeated exposure (Ursin *et al.*, 1978). Explanations for this pattern have been attributed to coping, or mastery over new situations which comes with experience.

Predictability

The effects of stimulus predictability have been investigated extensively. The basic pattern is that psycho-biological reactions tend to be more pronounced in the face of unpredictable events, even if the duration and intensity is the same as in a situation that is predictable. The same finding is true when the toleration of pain is considered. Explanations of the effects of predictability are varied but many are related to the notion of control which will be considered later.

Stress, behaviour and illness: the indirect route

The behavioural link between stress and illness is evident in many stressful situations such as when a family undergoes a divorce. According to Wallerstein (1983), in many cases following the break-up of a family, the parent who remains with the children is likely to be less available and less

responsive than she/he was before. The parent's behaviour often makes conditions in the family less healthy, for example by providing haphazard meals and less regular bedtimes. This behaviour has consequences for health. According to research conducted by Johnson (1986) and Quick and Quick (1984), children and adults who experience high levels of stress are more likely to suffer accidental injuries at home, during sporting activities, at work and whilst driving a car. Research by Wiebe and McCallum (1986) has also shown that people who experience high levels of stress consume more alcohol, cigarettes and coffee (Baer *et al.*, 1987), which in turn increases their chances of becoming ill. In addition stress can operate as a barrier preventing healthy behaviour.

The link between stress, behaviour and ill-health is mediated by a number of variables. These include individual differences in personality, the presence or absence of support and intimacy, and the capacity to use effective coping mechanisms. The work on personality types has focused upon typologies that increase the likelihood of illness as well as those that moderate the effects of stress and decrease the likelihood of ill-health.

Personality types, stress and illness

Type A behaviour pattern

In seeking to understand ways in which the experience of heightened levels of stress can cause ill-health, it is important to understand the complexities of the relationship. Since the original work of Friedman and Rosenman (1974) in the 1950s on the relationship between personality types and increased risk of ill-health, researchers in medicine and psychology have found evidence of psychological and behavioural stress factors to explain coronary heart disease (CHD) and coronary artery disease (CAD). People with type A behaviour pattern (TABP) are thought to react differently to stress than those with type B behaviour pattern (TBBP). Type A individuals react more quickly, more intensely, often interpreting stress as a threat to their personal control (Carver *et al.*, 1985). According to Bryne and Rosenman (1986), type A people seek out demanding situations in their lives; they have a greater level of resting arousal and high levels of reactivity (Mathews, 1986), which suggests that the tendency to high reactivity begins in childhood. TABP is complex and comprises three factors (Friedman and Rosenman, 1974; Chesney *et al.*, 1985):

- Competitive achievement orientation.
- A sense of urgency of time; they seem to be in a constant battle with the clock.
- Higher levels of anger and hostility; they tend to be easily aroused to anger and hostility, which may or may not be expressed outwardly.

In contrast, TBBP is characterised by low levels of competitiveness, time urgency and hostility. These individuals tend to be more easy-going, with a much more relaxed and philosophical outlook. In recent years the anger and hostility components of personality have emerged as the central personality factors in the aetiology of CHD and CAD. In a review of the literature, Gold and Johnston (1990) found numerous sources of evidence suggesting that anger is related to CHD.

Anger, hypertension and heart disease

Spielberger (1983) defined three separate aspects of the syndrome: anger, hostility and aggression, which he considered to be central to the development of CHD. Firstly, he defined anger as an emotional state characterised by increased arousal of negative feelings which may vary in intensity from mild irritation to rage. Secondly he considered hostility, which although involving elements of anger, refers to a complex set of attitudes which serves to motivate aggressive behaviour. Finally, aggression implies destructive behaviour directed at other people. The components of anger and hostility which have been assessed in CHD research include the frequency and intensity of the experience, angry feelings, the type of situations that an elicit angry response, the tendency of an individual to interpret situations as hostile, the way in which anger is expressed or suppressed once it is experienced, and finally the degree of guilt an individual feels after he or she has expressed anger.

In addition to the research on CHD and personality, attention has also been directed to hypertension. A number of studies have examined the relationship between blood pressure, anger expression and other traditional psychosocial risk factors such as race, sex and age (Harburg *et al.*, 1979; Johnson *et al.*, 1987). For example, Harburg *et al.* (1979) found that in the United States race is a risk factor for hypertension, with the black population having a greater proportion of hypertension than white people. In another study, Johnson *et al.* (1987) looked at blood pressure levels and anger expression in black and white adolescents. The results suggest that suppressed anger was the greatest predictor of hypertension in males, with the strongest association occurring in black males. Overall it appears that the suppression of anger is associated with elevated blood pressure. In summary it seems that the suppression of justifiable anger and the frequent experience and expression of unjustifiable anger both have deleterious effects on the cardiovascular system. The expression of appropriate anger which occurs infrequently may not be harmful.

Positive personality characteristics, stress and health

Research has focused not only upon personality factors that increase the likelihood of illness in the face of stress, but also on personality factors that moderate the effects of stress and increase the likelihood of healthy outcomes. The main areas that have come under scrutiny are hardiness, sense of coherence and resilience.

Hardiness

Kobasa's (1979) research has focused upon hardiness as a positive variable in the mediation of the impact of stress. Hardiness includes the following three characteristics:

- a strong sense of personal control
- a strong sense of commitment and purpose in life and relationships, which enable hardy people to turn to others for assistance and resist giving up in the face of threat
- a tendency to view change as an opportunity for growth rather than threat.

Related research confirms the findings of Kobasa (1979) and Kobasa *et al.* (1982). For example, Colerick (1985) scrutinised the personality of elderly people for what she called 'stamina', which closely resembles hardiness. This research was undertaken to determine how people deal with the death of a loved one and other significant life events. She found that elderly people with high stamina have a much more positive outlook in times of adversity. Additionally, they had more healthy past histories and more activities in their current lives which promoted personal growth.

Sense of coherence

Antonovsky (1979, 1987) developed the concept of a 'sense of coherence', which involves the tendency to see the world as comprehensible, manageable and meaningful. This tendency is linked to healthy styles of living and an enhanced capacity to deal effectively with stressful situations. Marks and Thomas (1992) have demonstrated that a high sense of coherence among severely disabled people correlates positively with effective coping and favourable adjustment in the community

Resilience

Beardslee (1989) proposed that resilient individuals have 'a total organizing insight into who they are and how they came to be'. This allows them self-understanding which is the key to resilience. The three crucial dimensions of self-understanding are:

- accurate cognitive appraisal of stressors over time
- realistic appraisal of capacities for, and the consequences of, action
- engagement and active involvement in the social and physical environment.

Hardiness, a sense of coherence, and resilience have a great deal in common and may well be different facets of the same phenomenon.

Pain, hospitalisation and illness as stressors

Stressful events may be causally linked to the development of ill-health; but ill-health itself can be viewed as a significant stressor. Being ill, facing medical interventions and becoming hospitalised are stressful events; indeed, going into hospital is often made more stressful by poor communication and treatment from health-care professionals. According to Wilson-Barnett (1986), diagnostic procedures account for a significant degree of stress because

threat, loss and challenge are integral aspects of the stress involved. For example, an individual may find a diagnostic procedure threatening because it is associated bodily harm, discomfort and loss of dignity. Loss may also be involved if the patient has to forgo pleasure, consciously take on the patient role and relinquish other responsibilities. Challenge is involved because some patients view investigations as a test of their tenacity and personal strength. For a detailed description of sources of stressors in the clinical setting, the reader is referred to Wilson-Barnett (1979, 1986).

Illness and injury are associated with the experience of threat and the experience of loss. The threat may refer to the immediate consequences of pain and immobility, and may also signify long-term effects such as losing control of events that affect one's life. In the sphere of illness and disability as stressors, the two main areas that have received much attention are firstly the short-term consequences of experiencing pain in the acute sector of medicine, such as the stress associated with major surgery and its repercussions. Secondly attention has been paid to the stress consequent upon living in the longer term with chronic illness.

Patient control in the health-care setting

A sense of personal control is seen to be an important determinant of healthy adjustment to acute pain as well as long-term illness and living with chronic pain. Thompson (1981) defined control as 'the belief that one has at one's disposal a response that can influence the aversiveness of an event'. As has already been noted, personal control is an important component of resilience and hardiness and thus mitigates against the harmful effects of stress in the development of disease. It is also relevant when considering the ways in which individuals cope with the negative effects of long-term disability and illness. Those individuals who have a greater sense of personal control are likely to cope better with the challenges of ill-health, pain and rehabilitation. Thompson (1981) has outlined five types of control: behavioural, cognitive, decisional, informational and retrospective control.

Coping with pain

A sense of personal control is particularly important in the context of coping with the impact of pain. The implications of research work (Miller,

1979, 1980, 1987) in this area are quite clear; those individuals who have a greater sense of personal control in all the areas outlined cope with pain more effectively and manage the challenges of their illness or disability more imaginatively. Therefore there have been a number of attempts (e.g. Hayward, 1975) to enhance the sense of personal control among patients in an attempt to facilitate healthy coping strategies. These attempts have been particularly effective in the area of pain control, in particular in the area of post-operative pain.

Pain and personal control

The uncontrollable aspects of pain lie in the fact that medical treatment, and traditional ways of dealing with pain (e.g. taking rest, avoidance of activities), often do not provide pain relief. Pain after an operation is felt to be beyond the influence of the patient, and this lack of control is a major source of suffering in itself. One factor common to anxiety and pain experience may be the sense the individual has of their uncontrollability; indeed, there is an abundance of human and animal studies which supports the link between perceived control, anxiety and painful or aversive events (Mandler and Watson, 1966). There are a number of ways in which researchers and clinicians in this field have attempted to increase the patient's sense of control over the experience of pain, these include the enhancement of cognitive, informational and behavioural control.

Cognitive control

A number of studies have looked at the effectiveness of 'reinterpretation' as a cognitive control strategy taught to patients before surgery. Reinterpretation interventions require the patient to focus selectively on the more positive, beneficial components of the procedure (for example, 'post-operative pain will be relieved by "painkillers" and it does not last long'). Ridgeway and Mathews (1982) found that among patients following hysterectomy, those who used reinterpretation reported less pain, required less oral and injected analgesia and had better sleep patterns than the untreated control group.

Informational control

Information given to patients before an operation allows them to interpret and understand their surroundings and circumstances. This in turn helps them to anticipate the events occurring during the post-operative period. The ability to understand and to anticipate events engenders a feeling of control and reduces helplessness (Mandler, 1972). Early work with surgical patients tended to use procedural information for relieving anxiety. Egbert et al. (1964) found that when patients were visited by the anaesthetist before surgery and given procedural information as well as instruction on breathing and leg exercises, there was a reduction in both the need for post-operative analgesia and length of stay in hospital. Similarly, Hayward (1975) compared the impact of detailed procedural information on post-operative pain experience among patients undergoing hernia operation and that of a no-treatment control. The results showed that the informed patients were less anxious and experienced less pain post-operatively than the control group. Although research evidence reveals that information reduces anxiety, it is more effective if it focuses upon what the patient is likely to experience rather than the objective nature of the procedure. Sensory information can be provided which includes details of common sensations that the patient is likely to feel, see, smell and hear. The terminology is ideally derived from patients themselves, because their vocabulary reflects both what is familiar to them and what is experienced. This is important because Byrne and Edeani (1983) found that several terms commonly used by staff were not understood by patients. Johnson et al. (1978) found that sensory information given in this way to patients undergoing cholecystectomy was superior in reducing the length of post-operative hospitalisation and the time patients first ventured from their homes after discharge.

Although information does give greater control, there is growing evidence which suggests that not all patients derive benefit from detailed information. Indeed it appears that such information can have the opposite effect. For example, Langer et al. (1975) reported that simple information had the effect of magnifying pain by causing patients to focus on the discomforting aspects of the experience they were about to undergo. Patients' coping style is an important moderator of how such detailed information will be utilised. Andrew (1970), for example, found that pre-operative information was detrimental to individuals who use denial as a coping strategy.

Since then many studies have looked at the interacting effects of individual differences and information. Miller (1980, 1987) found that pre-operative information is most effective for patients whose preferred strategy is to seek information ('monitors') or to ignore a threatening situation. Individuals who prefer to distract themselves ('blunters') experience a great deal of stress when given detailed information. This result supports Rogers and Reich's (1986) suggestion that the efficacy of psychological interventions could be significantly enhanced if they were tailored to meet the particular personality style of the patient.

Behavioural control

Behavioural control is perhaps the most obvious form of control available to the surgical patient faced with acute pain. The desire for control through action increases when patients have more information about the situation they are about to confront (Schorr and Rodin, 1984). For example, Cromwell *et al.* (1977) found that the most deleterious effects upon recovery occurred when patients had a great deal of information but no opportunity for control through action. Averill (1973) identified two types of behavioural control: firstly, control over the circumstances surrounding the experience of pain, and secondly the patient's capacity to modify the level of pain directly (through, for example the use of patient controlled analgesia, PCA). Several investigations have examined the impact of progressive muscular relaxation as a means of behavioural control, taught to patients prior to surgery. In a study using relaxation with 70 patients following cholecystectomy and hysterectomy , Wilson (1981) found that those taught to relax required less pain medication, showed better recovery and a quicker discharge than a no treatment control. In another study Flagherty and Fitzpatrick (1978) taught patients undergoing abdominal surgery to use relaxation on their first attempt to get out of bed after the operation. Patients using this technique were found to experience less pain and required less analgesia than a control group.

Controlling the actual level of pain, as, for example, in the use of self-administered pain medication via PCA, has been shown to be of enormous value in the management of post-operative pain (Sechzer, 1971). In a study of 164 patients following hysterectomy and chole-

csytectomy, Thomas (1991) found that this method provided better pain control, shorter length of stay and a reduction in the analgesic medication than with the use of conventional intramuscular injections. Other researchers (e.g. Notcutt and Morgan, 1990) have found similar results.

Why does control reduce pain?

Several theorists (e.g. Seligman, 1975) have proposed that behavioural control and information reduces pain and anxiety because they allow the person to predict some important aspects of the situation, such as when the painful experience will occur, when it will end and what it will feel like. Johnson's (1973) incongruency hypothesis suggests that increased control reduces pain because the patient's expectation of pain is more closely related to the actual experience of pain. According to this hypothesis anxiety and severe pain occur because of a discrepancy between what the patient expects to experience and what he or she does experience. Theories about the predictability of pain cannot adequately explain why many individuals are willing to tolerate more intense levels of pain when behavioural control is present. Nor can it explain the effects of the interaction between information and personality style.

Miller's (1979) minimax theory proposes that patients with control responses are able to minimise the impact of the most painful experience that might be anticipated, that is the maximum future danger. Specifically, the theory suggests that patients with control responses know that the post-operative situation will not become so painful that they cannot cope with it, because they can attribute the source of relief to stable internal factors, their own responses. This theory was developed to explain the effects of behavioural control, but it seems equally applicable to cognitive and informational control. With both behavioural and cognitive control, patients believe that the pain after surgery will not exceed the limits of what they can endure. Information is also effective because it confirms to the patient that the sensations they experience will not be unbearable. The minimax hypothesis also predicts that in some situations individuals will prefer to have no control, for example, when control is in the hands of another person who is seen to be minimising harm and pain (such as a skilled professional with a hypodermic needle).

Coping with long-term illness

There are many stresses inherent in living with long-term illness, for example the uncertainty of the future, living with chronic pain, living with the restrictions that the illness imposes, changes in social and work life and the repercussions on family and intimate relationships. Historically, the medical model of illness directed attention away from such variables in favour of emphasising physiological factors, but increasingly the psychological and social sequelae of long-term, chronic conditions are seen to be of crucial importance in planning health care. Research in this field has revealed wide variations of individual responses to living with chronic pain and long-term illness, in particular the range of factors which are known to moderate the impact of the stressful aspects. These factors include family relationships and social support, time, gaining information and enhanced control and maintaining normalcy in the face of disability.

Family relationships and social support

Communication and cooperation within a family are important in enhancing the ability to cope with a chronic illness. Parental agreement on a philosophy of child-rearing enables more positive coping with a child's chronic illness (Hymovich and Hagophian, 1991). In families of children with cancer, communication was found to be related to child happiness, closeness to parents and a non-defensive family atmosphere (Spineta and Maloney, 1978). More recent research by Hymovich (in 1990, cited in Hymovich and Hagophian, 1991) has found that open communication with children about parental chronic illness also facilitates family closeness.

Time

In the course of an illness many researchers have identified different stages, each associated with different coping strategies. During the initial phase attempts are made to minimise the impact of the event, including extensive denial of the seriousness of the condition and likely outcome. Following this there is gradual information-seeking about the condition. Early research looking at how parents cope with the impending death of their children (Chodoff *et al.*, 1964) found that the early phase included disbelief and denial, anger,

bitterness and disregard for needs of other family members. In the intermediate phase there was acceptance that they had to do what was required to meet all the needs of the sick child. In the final stage there is intense emotion and anticipatory grieving.

Seeking information

In order to cope with the challenges of chronic illness most people seek some degree of control through gaining information that enables them to understand better and to cope with the practical challenges. Patients and family members want information that is of prime importance to them at the time. For example, the mother of a newly diagnosed diabetic child will be concerned about how to administer insulin injections. Hymovich (1981) identified seeking and using information as a major coping strategy of parents of chronically ill children. Individuals may also need to acquire new skills in order to manage the condition. These skills are learned through experience and include such things as manipulating a wheelchair or giving an insulin injection. In the early stages skill acquisition requires enormous effort and concentration, but with time it becomes automatic. Once a skill becomes automatic, it can no longer be considered as a means of coping with a difficult problem because it no longer taxes resources (Hymovich and Hagopian, 1991).

Maintaining normalcy

Normalisation allows the family to acknowledge abnormality while minimising its social significance. Strategies for maintaining normalcy include minimising abnormalities in physical appearance, participating in usual activities, maintaining usual social ties, limiting contact with people with a similar condition and avoiding embarrassing situations. Normalisation is made easier when the condition becomes peripheral and is no longer the central organising theme in the person's life. There are many ways in which families seek to achieve higher levels of normalisation, for example, by assigning a chore to a chronically ill child, especially during adolescence, when this is normal practice. This may also be a significant way in which parents can convey a sense of competence to their disabled child.

Stress in nursing: understanding and confronting professional stress

What light does the preceding discussion on the nature of stress and the range of coping strategies throw upon the problems facing nurses, in training and after qualification, in the demands of their day-to-day work? Researchers in the field of stress among nurses (e.g. Hingley and Cooper 1986; Rentoul, 1989) acknowledge that they are confronted regularly with emotionally challenging and potentially distressing situations. The stresses are related to their closeness to pain, illness, serious threats to health, including threats to life itself, and dealing with death, bereavement and their sequelae. Marshall (1980) notes that 'most writers start by taking the existence of stress among nurses for granted'. This is not surprising when one considers that, among all professional groups, nursing has one of the highest rates of suicide and nurses top the list of psychiatric out-patient referrals (Gillespie and Gillespie, 1986). Bailey (1985) lists nurses as part of a group of health-care professionals who may be regarded as 'the casualties of caring'. The concept of the cost of caring is further developed by Skevington (1984) in her chapter on this topic.

Whilst nursing in general may be regarded as a stressful profession, it is important to recognise that nurses cannot be regarded as an homogenous category. Marshall (1980) points out that stressors may be different for different types of nurse, for different types of ward and for different types of hospital or community setting. Despite these differences she does conclude in her influential work on stress among nurses that 'the nurse's role is therefore implicitly and chiefly one of handling stress. She is the focus for the stress of the patient, relatives, and doctor as well as her own'.

Sources of stress among nurses

Research into occupational stress (for example, Cobb and Rose, 1973) has shown that work that exposes individuals to people, especially their suffering, is far more stressful than work with 'things'. One of the paradoxes for those entering the health-care professions is that a significant motivating force, and indeed a great potential source of satisfaction, is to help sick and distressed

people; however, it is also this arena, close contact with frightened, ill and dying patients and their relatives, that provokes the highest level of stress among health-care professionals. The rewards and stresses of taking care of sick and distressed people are closely intertwined. It is no longer disputed that hand in hand with the acceptance of holistic care and a more emotionally open stance towards patients and their families, nurses are increasingly exposed to the stress contingent upon this increased emotional burden. This observation is borne out by a huge and growing literature over the past 30 years (see, for example, Menzies, 1960b; Steffen, 1980; Jacobson, 1978; Marshall, 1980; Field, 1989; Tschudin, 1985; Rentoul, 1991). Other sources of stress which have been discussed in the literature include: the poor working conditions in many large hospitals (Lunn, 1973), the problems of shiftwork (Kemp, 1984), role conflict and ambiguity within the organisation (Rosse and Rosse, 1981), interpersonal relationships at work, including nurse–nurse problems (Jacobson and McGrath, 1983), nurse–doctor problems (Marshall, 1980), carer–patient/relative problems (Marshall, 1980), problems associated with the organisational structure and climate of the hospital (see, for example, the work of Hingley and Cooper, 1986; Jacobson and McGrath, 1983; Gray-Toft and Anderson, 1981; Rentoul, 1989) and finally home–work conflict.

Stresses associated with the client group

The prime focus of the nurse's responsibility is people rather than objects, and more than this, people who are likely to be vulnerable because of threats to their health. This kind of responsibility is more stressful than other kinds, such as responsibility for 'things'. Cobb and Rose (1973) have pointed out that those professional groups who have close professional responsibility for the lives of other people are more often victims of a range of stress-related diseases such as peptic ulcers, myocardial infarctions, hypertension and diabetes. Nurses are more likely than many other groups to be involved with people with problems, social, psychological or physical. Their day-to-day interactions are likely to focus upon matters which are dysfunctional or abnormal. The strain of dealing with clients face-to-face has been recognised in many groups of workers and is seen as one of the most important aspects of 'burnout'. Within the field of health, the stress created by such inter-actions can be exaggerated by the involvement with disability, deformity, physical suffering and sometimes death. In the words of Hingley (1984), 'Every day the nurse confronts stark suffering, grief and death as few other people do'. To cite his views further

> Many nursing tasks are mundane and unrewarding. Many are, by normal standards, distasteful, even disgusting. Patients are often difficult, frightened and resentful, and nurses can find themselves responding with a growing sense of irritability and frustration. Such 'unprofessional' feelings can arouse considerable anxiety and guilt.

The nature of the work is likely to arouse anxi-eties in the carer about, for example, his or her own mortality, or fears about sickness, mutilation or loss, a point emphasised by Menzies (1960a, b). The responsibility too that they may have to take for the health, welfare and ultimately, on occasions, the death of patients, marks them out from other profes-sional groups. A particular stress for nurses, too, is that their own stress may affect the very focus of their role, namely their patients. The issues of stress, therefore, become crucial for patient care itself.

Many people are drawn towards nursing be-cause of a long-standing need to care and make things better (see, for example, Cherniss, 1980). If this need is thwarted, and it may be for all sorts of reasons beyond the control of the nurse, then the consequent disappointment and sense of failure place great strain and stress upon the nurse. Particularly stressful in this area is the stress of dealing with dying patients and their relatives. The task of nursing inevitably involves dealing with death, dying and bereavement; how well the nurse copes with these demands is a major influence on the amount of stress likely to be experienced. Much of the literature on stress among nurses focuses upon the anxiety contingent upon high levels of exposure to death and dying patients (Steffen, 1980; Field, 1989; Rentoul, 1989; Jacobson, 1978). The degree of stress is likely to be high if the death is sudden (Jacobson, 1978), when it involves a certain category of patient, such as children (Schowalter, 1975), or a special patient with whom the nurse was closely involved (Glaser and Strauss, 1966).

Working conditions

There are many aspects of the working environ-ment which exacerbate the levels of stress experi-enced by nurses. These include lack of privacy, the difficulties in leaving the ward, which may at times be an emotionally charged and stressful environ-ment, ongoing commitments to a wide range of patients despite the distress associated with one patient. Few other professional groups have such high levels of client contact for such long stretches of time; if the ward environment becomes distressing there is often little or no opportunity for respite. There are also problems associated with shiftwork. Hingley and Cooper (1986) conclude from their review of the research evidence on the impact of shiftwork:

> From the evidence it would seem that nurses who are engaged in shift work must cope with an additional range of potential stressors. Not only are they subject to the well-documented physical and psychosocial ill-effects of this pattern of work but also they are likely to lose professional status and the respect of their immediate colleagues.

The grounds for this latter point is that it is often thought that the quality and calibre of nurses working night-shifts are less good than those on day-shifts, though there is no evidence to support this contention.

Role conflict and ambiguity within the organisation

Role conflict and ambiguity arise from a variety of sources, including unrealistic expectations from other professional groups, from patients and their families, from their own profession and from the individuals themselves, and lack of clarity in the roles and responsibilities within the nursing profession and among other health professional groups. Rosse and Rosse (1981) found that levels of role conflict and ambiguity were significantly related to job stress, organisational commitment, job satisfaction and intentions to leave the profession. One research study reveals that nurses feel that the problems associated with their role are poorly understood by many doctors and that communication problems arise as a consequence (Rentoul, 1989).

Interpersonal relationships at work

The quality of interpersonal relationships in the workplace has been found to be an important determinant of levels of individual stress and health. Interpersonal relations, both within professions and between professions, can be a source of stress for people at work. For nurses, lack of support from their own professional group has been cited as a source of conflict and stress (Rentoul, 1989; Bergh-Braam and de Wolff, 1988). Much, too, has been written about the problems of interpersonal relationships between nurses and doctors (see, for example, Rentoul, 1989; Marshall, 1980; Steffen, 1980; Hadley, 1977). The problems arise from lack of clarity with regard to professional boundaries, perceived differences in power and status, inadequate structures for communication, and a lack of understanding about the difficulties and stresses inherent in each professional role (Marshall, 1980; Rentoul, 1989). When different professional groups are working together under pressure the rewards of the work can be enjoyed if colleagues have positive and supportive working relationships. This entails some understanding of the nature of the demands and challenges of their respective work, an openness in communication and a supportive attitude.

Coping in nursing

When looking at stress in nursing it is important to consider not only the sources of stress but also the wide variety of ways in which nurses cope with the pressures of their work. The ways in which nurses moderate the impact of stress are manifold; some strategies are aimed mainly at short-term relief, others are long term. Some ways of coping with stress are adaptive but others may be less healthy, for example increased drinking, smoking and avoidance of difficult situations. Such ways of coping with stress are effective only because they lessen the awareness and psychological impact of stressors, but these strategies may have sub-optimal, even deleterious effects, on the care of patients because they may result in reduced effective communication with and support for patients. The impact of coping strategies must be assessed in terms of their impact on patients as well as nurses. Managing stress in an effective way is the focus of increasing concern among health-care professionals. Much of the literature on stress management tends to focus upon attempts to help individuals adopt more effective ways of dealing with stressful situations that they cannot avoid. Another approach is to look at the environment in which nurses work and look at structural ways within the organisation of nursing, and medicine

too, to reduce the levels of stress and increase the levels of support.

Support in nursing

One of the most important ways of combating stress in medicine and nursing is by the provision of a supportive working environment. This includes an open acknowledgement of the problems facing nurses and effective supervision and support in the stressful elements of their work, in Menzies' words (1990), to work in a **'talking culture'**, where it is appropriate to discuss regularly and openly the difficulties of work. In addition to this, in some settings it is deemed helpful to provide a regular staff support group (this is very common in mental health settings), occasional support groups following a particularly distressing episode or the opportunity for staff counselling as part of, or in addition to, the occupational health provision.

Stress among health-care professionals can also be alleviated by improving their conditions of work. Improved education about potential stressors, improved channels of communication to increase support, an effective mentorship scheme to ensure effective supervision in challenging work areas, and clear guidance on work role and responsibilities are all organisational means of moderating the impact of stress.

When reviewing the research literature on the ways in which health-care professionals are supported in dealing with stressful elements of their work, a number of themes emerge. Firstly, there is very little multidisciplinary research or programmes of support. There is a marked tendency in the literature to focus upon, for example, either medicine or nursing, despite many similarities in the stresses confronting these groups and the inadequacies of support for them. Secondly, research into ways of managing stress effectively has focused almost exclusively upon personal and interpersonal support, despite the fact that many problems might more usefully be addressed at an organisational level. Finally, what pervades the literature on stress in hospitals is a worrying picture of a failure to deal effectively with many of the problems described in the literature, despite a proliferation of research in the area. The magnitude of this failure should not be underestimated. Those studies which have specifically focused on the extent to which stress in the acute sector of nursing is being managed portray a rather bleak picture; not unrelenting, but nonetheless worrying. A picture of persisting stress remains. In reviewing the literature there is little evidence to suggest that managerial methods are being employed to combat stress and its sequelae, which is a sad indictment of a service committed to providing support for others, but apparently unable or unwilling to care for itself. The concluding comments of Hingley and Cooper (1986) go one step further and raise questions about the implications of this failure for patient care as well as the health of the professional concerned, 'If as a profession, they are unable or unwilling to care for themselves, can they in all honesty be expected or even trusted, to care for others?' If the value of clinical research is to be measured in terms of the changes that it brings about, then the achievements of the research on stress and support in medicine are unimpressive. Once again in the words of Hingley and Cooper (1986), 'Here we can only reiterate Menzies' (1970) astonishment at finding "how little basic and dynamic change has taken place".'

The empirical data on the related issues of stress and support for health-care professionals working in the acute sector of general medicine are unequivocal; many carers work under the shadow of high levels of stress and experience the support afforded to them as inadequate. The repercussions of this are worrying from the point of view of all concerned. Job satisfaction, the health and well-being of health-care professionals and their capacity to deliver high-quality care are all compromised. Firth and Morrison (1986) provided a disturbing account of some of the consequences for health professionals of feeling under unrelenting pressure. These included professional depression, emotional emptiness, and the avoidance of potentially worrying situations. Low staff morale is also worrying from the point of view of the patient. Indeed accounts of poor quality of care have been provided by patients and relatives in the areas of care of parasuicide patients on medical wards (Dunleavy, 1989) and bereaved relatives (Silvey, 1988; Wright *et al.*, 1988). From the point of view of the hospital, there are also problems arising from burnout (Tschudin, 1985), high staff turnover rates (Price and Bergen, 1977) and difficulties in recruiting and retaining staff.

There are some who might argue that some experience of stress is good, because it encourages efficient and healthy achievement. Indeed, there is some evidence to support this from, for example, the world of competitive sport. Much of the literature in nursing, however, argues strenuously against this. In the words of Wallis and de Wolff (1988) 'in our view the balance of research data argues overwhelmingly against the convenient supposition that occupational stress should ever be ignored, let alone encouraged'.

It is important to recognise that nursing offers a great opportunity for high levels of job satisfaction, and this must not be lost sight of when reviewing the literature on stress. When the challenges of nursing are addressed and dealt with positively, even if the situation is a distressing one, the nurse feels a sense of purpose and achievement. Problems arise when the challenges feel increasingly unmanageable, and there is neither understanding of this situation nor support for the nurse. Understanding stress in nursing can only be achieved by a comprehensive perspective, which takes account of the nursing task, including its highly rewarding elements, the environment in which it takes place, the organisational structure that provides a professional framework for working, and the personality of the individual nurse.

Conclusion

In this chapter we have reviewed the literature on stress, in particular the overlap between the general material on stress and the material applied to health, illness and nursing. Stress is seen to be a multifaceted phenomenon, which encompasses consideration of stressors, strain and the complex interactions that take place between them. Most researchers agree that stress should be conceptualised as a process, which can be understood at many levels from the physiological, psychological to the social. There have been a number of important influences during this century, for example the work of Bernard (1927) and the work of Cannon (1932) in the field of physiology, and the pioneering work of Selye (1956, 1976) bringing together physiological and behavioural components of stress. Since the early days of stress research, when the emphasis was largely upon understanding stress in terms of external demands on the biological organism, increasing attention has been paid in more recent years to the psychological variables which mediate the stress response. Seminal work in this context was carried out by Lazarus (1966) in the United States and Cox (1978) in Britain. Lazarus, in introducing the concept of 'cognitive appraisal', shifted attention to the meaning of external stressors and emphasised the active role of the individual in making sense of the changing demands of the environment. Cox (1978) emphasised the continuous adjustments that individuals make in negotiating challenges in the social and physical environment. He referred to these as on-going 'transactions', emphasising the way in which each interaction between the individual and stressors in the environment changes the situation and demands new solutions. The individual may be changed by the interaction and so may the environment. Sources of stress in contemporary Britain are manifold. They include large-scale tragedies, such as air crashes, and personal tragedies such as the death of a child. They include, too, the daily hassles of a tough working environment and the regular struggles of juggling child care, housework and professional demands as well as loneliness and isolation.

Of particular relevance to nursing are the complexities of the relationship between stress, health and illness. There is a great deal of recent research highlighting the ways in which heightened levels of stress in an individual can lead to health problems. A wide variety of disease processes are implicated, and include CHD, hypertension, cancer, asthma and skin diseases.

Illness and the consequent need for medical treatments and hospitalisation can also be viewed as highly stressful events challenging individual resources. Acute pain as a stressor has been the subject of much health research. Increasingly, behavioural interventions are proving to be highly beneficial in a health-care setting. Techniques, such as the introduction of PCA in pain control and personality assessments to ascertain the kind of patients who would most benefit from this approach, reflect the growing attempts in medicine and nursing to apply principles derived from stress research to the clinical setting to benefit patients. Living with chronic illness is also of concern to health psychologists and nurses interested in the long-term implications of stress. The impact, not just on the individuals, but also on all family members, especially children, is considered. As in the area of the control of pain in the acute setting,

behavioural means of dealing with stress in the long-term is also seen to be of great importance, these include stress management and the enhancement of personal control.

Finally, occupational stress in nursing is addressed. It is now recognised that nursing is potentially a highly challenging and rewarding profession that exposes its practitioner to a stressful environment. The key to working productively in this context is seen to lie in the area of good education, adequate preparation for the challenges of nursing, and satisfactory support and supervision; that is, to provide an open and supportive working environment where the daily challenges are acknowledged.

References

Ader, R. and Cohen, N. (1984). Behavior and the immune system. In Gentry, W. D. (ed.) *Handbook of Behavioral Medicine*, pp. 1171–1173. Guildford, New York.

Andrew, J. M. (1970). Recovery from surgery, with and without preparatory instruction for three coping styles. *Journal of Personality and Social Psychology*, 55, 513–520.

Anisman, H. and Sklar, L. S. (1984). Psychological insults and pathology. Contributions of neurochemical, hormonal and immunological mechanisms. In Steptoe, A. and Matthews, A. (eds) *Health Care and Human Behaviour*. Academic Press, London.

Antonovsky, A. (1979). *Health, Stress and Coping*. Jossey-Bass, San Francisco.

Antonovsky, A. (1987). *Unravelling the Mystery of Health*. Jossey-Bass, San Francisco.

Averill, J. R. (1973). Personal control over aversive stimuli and its relationship to stress. *Psychological Bulletin*, 80, 286–303.

Baer, P. E., Garmezy, L. B., McLaughlin, R. J., Pokorny, A. D. and Wernick, M. J. (1987). Stress, coping, family conflict and adolescent alcohol use. *Journal of Behavioural Medicine*, 10, 449–466.

Bailey, R. (1985). Autogenic regulation training (ART), sickness, absence, personal problems, time and the emotional–physical stress of student nurses in general training. PhD thesis, University of Hull.

Bailey, R. and Clark, M. (1989). *Stress and Coping in Nursing*. Chapman & Hall, London.

Beardslee, W. R. (1989). The role of self understanding in resilient individuals: the development of a perspective. *American Journal of Orthopsychiatry*, 59, 266–278.

Bergh-Braam, van der A. H. M. and de Wolff, Ch. J. (1988). Stress among ward sisters. In Wallis, D. and de Wolff, Ch. J. (eds) *Stress and Organizational Problems in Hospitals*. Croom Helm, London.

Bernard, C. (1927). *Introduction to the Study of Experimental Medicine* (translated by Green, H. C.). Macmillan Press, New York.

Boore, J. R. P. (1978). *Information: A Prescription for Recovery*. Royal College of Nursing, London.

Byrne, D. G. and Rosenman, R. H. (1986). The type A behaviour patterns as a precursor to stressful life events: a confluence of coronary risks. *British Journal of Medical Psychology*, 59, 75–82.

Byrne, T. J. and Edeani, D. (1983). Knowledge of medical terminology among hospital patients. *Nursing Research*, 33(3), 178–181.

Cannon, W. B. (1929). *Bodily Changes in Pain, Hunger, Fear and Rage*, 2nd edn. Appleton-Century-Crofts, New York.

Cannon, W. B. (1932). *The Wisdom of the Body*. Appleton-Century-Crofts, New York.

Carver, C. S., Diamond, E. L. and Humphries, C. (1985). Coronary prone behaviour. In Schneiderman, N. and Tapp, J. T. (eds) *Behavioral Medicine: The Biopsychosocial Approach*. Lawrence Erlbaum, Hillsdale, NJ.

Cherniss, C. (1980). *Staff Burnout: Job Stress in the Human Services*. Sage, London.

Chesney, M., Frautschi, N. M. and Rosenman, R. H. (1985). Modifying type A behaviour. In Rosen, J. C. and Solomon, L. J. (eds) *Prevention in Health Psychology*. University Press of New England, Hanover, NH.

Chodoff, P., Friedman, S. B. and Hamburg, D. A. (1964). Stress defenses and coping behaviour: observations in children with malignant disease. *American Journal of Psychiatry*, 120, 743–749.

Cobb, S. and Rose, R. M. (1973). Hypertension, peptic ulcer and diabetes in air traffic controllers. *Journal of the American Medical Association*, 224, 489–492.

Cohen, F. and Lazarus, R. S. (1979). Coping with the stresses of illness. In Stone, G. C., Cohen, F. and Adler, N. E. (eds) *Health Psychology – A Handbook*. Jossey-Bass, San Francisco.

Colerick, E. J. (1985). Stamina in later life. *Social Science and Medicine*, 21, 997–1006.

Cox, T. (1978). *Stress*. Macmillan Education, London.

Cromwell, R. L., Butterfield, E. C., Brayfield, F. M. and Curry, J. J. (1977). *Acute Myocardial Infarction: Reaction and Recovery*. C. V. Mosby, St Louis.

DeSilva, R. A. (1986). Psychological stress and sudden cardiac death. In Schmidt, T. H., Dembroski, T. M. and Blumchen, G. (eds) *Biological and Psychological Factors in Cardiovascular Disease*, pp. 155–183. Springer, Heidelberg.

Dunleavy, R. (1989). Exploration of parasuicide: patients' perception of the nursing care. Unpublished dissertation. Nursing Studies, King's College, London.

Dunlop, D. (1963). Eighty six cases of Addison's disease. *British Medical Journal*, ii, 887.

Egbert, L. D., Battit, G. E., Welch, C. E and Bartlet, M. K. (1964). Reduction of postoperative pain by encouragement and instruction of patients. *New England Journal of Medicine*, 270, 825–827.

Field, D. (1989). *Nursing the Dying*. Routledge, London.

Figley, C. (1986). *Trauma and its Wake*, Vol. 2. Brunner Mazel, New York.

Firth, J. and Morrison, L. (1986). What stress health professionals? A coding system for their answers. *British Journal of Clinical Psychology*, 25(4), 309–311.

Flagherty, G. G. and Fitzpatrick, J. J. (1978). Relaxation technique to increase comfort level for postoperative patients: a preliminary study. *Nursing Research*, 27, 352–355.

Folkman, S., Lazarus, R. S., Pimley, S. and Novacek, J. (1987). Age differences in stress and coping processes. *Psychology and Aging*, 2, 171–184.

Frankenhauser, M. (1975). Experimental approaches to the study of catecholamines and emotion. In Levi, L. (ed.) *Emotions: Their Parameters and Measurement*. Raven Press, New York.

Franklin, B. L. (1974). *Patient Anxiety on Admission to Hospital*. Royal College of Nursing, London.

Friedman, M. and Rosenman, R. H. (1974). *Type A Behavior and Your Heart*. Knopf, New York.

Gillespie, C. and Gillespie, V. (1986). Reading the danger signs. *Nursing Times*, 30 July, 24–27.

Glaser, B. G. and Strauss, A. L. (1966). *Awareness of Dying*. Weidenfeld & Nicholson, London.

Gold, A. E. and Johnston, D. W. (1990). Anger, hypertension and heart disease. In Bennett, P., Weinman, J. and Spurgeon, P. (eds) *Current Developments in Health Psychology*, pp. 105–128. Harwood Academic.

Gray-Toft, P. and Anderson, J. G. (1981). Stress among hospital nursing staff: its causes and effects. *Soc. Sci. Med.* 15a, 639–664.

Hadley, R. D. (1977). Staff nurse cites challenge satisfaction despite stress. *American Nurse*, 9, 6–11.

Harburg, E., Blakelock, J. R. and Roeper, J. (1979). Resentful and reflective coping with arbitrary authority and blood pressure: Detroit. *Psychosomatic Medicine*, 41, 189–202.

Hayward, J. (1975). *Information: A Prescription Against Pain*. The Study of Nursing Care Projects Report Series, Royal College of Nursing, London.

Heim, E. (1991). Coping and adaptation in cancer. In Cooper, C. L. and Watson, M. (eds) *Cancer and Stress: Psychological, Biological and Coping Studies*, pp. 197–235. John Wiley, Chichester.

Hingley, P. (1984). The human face of nursing. *Nursing Mirror*, December.

Hingley, P. and Cooper, C. (1986). *Stress and the Nurse Manager*. John Wiley, Chichester.

Holmes, T. H. and Masuda, M. (1974). Life change and illness susceptibility. In Dohrenwend, B. S. and Dohrebwend, B. P. (eds) *Stressful Life Events: Their Nature and Effects*. John Wiley, New York.

Holmes, T. H. and Rahe, R. H. (1967). The social readjustment rating scale. *Journal of Psychosomatic Research*, 11, 213–218.

Hymovich, D. P. (1981). *Chronic Childhood Illness: Family Impact and Parent Coping*. Association for Care of Children's Health, Toronto.

Hymovich, D. P. and Hagopain, G. A. (1991). *Chronic Illness in Children and Adults: A Psychosocial Approach*. W. B. Saunders, Philadelphia.

Jacobson, S. F. (1978). Stress and coping strategies of neonatal care unit nurses. Unpublished doctoral thesis, University of Minnesota.

Jacobson, S. F. and McGrath, H. M. (1983). *Nurses Under Stress*. John Wiley, New York.

Jemmot, J. B. and Locke, S. E. (1984). Psychosocial factors, immunologic mediation and human susceptibility to infectious diseases: how much do we know? *Psychological Bulletin*, 95, 78–108.

Johnson, J. E. (1973). Effects of accurate expectation about sensations on the sensory and distress components of pain. *Journal of Personality and Social Pyschology*, 27, 261–275.

Johnson, J. E. (1983). Preparing patients to cope with stress while hospitalized. In Wilson-Barnett, J. (ed.) *Patient Teaching*. Churchill Livingstone, Edinburgh.

Johnson, J. E., Rice, V. H., Fuller, S. S. and Endress, M. P. (1978). Sensory information instruction in coping strategy and recovery from surgery. *Research in Nursing and Health*, 1, 4–17.

Johnson, J. H. (1986). *Life Events as Stressors in Childhood and Adolescence*. Sage, Newbury Park, CA.

Johnson, E. H., Spielberger, C. D., Worden, T. and Jacobs, E. H. (1987). The emotional and familial determinants of elevated blood pressure in black and white adolescent males. *Journal of Psychosomatic Research*, 31, 287–300.

Johnson, E. O., Kamilaris, T. C., Chrousos, G. P. and Gold, P. W. (1992). Mechanisms of stress: a dynamic overview of hormonal and behavioural homeostasis. *Neuroscience and Behavioral Reviews*, 16, 115–130.

Kanner, A. D., Coyne, J. C., Schaeefer, C. and Lazarus, R. S. (1981). Comparison of two modes of stress measurement: daily hassles and uplifts versus major life events. *Journal of Behavioural Medicine*, 4, 1–39.

Kasl, S. V. (1984). Chronic life stress and health. In Steptoe, A. and Matthews, A. (eds) *Health Care and Human Behaviour*. Academic Press, London.

Kemp, J. (1984). Nursing at night. *Journal of Advanced Nursing*, 9, 217–223.

Kobasa, S. C. (1979). Stressful life events and health: an inquiry into hardiness. *Journal of Personality and Social Psychology*, 37, 1–11.

Kobasa, S. C., Maddi, S. R. and Puccetti, M. C. (1982). Personality and exercise buffers in stress–illness relationship. *Journal of Behavioural Medicine*, 5, 391–401.

Langer, E. J., Janis, I. L. and Wolfer, J. A. (1975). Reduction of psychological stress in surgical patients. *Journal of Experimental and Social Psychology*, 11, 155–165.

Lazarus, R. S. (1966). *Psychological Stress and the Coping Process*. McGraw-Hill, New York.

Lazarus, R. S. (1976). *Patterns of Adjustment*. McGraw-Hill, New York.

Lazarus, R. S. and Folkman, S. (1984a). *Stress Appraisal and Coping*. Springer, New York.

Lazarus, R. S. and Folkman, S. (1984b). Coping and adaptation. In Gentry, W. D. (ed.) *Handbook of Behavioral Medicine*. Guildford, New York.

Lazarus, R. S. and Launier, R. (1978). Stress related transactions between person and environment. In Pervin and Lewis (eds) *Perspectives in Interactive Psychology*. Plenum Press, New York.

Levy, S. M. (1985). *Behavior and Cancer*. Jossey-Bass, San Francisco.

Lewinsohn, P. H., Mermelstein, R. M., Alexander, C. and MacPhillamy, D. J. (1985). The unpleasant event schedule: a scale for the measurement of aversive events. *Journal of Clinical Psychology*, 41, 483–498.

Lunn, J. A. (1973). Hospital hazards. *The Practitioner* 210, April.

McKinney, M. E., Hofschire, P. J., Buell, J. C. and Elliot, R. S. (1984). Hemodynamic and biochemical responses to stress: the necessary link between type A behavior and cardiovascular disease. *Behavioral Medicine Update*, 6(4), 16–21.

Mandler, G. (1972). Helplessness : theory and research in anxiety. In Spielberger, C. D. (ed.) *Anxiety, Current Trends in Theory and Research 2*, pp. 79–94. Academic Press, New York.

Mandler, G. and Watson, D. L. (1966). Anxiety and the interruption of behavior. In Spielberger, C. D. (ed.) *Anxiety and Behavior*. Academic Press, New York.

Marks, D. and Thomas, S. (1992). Psychosocial factors and well-being in people with disabilities and their carers. Book of abstracts – *Proceedings of the Annual BPS Health Psychology Section*.

Marshall, J. (1980). Stress among nurses. In Cooper, C. L. and Marshall, J. (eds) *White Collar and Professional Stress*. John Wiley, Chichester.

Mason, J. W. (1971). A re-evaluation of the concept of 'nonspecificity' in stress theory. *Journal of Psychiatric Research*, 8, 323–333.

Mathews, K. A. (1986). Summary, conclusions and implications. In Matthews, K. A., Weiss, S. M., Detre, T., Dembroski, T. M., Falkner, B., Manuck, S. B. and Williams, R. B. (eds) *Handbook of Stress, Reactivity, and Cardiovascular Disease*. John Wiley, New York.

Menzies, I. E. P. (1960a). A case study in the functioning of social systems as a defence against anxiety. *Human Relation*, 13, 95–121.

Menzies, I. E. P. (1960b). Nurses under stress: a social system functioning as a defence against anxiety. *International Nursing Review*, 7, 9–16.

Menzies, I. E. P. (1970). *The Functioning of Social Systems as a Defence Against Anxiety*. Tavistock Institute, London.

Menzies, I. E. P. (1990). Personal communication, Oxford.

Miller, S. M. (1979). Controllability and human stress: methods, evidence and theory. *Behaviour Research and Theory*, 17, 287–304.

Miller, S. M. (1980). Why having control reduces stress: If I can stop the roller coaster I don't want to get off. In Seligman, M. and Garber, J. (eds) *Human Helplessness: Theory and Application*, pp. 71–95.

Miller, S. M. (1987). Monitoring and blunting: validation of a questionnaire, to assess different styles of coping with stress. *Journal of Personality and Social Psychology*, 52, 345–353.

Money, J. (1977). The syndrome of abuse dwarfism. *Am. J. Dist. Child.*, 131, 508–513.

Munck, A., Guyre, P. M. and Holbrook, N. J. (1984). Physiological functions of gluco-corticoids in stress and their relation to pharmacological actions. *Endocrine Review*, 5, 25–44.

Notcutt, W. and Morgan, R. J. M. (1990). Introducing patient controlled analgesia for postoperative pain into a district general hospital. *Anesthesia*, 45, 401–406.

Price, T. R. and Bergen, B. T. (1977). The relationship to death as a source of stress for nurses on a coronary care unit. *Omega: Journal of Death and Dying*, 8, 229–238.

Quick, J. C. and Quick, J. D. (1984). *Organizational Stress and Preventive Management*. McGraw-Hill, New York.

Rahe, R. H. (1987). Recent life changes, emotions and behaviors in coronary heart disease. In Baum, A. and Singer, J. A. (eds) *Handbook of Psychology and Health*, Vol. 5. Lawrence Erlbaum, Hillsdale, NJ.

Rentoul, L. P. (1989). Caring for bereaved relatives: problems and possibilities. Paper presented at the *Third Annual Macmillan Conference on Nursing Research and Palliative Care*. King's College, London.

Rentoul, L. P. (1991). Stress among nurses and junior doctors; a qualitative study. Paper presented at the *Death and Dying Group Annual Conference (Medical Sociology)*, Leicester.

Ridgeway, V. and Mathews, A. (1982). Psychological preparation for surgery: A comparison of two methods. *British Journal of Clinical Psychology*, 21, 271–280.

Rogers, M. and Reich, P. (1986). Psychological interventions with surgical patients: Evaluation outcome. *Advances in Psychosomatic Medicine*, 15, 23–50.

Rosse, J. G. and Rosse, P. H. (1981). Role conflict and ambiguity: an empirical investigation of nursing personnel. *Eval. Health Prof.*, 385–405.

Sarafino, E. P. (1990). *Health Psychology: Biopsychosocial Interactions*. John Wiley, New York.

Schleifer, S. J., Scott, B., Stein, M. and Keller, S. E. (1986). Behavioural and developmental aspects of immunity. *Journal of the American Academy of Child Psychiatry*, 26, 751–763.

Schorr, D. and Rodin, J. (1984). Motivation to control ones' environment in individuals with obsessive compulsive, depressive and normal personality traits. *Journal of Personality and Social Psychology*, 46, 1148–1161.

Schowalter, J. E. (1975). Paediatric nurses dream of death. *Journal of Thanatology*, 3, 223–321.

Sechzer, P. H. (1971). Studies in pain with the analgesic demand system. *Anaesthesia and Analgesia*, 50, 1–10.

Seligman, M. (1975). *On Depression, Development and Death*. W. H. Freeman, San Francisco.

Selye, H. (1956). *The Stress of Life*. McGraw-Hill, New York.

Selye, H. (1975). Confusion and controversy in the stress field. *Journal of Human Stress*, 1, 37.

Selye, H. (1976). *The Stress of Life*, 2nd edn. McGraw-Hill, New York.

Selye, H. (1985). History and present status of the stress concept. In Monat, A. and Lazarus, R. S. (eds) *Stress and Coping*, 2nd edn. Columbia University Press, New York.

Silvey, S. (1988). An exploration of the feelings and attitudes of recently bereaved relatives to the care and support of hospital nurses. Unpublished thesis, Nursing Studies, King's College, London.

Skevington, S. (1984). *Understanding Nurses: The Social Psychology of Nursing*. John Wiley, Chichester.

Snowley, G. (1992). Stress, pain, and the individual. In Kenworthy, N., Snowley, G. and Gilling, C. (eds) *Common Foundation Studies in Nursing*, Chapter 4. Churchill Livingstone.

Spielberger, C. D. (1983). Assessment of anger: the state trait anger scale. In Butcher, J. N. and Spielberger, C. D. (eds) *Advances in Personality Assessment*, pp. 159–187. Lawrence Erlbaum, Hillsdale, NJ.

Spinetta, J. J. and Maloney, L. J. (1978). The child with cancer: Patterns of communication and denial. *Journal of Consulting and Clinical Psychology*, 46(6), 1540–1541.

Steffen, S. M. (1980). Perceptions of stress. In Claus, K. E. and Bailey, J. T. (eds) *Living with Stress and Promoting Well Being*. C. V. Mosby, St Louis.

Steptoe, A. (1990). Psychobiological stress responses In Johnston, M. and Wallace, L. (eds) (1990). *Stress and Medical Procedures*. Oxford University Press, Oxford.

Tapp, J. T. (eds) *Behavioral Medicine: The Biopsychosocial Approach*. Lawrence Erlbaum, Hillsdale, NJ.

Tennes, K. and Kreye, M. (1985). Children's adrenocortical responses to classroom activities and tests in elementary school. *Psychosocial Medicine*, 47, 451–460.

Thomas, V. J. (1991). Personality characteristics of patients and the effectiveness of patient controlled analgesia. Unpublished PhD thesis, Goldsmiths' College, University of London.

Thompson, S. C. (1981). Will it hurt less if I can control it? A complex answer to a simple question. *Psychological Bulletin*, 90, 89–101.

Tschudin, V. (1985). Ethics and management of support for nursing staff. Unpublished dissertation, North East London Polytechnic.

Ursin, H., Baade, E. and Levine, S. (1978). *Psychobiology of Stress*. Academic Press, London.

Vogele, C. and Steptoe, A. (1986). Physiological and subjective stress responses in surgical patients. *Journal of Psychosomatic Research*, 30, 205–215.

Volicer, B. J. and Bonhannon, M. W. (1975). A hospital stress rating scale. *Nursing Research*, 24(5), 352–359.

Wallerstein, J. S. (1983). Children of divorce: stress and developmental tasks. In Garmezy, N. and Rutter, M. (eds) *Stress Coping and Development in Children*. McGraw-Hill, New York.

Wallis, D. and de Wolff, Ch. J. (1988). *Stress and Organizational Problems*. Croom Helm, London.

Wells, J. F., Howard, G. S., Nowlin, W. F. and Vargas, M. J. (1986). Presurgical anxiety and postsurgical pain and adjustment: effects of stress inoculation procedure. *Journal of Consulting Psychology*, 54, 831–835.

Wiebe, D. J. and McCallum, D. M. (1986). Health practices and hardiness as mediators in stress–illness relationship. *Health Psychology*, 5, 425–438.

Willis, L., Thomas, P., Garry, P. J. and Goodwin, J. S. (1987). A prospective study of response to stressful events in initially healthy elders. *Journal of Gerontology*, 42, 627–630.

Wilson, J. F. (1981). Behavioural preparation for surgery: benefit or harm? *Journal of Behavioural Medicine*, 4, 79–102.

Wilson-Barnett, J. (1979). *Stress in Hospital: Patients' Psychological Reactions to Illness and Health Care*. Churchill Livingstone, Edinburgh.

Wilson-Barnett, J. (1984). Interventions to alleviate patients' stress: a review. *Journal of Psychosomatic Research*, 28(1), 63–72.

Wilson-Barnett, J. (1986). Reducing stress in hospital. In Tierney, A. (ed.) *Clinical Nursing Practice: Recent Advances in Nursing*, Vol. 14. Churchill Livingstone, Edinburgh.

Wilson-Barnett, J. and Carrigy, A. (1978). Factors affecting patients' responses to hospitalization. *Journal of Advanced Nursing*, 3(3), 221–228.

Wright *et al.* (1988). Matters of death and life. King's Fund Project Paper No. 77. King Edward's Hospital Fund, London.

Zautra, A. J., Okun, M. A., Robinson, S. E., Lee, D., Roth, S. H. and Emmanual, J. (1989). Life stress and lymphocyte alterations among patients with rheumatoid arthritis. *Health Psychology*, 8, 1–14.

8

SELF-CARE – THE ULTIMATE HEALTH OBJECTIVE?

Jane Bayliss

Introduction

Individuals have been carrying out self-care for ill-health and health maintenance probably since the origins of humanity, but until quite recently very little information has been available on the subject. In this chapter I will explore the rising interest in self-care and its relevance to modern nursing practice.

> ### Reflective point
> Take a few minutes to write down what you believe self-care to be.

You may have come up with several possibilities but the main theme running through them all should be that self-care is what individuals do for or to themselves or their families in order to keep them healthy or help them recover if they are unwell.

This might appear obvious but a popular assumption that is often made is that if individuals feel unwell and are experiencing distressing symptoms they will invariably consult a doctor (Scambler, 1986). Research has indicated, however, that this is not so. Scambler et al. (1981) cited by Scambler (1986) found that the most frequent symptoms of illness did not result in formal medical consultation. This was observed in health diaries kept by 79 London women between the ages of 16 and 44. Even the least common symptom, a sore throat, only produced one consultation out of nine reported episodes. Similarly other investigations in the

United Kingdom and the United States [cited by Sorofman et al. (1990)] suggest that during episodes of illness, the use of self-care alone may be as high as 76 percent. Other recent research comparing self-care among older adults in the United States and Japan (Haug et al., 1991) reflects the hidden complexities that exist in self-care. Culture was seen to play an important part in self-care behaviour both in terms of the reporting of symptoms and in the actual response to those symptoms. All of these findings have important implications for nurse–patient interactions.

> ### Reflective point
> Discuss with colleagues and friends, ideally from a range of cultural backgrounds, some common self-care activities for a variety of situations.

You have probably thought of many different activities too numerous to include here, but some of the more common ones may be a hot toddy of lemon or lime juice, honey and possibly some alcohol for colds and 'flu', lying down and resting for a whole range of symptoms, dock leaves for nettle stings, a variety of herbal teas for a range of situations, self-medication with proprietary medicines, e.g. aspirin and paracetamol; the list could go on. These activities are all disease- or illness-based but there are some self-care behaviours which can be classed as health promoting. For example breast and testicular self-examination, immunisation, self-monitoring of urine or blood glucose, or merely following a 'healthy' diet and taking regular exercise; these could all be interpreted as positive self-care activities.

A comparison of self-care in nursing and medicine

Self-care cannot be generalised and is interpreted differently by different disciplines, e.g. medicine, nursing, psychology, sociology and public health. All these disciplines do agree on a number of characteristics that are common to the self-care concept as stated by Gantz (1990)

The concept

- is situation and culture specific
- involves the capacity to act and to make choices
- is influenced by knowledge, skills, values, motivation, locus of control, and efficacy; and
- focuses on aspects of health care under individual control (as opposed to social policy or legislation) (p. 2).

All of the disciplines mentioned are important to the concept of self-care but only nursing and medicine will be compared here.

Medical self-care focuses on the transfer of responsibility of certain types of care from the practitioner to the patient. For example self-assessment (of blood pressure or temperature), self-monitoring (of blood glucose), self-treatment [using over-the-counter (OTC) medications or first aid] and prevention (e.g. breast or testicular self-examination). It is obvious that many of these activities are not solely the domain of physicians as many of them are taught by nurses and other health-care personnel. Self-care in this context can be seen as a specific set of learned activities or protocols encouraging individuals to act in a particular way in a given situation. Patients are expected to modify their behaviour to cope with a disease or condition; the physician does not usually modify the treatment recommendations to fit in with the patient (there may be occasions, however, when treatment may be adapted, depending on the social circumstances of the patient, e.g. transplantation versus dialysis for a person with chronic renal failure).

Self-care in the context of nursing has a very different focus; where possible, patients are involved at all stages of care management. Nurses identify and assess self-care needs *with* individuals, interventions are then planned which should meet those needs, evaluation is carried out *with* the individual to assess the effectiveness of the interventions and then an understanding is gained as to how patient needs determine further nursing actions. In other words nurses modify their behaviour to fit in with the patient's needs and capabilities – a complete contrast to self-care in the medical context.

Orem's self-care deficit theory of nursing

In 1958 Dorothea Orem had a spontaneous insight which enabled her to develop her theory of nursing based on the concept of self-care. In the most recent edition, Orem (1991) defines self-care as 'the practice of activities that individuals initiate and perform on their own behalf in maintaining life, health and well-being' (p. 117).

Within this model, emphasis is placed on personal responsibility for health, but it recognises that self-care is dependent on a variety of factors, e.g. age, stage of development, life experiences, socio-cultural background, availability of resources and state of health (Ham, 1993). The theory states that all individuals have a 'therapeutic self-care demand', i.e. everyone has self-care needs which they have a right to meet themselves providing they have adequate knowledge and skills to do so; individuals also need an understanding of the actions required to initiate and maintain self-care and how these actions relate to health and disease. The person providing the self-care is known as the 'self-c are agent' and in a normal, healthy adult this would be the person themselves; but there are other situations where the self-care agent is someone other than the individual, e.g. infants, children and individuals who are dependent in some way have varying degrees of self-care agency resulting in a 'self-care deficit'. In this situation the self-care agent would be another individual, e.g. a parent, carer or nurse.

There are several universal self-care requisites identified by Orem which are common to all human beings and are related to normal functioning and life processes:

- an adequate air intake
- an adequate water intake
- an adequate food intake
- an adequate functioning of the processes of elimination
- an appropriate level of activity balanced with adequate rest
- a balanced amount of time spent alone and with others
- preventing situations hazardous to the self
- promoting normal human functioning.

Orem also identifies two more categories of self-care requisites. These relate to events which affect the universal self-care requisites (as stated above):

- developmental self-care requisites are dependent on the stage of development of the individual and the effects of the environment on that individual with regard to his or her development. They can be related to stages of the lifecycle or life changes experienced by the individual
- health deviation self-care requisites develop as a result of disease, disability or injury and are recognised by a change in self-care behaviour. This self-care requisite can also be precipitated by medical intervention, e.g. surgery.

Where a self-care deficit exists and an individual is unable to adapt unaided to address this deficit, then nursing care may be needed. The goals of nursing in this model are to enable individuals to attain their own therapeutic self-care demands and this can be achieved by using one of three nursing systems:

- **wholly compensatory nursing systems.** Here the nurse takes full responsibility for the activities required to meet self-care needs
- **partly compensatory systems.** Self-care needs are met by both nurse and patient
- **educative–supportive systems.** In these situations patients are able to perform or can learn to perform different aspects of self-care but need help to carry them out.

Orem also identifies five methods by which nurses assist patients and five areas of activity where these methods of assistance can be implemented. The five methods of assistance are:

- acting or doing for
- guiding

- teaching
- supporting
- providing a developmental environment (Orem 1991, p. 286).

The five areas of activity where implementation can take place also reflect the advanced holistic nursing role which is becoming increasingly important. These areas are listed below:

- the continuation of relationships with individuals, families or groups until patients are ready to be discharged from nursing care
- assessing if and how patients could be helped through nursing
- responding to patients' requests, needs and wants for nursing contact
- the provision of nursing care as a way of prescribing, providing and regulating direct help to patients and their families and friends
- ensuring that their nursing care is coordinated and integrated with any other care they might need or be receiving, either health, social or educational.

Orem's self-care deficit theory of nursing has generally been favourably received within nursing. The principles of the theory have been successfully applied in many different situations of both primary and secondary care, e.g. the care of patients with diabetes, within general practice (Ham, 1993); community health promotion programmes (Nowakowski, 1980); acute care units (Mulli, 1980); within care programmes for adolescents with alcohol-abuse problems (Michael and Sewall, 1980) and many more (Eben *et al.*, 1989).

The historical perspective

There has been a recent upsurge in interest in 'self-care' and various ideas have been put forward to explain this so-called social movement. It is vital, however, to look at self-care in an historical context to put it into perspective.

Self-care as the 'norm'

Prior to the Industrial Revolution the home was the centre of productive activity; men and women had equal and complementary, though different, roles.

Generally it was the elder women who carried (and handed down) the knowledge of healing and caring for the sick; it was also women as the child-bearers who acted as midwives (Ehrernreich and English cited by O'Connor, 1987). Essentially men and women were seen as having the same health requisites with the obvious exception of childbirth and its associated health needs. The majority of health care at that time was based on the collective knowledge of herbal remedies and simple surgical techniques (e.g. bone setting and suturing) that had been handed down through generations. Self-care was more or less the only form of health care available but as the society was more close-knit, information was much more easily passed on. Obviously there were those individuals who carried the specialist knowledge, the wise women and to some extent the monks, but many of the more common herbal remedies were widely known and used.

The 13th century saw the establishment of the universities in Europe and they actively prohibited the entry of women into higher education including medicine. Thus the separatist, élitist medical care system was born. Collectively the church, the state and social convention were used to eradicate the lay health-care system which was in operation at that time. This resulted in a hoarding of medical knowledge by the élite (male) few as opposed to the sharing and mutual support that the lay (female) health providers had been giving until this time. There is perhaps an interesting parallel here with today's health-care system: the holistic nursing approach versus the disease-oriented medical approach.

It is an oversimplification to assume that the establishment of the scientific model of medicine totally eradicated the self-care system of health provision that was already in place. The church and the state, however, were very successful with their witch-hunts of the 15th and 16th centuries and many respectable female herbalist healers and especially midwives were burned for practising their skills (O'Connor, 1987). Thus self-care became very unfashionable and with the growing body of scientific knowledge in the 17th and 18th centuries the art of healing and caring was overtaken by the mechanistic view of the universe. Biology and medicine were seen in this same context and so disease was viewed as the breakdown of a biological machine which needed to be repaired by the physician (Laffan, 1993).

By the middle of the 19th century the industrialisation of the western world was at its height. This was very closely linked to the division of labour by gender based on theories of evolution and biological determinism (Jordanova, 1980; MacCormack, 1980) – women were seen as the 'natural' homemakers, only suitable for domestic activities. At the turn of the century, however, women in the 20–35 age group outnumbered men and therefore had to find work to survive. The employment seen as suitable for these women was teaching and nursing – extensions of the socially acceptable domestic role. Nursing was perceived as mothering of the adult who reverted to a child-like status as a result of illness. Similarly the carrying out of the physician's orders was seen as a good preparation for marriage, as the obedient wife must obey the wishes of her husband (O'Connor, 1987). This paternalistic approach to medicine and health care served to encourage passivity in patients as well as nurses, although there was a strict economic division in the provision of that health care. Medical care had to be paid for and thus, although in the middle and upper classes, care by a physician was the norm, in the working classes visits to the doctor were rare – self-care and self-medication, usually provided by the women of the household, remained the mainstay of health care at that time. Interestingly women in the working classes were viewed as being of different stock from women of the higher classes and thus employment of all kinds was considered suitable.

As the body of scientific knowledge grew medicine began to achieve great things. The invention of the microscope and the germ theory of disease helped to revolutionise health care but with these great advantages there has appeared a subtle shift in attitude towards the medical profession. The more technological it has become the more dissatisfied are the population with the treatment they are receiving; a possible explanation for the growing interest in 'alternative' therapies and an increasing readiness to apportion blame when things go wrong (highlighted by the growing number of cases for litigation).

The 'new' self-care movement

In the middle of the 1970s the academic world suddenly 'discovered' that individuals actually do look after themselves (Kickbush, 1989). Until this time, although it was recognised that self-care existed, it was not considered worthy of scientific interest. About the same time there was a growing criticism of the imbalance of power inherent in the doctor–patient relationship; the concept of 'medicalisation' was developed, principally by Ivan Illich (cited by Porter, 1984; Kickbush, 1989; and DeFriese et al., 1989), in which medicine was perceived to 'take over' the individual, treating him or her as a set of diseases (the mechanistic approach) or at best reduced to the status of patient and hence passivity. There was also a growing criticism, particularly in the United States, that the cost of medical care was increasing far too rapidly. The late 1960s and early 1970s were a time of great social upheaval, reflected by the emergence of the Civil Rights Movement and the Women's Movement; both movements were characterised by their questioning of authority and the correctness of the establishment.

The Women's Movement was particularly active in the criticism of the medical establishment in the area of childbirth and women's health. The medicalisation of human reproduction became the key issue and the feminist self-care ideal was complete autonomy, self-determination and independence from the male-dominated medical system (Kickbush, 1989).

Throughout the 1970s the popularity of self-care increased dramatically, especially in the United States, where large numbers of self-care educational programmes and self-help organisations sprang up. At the same time a debate developed about the differences between self-care and self-help. Self-help was considered to be more political than self-care, probably because of its group structure and organisation. It was also being examined closely by sociologists, not least because of its challenge to the established order of society. Politically, however, the self-care movement was met with suspicion especially in Europe. Here it was seen as a potential conservative weapon for the dismantling of the welfare state (Kickbush, 1989), an interesting observation when looking at the changes in social and health-care provision in Britain in the 1990s.

In the mid-1970s, the self-care movement in the United States attracted support from the two extremes of the political divide, both conservative and progressive elements (DeFriese et al., 1989). On the one hand self-care was seen as a self-reliant mode of behaviour, reducing the spiralling costs produced by dependence on professional health care. The other extreme saw it as a self-reliant mode of behaviour to hasten the 'demedicalisation' of society and end the uneven power balance between professional and lay person. By the end of the 1970s there was a polarisation of the differences between the two extremes. The viewpoint put forward by Levin and Barofsky [both cited by DeFriese et al. (1989) and by Kronenfeld (1979)] was that self-care should be employed as a protection against the perceived negative effects of modern health care (iatrogenesis and medicalisation). Whereas the other view was that self-care could be learned as an extended form of 'first aid', a self-enhancement programme to be used until the doctor arrived (DeFriese et al., 1989). Interestingly the underlying philosophy of both groups was that individuals possess the resources necessary to cope with self-care, a phenomenon that had not been recognised prior to the 1970s. The difference between the two groups underpins the different attitudes to self-care – the health professionals viewed self-care as an intervention engineered by themselves to improve the competence of individuals to perform tasks within the health-care domain. The other view was that self-care was the primary health intervention within the whole spectrum of health provision, and professional intervention was seen in a supportive role, secondary to individual self-care.

Ironically the main critics of the self-care movement, the health professionals, were the very people who went on to develop the main self-care educational programmes that were set up in the United States during the 1980s (DeFriese et al., 1989).

Since the mid-1980s, particularly in the United States, there has been a decline in interest in self-care in the sociological arena, evidenced by an absence of writing on the topic. The decline has been less apparent in Europe (Kickbush, 1989; DeFriese et al., 1989; Dean, 1986) and offset in the USA by an upsurge of writing in the clinical and research literature of nursing and medicine. There is probably no cause for alarm that this change has taken place. The changes in society, particularly evident in the United States, have shown a shift in attitude towards 'wellness' and health promotion; a shift which is supported by the main purchasers and providers of health care. This may well be linked to the realisation within medicine that further improvements to health will not be provided by greater and greater technological interventions but by a dramatic alteration of lifestyle to reduce the effects of the main risk factors which lead to the major chronic diseases of the 1990s.

The danger here is that just as the important health improvements that occurred in the first half of this century were largely attributable to improvements in sanitation, housing and public health measures, the expected improvements in mortality and morbidity from the 'modern' chronic diseases will probably only be achievable by a partnership approach. Individuals need to take responsibility for their own health but they need to be in an environment which allows this and actively promotes the health of the population as a whole.

Nursing and paternalism

Traditionally nursing has been based on the medical model of care. Put simplistically, individuals perceive themselves as ill and adopt the 'sick role'; they seek help from the 'expert', i.e. the physician, who takes over the decision making for them. The illness is treated primarily using clinical procedures (e.g. by drugs and/or surgery) and only trained professionals have sufficient knowledge to carry out the diagnosis and treatment of illness [DeJong cited by Roberts and Krouse (1990)]. Until recently nursing has tended to react in a similar way, nurses perceiving themselves as the expert care-givers, deciding what is best for 'their' patients. Current trends in nursing revolve around such themes as empowerment, power-sharing and 'holistic' nursing, but are nurses ready for these shifts in thinking?

Nurses and patients as partners

> **Reflective point**
> Consider a situation in which a woman has spoken to you about a small lump in her breast. She has been persuaded to have a biopsy, although reluctantly, and the lump is found to be malignant. The woman decides to have no further investigations or treatment.
>
> What are your feelings about this situation? What would you say to the woman?

Initially this situation may appear to be concerned more with 'self-neglect' than with self-care. How could this woman ignore the fact that she has a readily treatable condition which, with close follow-up, might be totally eradicated?

Looking again at Orem's definition which states that self-care is: 'the practice of activities that individuals initiate and perform on their own behalf in maintaining life, health and well being' (Orem, 1991, p. 117), there are several key words which are crucial to this situation. The maintenance of life, health and well-being are subjective qualities – what the 'expert' nurse perceives as important to maintain may not coincide with the woman's perception in the same situation.

Levin (1981) sees self-care as involving empowerment and encouraging self-reliance in health care. Nurses often perceive that self-care involves empowering their patients but is empowerment within a medical model framework of health provision really empowerment? It is very easy to fall into the trap of believing that power is being shared with patients when in fact we, as professionals, are saying 'I am the powerful person in this interaction but because I provide care for you I am willing to relinquish some of my power to you. In return, however, you must do as I say and you must realise that the power was all mine to give in the first place and is only being handed over as an act of beneficence' (adapted from Clifton, 1993). This beneficence is also reflected in some of the terms that remain in common use within nursing. One such term 'weekend leave' is used by Clifton (1992) to illustrate the paradox that exists in modern nursing practice. The use of the word 'leave' implies that someone has been given permission to go, but who has the right to grant, or withhold that permission? If treatment is suspended, for whatever reason, over a weekend and the patient is well enough to leave, then they should be free to choose to go home (or anywhere else for that matter). The term 'weekend leave' is then inappropriate, since it ignores the patient as an individual and reduces him or her to the role of passive dependent. In order for nurses really to achieve empowerment in their interactions with patients, and thereby enhance the process of self-care, a paradigm shift needs to take place.

Roberts and Krouse (1988) have developed a negotiation model for nursing, based on work carried out by Eisenthal and Lazare (1976, cited by

Roberts and Krouse, 1990). This model consists of three phases:

1. finding out the patient's perspective of the problem as well as their goals and expectations and sharing the nurse's perspective with the patient
2. active interaction between the nurse and patient in which the nurse tells the patient about his or her initial assessment of the problem and summarises the plan of action, at the same time encouraging the patient to question and respond to it
3. the patient and nurse negotiate which part of each person's perspectives will be used when making the final decision about care. The goal being to arrive at a decision which is agreeable to both individuals.

The process ensures that the patient's perspective of the situation is acknowledged and that their goals for the encounter are made explicit. Patients then feel that their views are important and their opinions are valued. At the same time the patient is made aware of the nurse's thoughts and opinions. In this way nurse and patient are able to discuss and negotiate solutions based on a shared view of the problems involved.

Although this may appear to be a simple model, these behaviours do not come easily either to the nurse or the patient. As already discussed, nursing has grown up based on the medical model and hence nurses have been encouraged to think of themselves as the experts. Research carried out by Kappeli (1986) on the extent to which nurses facilitated self-care behaviour indicated that overall, they did not enable patients as much as might have been expected. An analysis of the nurses' activity highlighted nine types of behaviour which could be divided into accepting and non-accepting. Nurses showed a strong paternalistic/medical tendency by displaying directive and coercive behaviours, while the behaviours to encourage patient growth and enablement were episodic in nature. Patients have also been socialised into believing themselves to be at best, passive recipients of professional intervention and at worst unwilling subjects for professional domination. This process of interaction based on power-sharing and negotiation needs practice and reinforcement (Roberts and Krouse, 1990).

Many of the behaviours involved in this negotiation model of nursing form the basis of the skills required by the advanced practitioner of nursing. In order to elicit information from patients to build a negotiation strategy, effective communication must exist between nurse and patient; but part of this effective communication must be based on the nurse's reflection on his or her own beliefs and attitudes. Before we can advise and support patients we need to understand our own feelings about power and whether we are able to share it effectively.

Are patients ready to be 'activated'?

This ground swell of interest in the development of partnerships with patients can sometimes neglect those individuals central to the debate – the patients themselves. Do patients want to be partners in their care or do they actually prefer passivity?

Reflective point
Consider a patient who has recently had surgery which has resulted in the formation of a permanent colostomy. The patient is now several days post-operation but refuses to have anything to do with the care of the stoma. How would you care for this patient?

In order for this patient to function independently within his own environment he will need to be able to care for the colostomy. How can this be achieved?

Muetzel (1988) believes that the nurse–patient relationship has always been a partnership but without equality or a true sharing of power. She also believes, however, that in order for the interaction to be therapeutic then intimacy and reciprocity must be inherent in the situation. An intimate partnership is based on the concepts of security and freedom; patients need an environment that is secure both physically and emotionally (Bayntun-Lees, 1992). In order to achieve this, Muetzel believes that the nurse must possess 'self-awareness' and hence be able to use 'the self' effectively to promote feelings of warmth, sympathy and acceptance of the patient. The patient is then perceived as an individual who has beliefs and feelings that are worthwhile. Peplau (1969) also argues that nurses must believe in the moral right of another individual to exercise choice and control in order to avoid the trap of directive manipulation of behavioural change. The individual is thereby trusted to make decisions for and by themselves.

Considering the exercise again can help put this into perspective. The patient with the colostomy is unable to cope with this new aspect of himself. Within a relationship that values his beliefs and attitudes this patient should feel safe enough to verbalise these anxieties. While the care of the colostomy is being maintained by the nurse she can provide comprehensive information about the need for the surgical procedure, the way the colostomy functions and the importance of the daily care routine. During this process any questions should be answered accurately and truthfully, thereby building a trusting relationship. Written material and possibly audio-visual aids can also be used to provide further knowledge, thus enabling the patient and enhancing his autonomy. The nurse can encourage participation in the physical care of the colostomy, reinforcing any participation with praise and reassurance, stating that she will be there to help if necessary. Clearly this example reflects the development of a therapeutic nurse–patient interaction in which care is individualised to achieve beneficial outcomes for the patient (McMahon, 1991). Within this situation the patient should feel valued and eventually safe enough to carry out his own self-care of the colostomy (Kyle and Pitzer, 1990).

There are obviously situations in which patients do not possess the skills necessary to participate in their own health care. They may never before have been asked or expected to contribute to decisions affecting their lives. It is very easy in this situation to perpetuate the suffocating paternalism that has ruled some people's lives and continue to exclude them from any decision making. By democratically encouraging and developing their participation skills and enabling them to express their attitudes and beliefs in their own words, they are given an opportunity to examine those beliefs more objectively (Bayntun-Lees, 1992).

This still does not answer the question of whether patients want to be more 'active' in their care or not. Perhaps this is the wrong question. Seedhouse (1988) defines autonomy as 'a person's capacity to choose freely for himself, and to be able to direct his own life' (p. 130). Personal autonomy is dependent on several factors: to be able physically to carry out one's wishes; to be in an environment which allows this; to have sufficient knowledge to be able to carry them out; to be able to use the knowledge appropriately, being aware of any drawbacks and options available; and the ability to choose outcomes that are appropriate to that person, sometimes called rationality (Seedhouse, 1988). For the patient, being an autonomous participant within a therapeutic environment does not necessarily mean that they will have to make decisions all of the time, rather it is having a choice. They have the power to choose whether they make the decisions or whether they allow someone else to decide on their behalf (Bayntun-Lees, 1992). This situation cannot exist, however, unless the practitioner really does interact with the patient as an equal partner – rather than providing care to or for the patient.

Reflective point

Are there any situations where you believe information should not be given to a patient?

Patient self-care is based upon the tenets of patient autonomy, patient participation, power-sharing and partnerships in care. The therapeutic environment is dependent on trust and a feeling of 'being safe' (both physically and emotionally) for the patient. If that trust is broken by telling lies or by not telling the whole truth, i.e. withholding information, then why should patients trust their carers at all?

There are obviously situations where all the facts may not yet be known or where evaluation has to take place; patients must then be made aware that these are the reasons why information is being withheld. There are other situations, however, where the practitioner (doctor or nurse) makes the decision not to tell the truth, as they perceive it may be harmful to the patient.

When a patient seeks treatment they are, in effect, surrendering their body into the care of another person. Unless they make it clear that they are surrendering their autonomy as well or they are in a position where they are unable to act autonomously (they may be unconscious) then that autonomy should be respected (Martin, 1993). If a patient actively states that he or she does not wish to be included in the decision making or does not wish to be told the diagnosis, then that person has made that choice him- or herself and this choice should also be respected. Withholding information or forcing information onto patients when they have specifically asked not to know is withdrawing their equal status from the relationship – they are then no longer partners in their care.

Nurses and the practice of self-care

As nurses we are often very good at saying 'do as I say, not as I do'. This is evidenced in the high numbers of nurses that still smoke cigarettes (around one in three) while advocating smoking cessation and health promotion for their patients (Day, 1994; Lorenzo and Drick, 1990). A study by Adriaanse *et al.* (1991) into the smoking habits of nurses worldwide, suggests that the major contributory factors are stress, a lack of control over their working environment and the existence of an occupational subculture. These are hardly ideal situations for the promotion of empowerment, a prerequisite for the development of self-care!

The traditional model for nurse education was very hierarchical in structure; nurses were taught about disease processes, about how to carry out numerous procedures but above all nurses were taught to do as they were told! Hardly a good starting point for the development of a power-sharing relationship. Modern nurse education has, hopefully, moved away from this didactic approach, but to what extent are nursing students actively encouraged to develop their own self-care abilities in relation to the development of their professional identity? Nursing students are being encouraged to view their patients holistically but it is often the case that the student is not viewed from the same perspective (Lorenzo and Drick, 1990). Nurses are educated into the role of professional and taught to care for others, it is then often assumed that they can apply these skills when caring for themselves. Ideally nursing curricula should offer the opportunity for nursing students to reflect on their own self-care concepts, thus providing a sound basis for encouraging the development of self-care abilities in their patients. Even with the introduction of Project 2000, nursing students may still experience a heavy work schedule of class and clinical teaching time, plus coursework. This, together with expectations from teaching staff, may leave little time for activities outside academic life. These demands placed upon students could be conveying the wrong messages – that taking time to care for oneself is not important. Obviously there are time restrictions on academic courses and there are always deadlines that need to be met, but involving students in the decision-making process and the setting of goals for learning achievement are ways of encouraging the development of healthy self-care attitudes.

A good example of student involvement has been set up by the Mid Trent College of Nursing and Midwifery. Students are encouraged to participate in the curriculum planning groups, there is regular student evaluation of the course, student handbooks and a student counselling service are available and a student charter has been implemented (believed to be one of the first of its kind in a college of nursing and midwifery) (Hollingsworth *et al.*, 1994).

Health promotion and self-care

Health promotion and the health of the nation

> ### Reflective point
> *Write down what you believe health promotion to be.*

You may have thought of several areas: stopping smoking; reducing alcohol intake; eating a healthy diet; breast and cervical screening programmes and so on.

Many of these activities are potentially ideally suited to the process of self-care and health promotion might be viewed as an ideal medium for the development of self-care strategies. At its simplest level, individuals are given lots of information about how to make healthy choices, educated about healthier lifestyles and encouraged to go forth and improve the nation's health. This is a very individualistic approach to health promotion.

In the early 1980s, the World Health Organization (WHO) introduced a new programme in

Europe on 'Lay, community and alternative health care' as part of a wider strategy looking at lifestyles and health (Hatch and Kickbush, 1983; Kickbush, 1989). The main outcome of this programme was the decision that self-care needs to be looked at in the context of the social system in which it is functioning, i.e. people carry out self-care against the background of their everyday lives. Lifestyle is then observed as a phenomenon related to the conditions in which people live and is based on both collective *and* individual experiences (Kickbush, 1986). From this perspective, health is then perceived as a 'social project' and self-care and self-help are social phenomena (Kickbush, 1989). The lifestyles that people adopt are dependent upon their socio-economic circumstances, their cultural background (and therefore their health beliefs), and how easy it is for them to choose between the options available. The UK pledged its support to the strategy developed in 1984 by the European region of the WHO to attain 'Health for All by the Year 2000'. The aims of the strategy included a reduction in health inequalities and an increased emphasis on health promotion to at least equal that of treating acute disease.

Much of recent health promotion activity has been focused on individuals whilst largely ignoring the environment in which these individuals function. The recent *Health of the Nation* White Paper (Department of Health, 1992) identifies five key areas for action to improve the nation's health, with national targets for the reduction of mortality and morbidity by the year 2000. The five key areas are:

- coronary heart disease and stroke
- cancers
- mental illness
- HIV/AIDS and sexual health
- accidents.

Although this document advocates the development of healthy alliances between individuals and larger groups, e.g. schools, employers, local government agencies, the main effort to attain these targets is expected to come from individual behaviour change. Obviously this is a great opportunity for the development of increased self-reliance and self-care – encouraging people to take a greater responsibility for their own health – the problem arises should the targets not be achieved; there is then a great danger of employing a 'victim blaming' response. Individuals will have been provided with vast quantities of information, they should then be in a position to make

informed healthy choices – if they do not choose the healthy option it is their fault that they are ill? Should they then be entitled to receive health care to treat their self-inflicted illness, thus preventing someone 'more worthy' from receiving care? This situation may seem unlikely but recent cases highlighted in the media have shown that within the market-led economy of the National Health Service (NHS), clinical decisions are being made not to treat patients for certain conditions if they continue to smoke or refuse to lose weight. There are often good clinical reasons for taking this line. For example patients are more likely to develop chest infections post-operatively if they smoke and are then more likely to suffer delayed healing and wound break-down. However, is this attitude really empowering patients to participate in their care? Or is it just a perpetuation of paternalism: 'I the expert, know what is best for you. If you do not do as I say then I shall withhold treatment'?

The WHO definition of health promotion in the Ottawa Charter (1986) as cited by Kickbush (1989) states that it is a process which enables people to increase the control they have over, and therefore improve, their health. It also states that in order to attain health, people 'must be able to identify and to realise aspirations, to satisfy needs, and to change or cope with the environment' (p. iii). *The Health of the Nation* document (Department of Health, 1992) acknowledges the WHO approach of 'Health for All by the Year 2000' and incorporates some of its philosophy into the targets for health improvement in the UK. Unfortunately the implementation of action to achieve those targets does not necessarily tie in with the WHO philosophy of health promotion. To a great extent, the attainment of the targets is to be achieved by action at an individual level, i.e. by behaviour change (see below). This is to be brought about by raising awareness and the encouragement of individuals to make 'healthy choices'. Nowhere, however, does it indicate how individuals might be empowered to exercise a greater degree of control over, and, therefore, cope with or change their environment to attain better health – an integral part of the WHO philosophy.

Within primary care, 1993 saw the introduction of a new system of health promotion which was based upon *The Health of the Nation* targets. This system initially focuses on three main areas: smoking cessation, coronary heart disease and stroke. The way in which general practitioners are funded for health promotion activities is based on a system of banding with an ascending scale of remuneration.

- Band 1 is concerned with monitoring and advising patients to stop smoking
- Band 2 is designed to minimise the mortality and morbidity of patients with hypertension, coronary heart disease and stroke
- Band 3 is designed to reduce the incidence of coronary heart disease and stroke by identifying those people with risk factors.

This system of organising health promotion activities appears to be more flexible and 'user-friendly' than the previous system. The old system consisted of a series of health-promotion clinics run at a specific time, concerned with a wide range of health and chronic disease management issues. One of the main problems with such a system was that the emphasis was on quantity rather than quality, as remuneration was based on the numbers of patients seen. Also the patients who could attend at rigid clinic times were not necessarily the ones who most needed health-promotion input (Eveleigh, 1993). The new arrangements can be carried out opportunistically and patients do not necessarily need to be seen in a clinic setting; in fact practices will be expected to reach those patients who do not attend the surgery. There are disadvantages in the new system, which again relies heavily on individual behaviour modification and which has to be achieved through intervention by health professionals. In certain primary health-care settings the new system is in effect reducing the opportunities for a more comprehensive 'well-person health check', and hence patient choice, as resources have to be concentrated on coronary heart disease prevention programmes.

There is another drawback which can be seen when the requirements are looked at more closely. In the first year general practitioners (GPs) are asked to screen differing percentages of their target population (15–74 years old) depending on the band they have applied to be remunerated for: 30 percent for Band 1 and 20 percent for Bands 2 and 3. This percentage will increase each year by 15 percent to a maximum of 80, 90 and 75 percent, respectively, and will be monitored by annual and half-yearly reports (Eveleigh, 1993). The gathering of this information is relatively easy when registering a new patient as it can form part of a routine health check, but it can be more difficult

for patients attending for problems which are totally unconnected with the data required, e.g. a patient who attends the GP surgery following the death of a spouse does not want the intrusion into her grief which would be necessary in order to obtain all the data for Band 3 (smoking habits, blood pressure, alcohol intake, family history, body mass index, diet and exercise). Health professionals therefore need to be sensitive to the needs of patients and effective communication must form the basis of good practitioner–patient interactions.

Nursing and health promotion

As discussed earlier, Orem's self-care deficit theory of nursing (1991) recognises the importance of promoting and maintaining health for the individual. More than this, Orem's theory is based on the fundamental right of the individual to meet his or her own self-care needs providing he or she has the ability to do so. Within the model the nursing system which provides the closest correlation with health promotion is the 'educative–supportive system' – where nurses are required to assist with decision making, behaviour control and the acquisition of skills and knowledge by the patient (Ham, 1993). For nurses to participate effectively in health promotion therefore, a system of negotiation with the patient must again be developed (Roberts and Krouse, 1990).

Nurses are often involved in teaching health promotion activities, but when patients fail to adopt healthy behaviours it is all to easy to say 'I tried but the patient just wasn't motivated' (Williams Utz, 1990). This view of motivation is very paternalistic: the patient should listen to the 'expert' and take his or her advice on how to behave healthily. If they choose to ignore that advice then they are labelled as 'non-compliant'. Motivation must be viewed, therefore, from a more holistic perspective in order that nurses may truly carry out their duty of care. In Orem's theory (1991), motivation is described as one of the power components of self-care that nurses can use to help patients harness their energies. Motivation from this perspective allows a much more positive view of the patient, thus ensuring a respect for autonomy and decision making by the individual. Health beliefs and perceptions are respected and goal-setting and priorities are discussed and agreed with the full participation of the patient. Orem (1991) identifies three phases of self-care motivation which the nurse needs to be able to recognise within the patient – estimative, transitional and productive:

- the estimative phase involves patients exploring and developing knowledge about themselves, their condition and their environment
- the transitional phase involves patients reflecting on what they would prefer to do and then deciding on a course of action; and
- the productive phase is where patients prepare for and carry out self-care functions, monitor and reflect on the results and thereby affirm their judgement about their actions.

There is evidence that in order for individuals to feel motivated to change health behaviours several criteria must be met: the person must believe that the problem can be solved (Ditto *et al.*, 1988); possible solutions must be viewed as attractive (Briody, 1984); they need to feel competent to carry out the behaviour successfully (Brown, 1989); and they need to experience positive feedback and favourable consequences (Girdano and Dusek, 1988). In other words, nurses have a vital role to play in promoting healthy self-care behaviour: providing appropriate information and guidance; valuing the patient's understanding of situations and therefore enabling him or her to understand the cause of the health problem; respecting the autonomy of the individual, while at the same time assisting them to set achievable goals and commit themselves to an agreed course of action. Perhaps the most important function that nursing can provide for patients is to enable them to develop self-management skills. In this way patients really do become empowered and are able to recognise and control their own behaviours, which they see are influenced by thoughts, feelings, their internal state, environmental factors and consequences (Williams Utz, 1990). Skilful nursing enables the patient to become a reflective individual who can examine his or her own behaviour and take charge of situations thus maintaining motivation.

Orem's model for health-promoting activity, by definition, is restricted to individual behaviour change. There remains, however, the need for promoting healthy behaviour on a much greater scale and there is no reason why nurses cannot be involved at the macro as well as the micro level. Jowett (1992) suggests a model for health pro-

motion developed by Tannahill (1985) which encompasses the whole range of aspects of health promotion. The model is characterised by three overlapping spheres of activity – health education, health protection and prevention, none of which are mutually exclusive.

Health education within this model is not seen to be restricted to the traditional situation of a nurse teaching a patient about a specific condition or procedure, although that remains important, it also involves raising the awareness of policy makers at different levels. Nurses can continue to participate in this, not only through their professional organisations, but also by joining with other nurses at a local level to lobby policy-makers and make their feelings known.

Prevention in Tannahill's model is seen as those activities designed to reduce the risk of disease occurring; perhaps the most commonly recognised terms for nurses are primary, secondary and tertiary prevention. Generally these activities need to be carried out by nurses on an individual or group basis, although there is always opportunity for nurses to try and influence for example, immunisation and breast screening programmes.

The third area of the model is health protection which has the aim of reducing possible health hazards in the environment thus enabling individuals to adopt healthy behaviours. Examples of this might be the lobbying of parliament to ban tobacco advertising, or on a more local level the lobbying of local authorities to improve exercise facilities for their employees and the local community. This model is useful in that it emphasises the need for a broad approach to health promotion, while at the same time recognising that nurses can and should become involved at all levels in order to achieve health enhancement for the community.

Denmark is one European country which seems to be trying to address the need for effective self-care enhancement by looking at innovative schemes within their primary health-care system. One such scheme was set up at the Billund Health Centre (Krasnik, 1986). Billund is a small township in Jutland where the Health Centre serves a population of 7000. Here they have been putting into practice many of the theories already discussed – the philosophy of the primary health-care team at the centre is to enable people to mobilise their own resources and to enhance their abilities to lead healthy lives. The key process in this philosophy is the interaction with the patient as an equal within the relationship, but the philosophy also recognises that disease is a phenomenon not only of the individual but also of their social situation.

There are many situations reported in the nursing press of nurses being involved in community health initiatives, examples include a primary health-care clinic geared to the needs of homeless people (Gibb and Lucas, 1993); the setting up of a coronary heart disease prevention programme in an inner city area (Cook, 1993); a centre in Nottingham where women are empowered to make better decisions about their own and their children's health (Rowe and Miles, 1994) and a scheme run by a district nurse that offers exercise programmes on prescription from local GPs (Turner, 1994). All of these initiatives serve to underline the valuable contribution nurses can make to health promotion at all levels.

Self-care and chronic or terminal illness

Within the industrialised societies of the world a large proportion of health-care expenditure occurs on the care and treatment of individuals with chronic diseases, e.g. heart disease, diabetes, hypertension and cancer. Although individuals are living longer the quality of life in later years is often reduced by these diseases. Data presented in *The Health of the Nation* (Department of Health, 1992) show that in the last sixty years deaths from circulatory disease have risen from 26 to 46 percent of the total number of deaths, and deaths from cancers have risen from 13 to 25 percent. With the great improvements in early detection and management of such diseases the likelihood is that morbidity has also increased dramatically and will probably continue to rise. Where does self-care feature in these situations which are often characterised by extensive medicalisation? At first there may seem to be little room for the exercise of autonomy and self-direction but, as with any illness, it is the care people carry out for themselves which can provide the primary resource.

Cancer therapies and self-care

The diagnosis of cancer can have a devastating

effect on the life of an individual. Gammon (1991) makes the observation that as the incidence of cancer is high and the survival rates, once the disease is diagnosed, are increasing (Cancer Research Campaign, 1990) then it becomes important to examine how individuals are coping. Individuals with cancer often have to learn to cope with demands that are not part of their normal repertoire of skills and knowledge (Richardson, 1991). The coping skills required for cancer are also different from those necessary to cope with more acute or self-limiting illnesses (Gammon, 1991). A model proposed by Craig and Edwards (1983) suggests that individuals cope with the crises of their disease by problem-solving techniques, the main focus of the model being on the individual and his or her family within a nursing context – a basic component of self-care. There appear to be other good indicators of coping, highlighted by various pieces of research [all cited by Gammon (1991)], including self-esteem, levels of anxiety and depression, feelings of control and meaningfulness, and extent of acceptance or recovery after the crisis. Research carried out by Gammon (1991) shows that there seems to be a strong correlation between coping with cancer and a high self-care agency. Self-care also seems to be linked to a higher self-esteem, improved feelings of control and lower depression and anxiety. Consequently there would appear to be a role here for nurses to develop further their 'educative-supportive' role (Orem, 1991) when caring for patients with cancer.

One of the most distressing problems faced by individuals with cancer is the side-effects from the treatment they receive. These can sometimes be so severe as to overshadow the disease itself (Richardson, 1991). Nausea and vomiting are reported to be two of the most distressing side-effects of chemotherapy. Although there is a wealth of information on pharmacological and behavioural methods of dealing with the problems, little attention seems to have been given to self-care interventions (Richardson, 1991). Research in the USA also indicates that patients who experience more severe side-effects from chemotherapy are at risk from a reduction in self-care ability (Musci and Dodd, 1990). There is therefore, an important role here for nurses to intervene to ensure that adequate symptom control is being achieved with whatever method the patient feels most comfortable.

One of the major difficulties that nurses (and doctors) often experience with advanced cancer is coming to terms with the notion that the disease is no longer curable. Within a health culture that is based on the apparent ability to provide a cure for every ill, having to recognise that 'nothing more can be done' for the patient, can be very difficult to accept. This belief is in fact inaccurate as a great deal can be achieved for and with the patient and the family to ensure the best possible quality of life for the time that is left. The aim of care at this time is to ensure the patient has autonomy and control over his or her life for as long as possible, while at the same time consulting and considering his or her wishes on all aspects of care management (Marks, 1993).

An area in which there is a growing interest amongst both lay and health-care personnel is the use of complementary therapies, e.g. aromatherapy, massage, reflexology, relaxation and meditation, acupuncture. Some of these methods, such as acupuncture and the various relaxation techniques, are becoming more widely accepted amongst practitioners of conventional medicine, but many of the other procedures remain at the fringe of health care.

Within the area of palliative care for patients with a terminal illness one of the prime considerations must be the control of pain. Pain in these situations can be experienced as 'total pain', i.e. emotional, spiritual, social and physical pain (Marks, 1993). Obviously there are conventional methods of dealing with physical pain, primarily analgesia of varying strengths, but methods which can improve the experience of the whole range of pain in these situations is an absolute necessity. The human body produces its own morphine-like analgesic substances called enkephalins and endorphins. These have been found throughout the nervous system and can be produced in response to treatments such as acupuncture, transcutaneous electrical nerve stimulation (TENS) and aromatherapy (Sanderson and Carter, 1994). Interestingly, psychological state also influences endorphin levels – negative emotions such as fear and anxiety cause a decrease in endorphin levels whereas they show an increase under positive influences. There is evidence to suggest that some of the 'fringe' complementary therapies do have a positive effect on mood, psychological state and wound healing (Sanderson and Carter, 1994; Sayre-Adams, 1994; Heidt, 1981). It seems reasonable to assume, therefore, that this beneficial effect may be useful, not only in palliative care, but also in a wide range of other stressful situations. There is obviously scope for extensive research into the use and effects of complementary therapies within the more conventional health-care system. Within the context of self-care and terminal illness, however, if the prime consideration is to maximise patient autonomy and control that then any process which improves quality of life must be worthy of consideration.

Self-care in relation to chronic illness

Reflective point
Using your own experience reflect on the statement 'it is possible to be well while at the same time experiencing an illness'.

The concept of health and wellness was defined by the WHO at its inception at the end of the Second World War. Health was defined as 'a state of complete physical, mental and social well-being, not just the absence of disease or infirmity' (Townsend and Davidson, 1988, p. 34). An interesting observation made by Brooks (1984) is that many of the lifestyle management programmes aimed at promoting health for the majority of the population are very similar to those self-care regimes developed by individuals with a chronic disability. There are four themes which Brooks sees as common to both situations:

- individual responsibility for self-care
- a comprehensive concept of health
- the ability to achieve the highest potential for that individual
- the recognition of the social aspect of health maintenance.

The recent trend, both in the UK and the USA, is to encourage and enable people with chronic disabilities to participate more in the management of their care and be more self-directing, rather than being passive recipients of rehabilitation programmes. This is obviously the development of self-care, but what about those individuals who are experiencing a chronic disease? Should they be encouraged to manage their own illness?

A growing number of individuals who are seen to experience more chronic illness are older adults. Often health-promotion efforts are aimed at young or middle-aged people, based on the reasoning that early prevention may offset problems later on. In our society older people are often dismissed, ignored or ridiculed; we are experiencing a youth culture and it is assumed that older people are usually unable or unwilling to learn new ideas or behaviours. Yet it is these older persons who show an increased risk from chronic illnesses such as diabetes, high blood pressure and congestive heart failure – strategies for health promotion and illness prevention are therefore vital for this age group. As already discussed, health-promoting activities often involve behaviour change which requires motivation. Elderly people are often very firm about what they can and cannot do and may need a lot of encouragement to change behaviours or realise potential skills (Moore, 1990).

The aim of teaching self-care to any individual is maintenance of health and to improve quality of life. Diabetes is an 'ideal' disease for self-care management as there are a large number of daily activities necessary to maintain good control, i.e. prevention of hypo- and hyperglycaemia, skin care, foot care and regular dental care. Once diagnosed, the routine for diabetes management is basically the same for both young and older people alike. Education about the disease is the first stage in helping older people adjust to the diagnosis (Dellasega, 1990). As already discussed, in order to teach individuals of any age effectively, there must first be an assessment of their knowledge base, motivation and abilities to communicate. The main difference when teaching older people is the importance of recognising and compensating for any changes due to the ageing process which might affect learning ability. These changes might be deteriorating sight and/or hearing, reduced short-term memory and reduced dexterity because of joint stiffness. Teaching methods, therefore, need to be tailored to meet the needs of the individual client. The presentation of small amounts of material at a slow pace enhances retention of the information; the provision of written or verbal cues to remind the individual about the key points helps to overcome short-term memory problems. Encouraging feedback at the end of one teaching session and at the beginning of a new session may highlight areas that need further attention (Dellasega, 1990). Perhaps the most important aspect of teaching diabetic care is stressing the need for individual responsibility for

the daily management of the condition. Dieticians, nurses and other health-care professionals can teach patients how to care for themselves but it is up to the individual whether he or she chooses to implement their knowledge and comply with the information and advice.

It has been shown that compliance with therapeutic regimes is inversely related to their complexity (Haynes, 1976; Runyan, 1975), i.e. the more complex the regime is, the less likely individuals are to follow it. Bushnell (1992) cites two studies on the self-care of older adults with congestive heart failure (CHF). One study on 100 elderly patients found that those individuals who knew about their condition and had a positive perception of the benefits of treatment were more likely to comply with their advised diet and medication, smoking cessation programme and the avoidance of stressful situations (Lacy, 1988). The other study concluded that those patients with CHF who received teaching about their condition at home were significantly less likely to be re-admitted to acute care hospitals than those who received no additional teaching (McKee, 1971). The old adage then that 'you cannot teach an old dog new tricks' holds no truth. Ageing is a part of development and as with any stage there are advantages and disadvantages within the process. It must be the goal of nurses when educating towards self-care to recognise the strengths and capabilities that older people possess, so that they too can be partners in, and not just objects of, care (Moore, 1990).

Self-care – the future?

In order to consider the future of health care, and self-care in particular, it is necessary to look at the past, the current trends can then be put into context. The present system of social welfare, including the NHS, was based on the Beveridge report (House of Commons, 1942). This report had the central assumption that there was a finite pool of illness which, with the introduction of a free health service, would be gradually reduced. Consequently service provision could also eventually be reduced. When the NHS came into existence in 1948 there was a tremendous inequality in the allocation of resources. The south was better provided for than the north; urban areas were better off than rural; and richer areas had better resources than poorer ones (Masterson, 1993). This division appears to have persisted (Townsend and Davidson, 1988) and as early as 1953 it was recognised by the Guillebaud Committee of Enquiry that the hospital sector was consuming the most funds, whilst seeing the least number of patients (Masterson, 1993). The initial intention to provide good primary health care, and therefore prevention, had already been lost to the politically more powerful hospital and specialist services sector of the tripartite system of administration.

Since the 1970s it has been recognised, both in professional and academic circles, that a greater emphasis should be placed on health promotion. Government policy has also recognised this to some extent, as there has been guidance that priority should be given to preventive services and community care. Even as recently as 1989, however, hospital services still accounted for the greater proportion of health expenditure (Ham, 1992). There have been attempts made to re-allocate resources more fairly since 1976, when the Resource Allocation Working Party recom-mended that money should be diverted away from the four Thames regions to the rest of the country. More recently, resources have been allocated to regions based on a formula which takes into account not only the population size but also such weighting factors as age distribution and amount of illness. It would seem, however, that it has made little difference, partly because of general financial constraints and partly through the major potential losers, the large teaching hospitals, having the ability to mobilise an effective opposition to the proposals (LeGrand, 1982).

Obviously the fundamental assumption made by Beveridge was incorrect. There is no finite demand for health care and there can never be a maximum level of health-care provision. Thus the provision of health care has to be negotiated with the interested parties against a backdrop of affordability and political acceptability. The emphasis for too long seems to have been on the treatment of disease at the expense of health promotion and this, in turn, has led to unrealistic expectations of the medical system. If as individuals we believe that medicine, which is essentially curative, can be called upon to deal with all the problems we encounter in life, then we neglect to appreciate many of the situations which make us sick in the first place. This can result in us not employing the social and personal preventive measures which are available (Porter, 1984).

The Health of the Nation (Department of Health, 1992) was thus produced with the realisation that further improvements to the health of the population could only be achieved by a strategic approach. The emphasis must be on health not just health care. Technological advances in medicine obviously still hold an important position. The high cost of such advances, however, balanced against the number of individuals that might benefit, brings into question the validity of allocating so large a portion of the finite resources to their further development. Consequently, with the recent reforms in the NHS, there has come an increased emphasis on health promotion and disease prevention. Thus the future health of the nation looks to be secure – or does it? As already discussed above there is a high expectation within the White Paper that the majority of the changes necessary to improve health will need to be made at the level of the individual. For many this is achievable, if not always acceptable, but there are many others for which the expected behavioural change is impossible.

Reflective point

Take a few minutes to reflect on the health needs of this patient: an unsupported lone mother of one child, aged 2, who lives in an inner city area. Her GP is a single-handed practitioner whose surgery is three miles away; there is no health authority clinic near by. Her only income is income support plus child benefit. The property she lives in is a large, old house which has been converted into flats; there is central heating but it is very expensive to run. She has been treated for anxiety and depression and she smokes 10 cigarettes per day. Her child suffers from frequent coughs and colds.

For anyone who works in primary health care in an inner city area this is a fairly common scenario. There are several other situations which could have been used as examples – the recently discharged patient who has mental health problems and who is living in a hostel; the growing numbers of people who are living on the streets and have no permanent address (and therefore cannot even register with a GP); the elderly person who has no surviving relatives and exists on the basic pension. All of these examples have several things in common – the people involved usually feel powerless, are often not respected and are poor, sometimes extremely poor. The health attainment targets proposed for the year 2000 do not mean very much if the only clothes you have are full of holes and you are not sure where you are going to sleep tonight. Maslow's hierarchy of need has become familiar to many; he believed that the basic necessities must come first – shelter, safety, warmth, physical needs, clothing and money in the pocket – before self-actualisation can be achieved (Allen, 1993). There seems to be a dichotomy of interest – on one side there is a great emphasis on the empowerment of the individual to improve his or her health status, eat healthy food, take regular exercise, enact healthy behaviours, while on the other side there are a growing number of individuals who are economically or socially unable even to consider improving their health. Through the media there have been political calls for society to become more caring and to be less self-oriented, while at the same time efforts are being made to reduce state benefits to vulnerable groups. Obviously there can never be unlimited resources for health and social services. If there is to be true health for all, however, then individuals must have sufficient resources to enable them to choose freely and have access to opportunities to live more satisfying, valued and healthy lives.

Should self-care, therefore, be the ultimate health objective?

Summary

- Self-care is what individuals do for themselves or their families in order to keep healthy or recover if unwell.
- Self-care in medicine involves the transfer of responsibility for certain types of care from the practitioner to the patient. The patient is expected to modify his or her behaviour to fit in with the treatment.
- Self-care in nursing is based on the total involvement of the patient and ways of tailoring nursing interventions to patient needs.
- Orem's self-care deficit theory of nursing has three main components: a theory of self-care; a theory of self-care deficit; and a theory of nursing systems.
- The mechanistic view of the universe developed in the 17th century influenced biology and medicine. This resulted in disease being viewed as the breakdown of a biological machine in need of repair by the physician.
- Theories of evolution and biological determinism of the 19th century underpinned the paternalism of medicine and the development of nursing as an extension of the dependent domestic role of women.
- The upsurge of the self-care movement was linked with the Women's Movement in the 1960s and 1970s. This resulted in a backlash against the medicalisation of life events.
- Self-care can be viewed as the primary health intervention with professional care in a secondary role. Or the view that is held by some health professionals is that self-care is brought about by their intervention, teaching individuals to carry out activities that are normally part of the health-care domain.
- Can nurses really empower individuals when working within a medical model of care?
- Patients have been socialised into a passive role. There is a need for the development of autonomy to enable patients to make informed choices.
- How effective can health promotion be if it is based only on an individualistic approach? Are social and environmental factors also of importance?
- Nurses have a valuable role in promoting healthy behaviour. Firstly as role models but also by providing information, understanding and encouragement to patients.
- Nurses also have a wider role in promoting health by influencing health strategy and policy making.
- There is a vital role that self-care and the development of autonomy have in helping patients cope with terminal illness.
- The value that self-care has for elderly people and individuals with a chronic illness is vital in helping them to achieve their maximum potential.
- In the present economic climate is self-care the way forward to improve the health of the nation? Or is there too great a danger of victim blaming and neglecting those people most in need in our society?

References

Adriaanse, H., Van Reek, J., Zandbelt, L. and Evers, G. (1991). Nurses' smoking worldwide. A review of 73 surveys on nurses' tobacco consumption in 21 countries in the period 1959–1988. *International Journal of Nursing Studies*, 28(4), 361–375.

Allen, C. (1993). Powerless to be empowered. *Nursing Standard*, 20 January, 7(18), 44–45.

Bayntun-Lees, D. (1992) Reviewing the nurse–patient relationship. *Nursing Standard*, 8 July, 6(42), 36–39.

Briody, M. E. (1984). The role of the nurse in modification of cardiac risk factors. *Nursing Clinics of North America*, 19, 387–395.

Brooks, N. A. (1984). Opportunities for health promotion: including the chronically sick and disabled. *Social Science and Medicine*, 19(4), 405–409.

Brown, S. J. (1989). Perceived self efficacy and recovery from cardiac illness. *Research Review: Studies for Nursing Practice*, 5(4), 2.

Bushnell, K. L. (1992). Self-care teaching for congestive heart failure patients. *Journal of Gerontological Nursing*, 18(10), 27–32.

Cancer Research Campaign (1990). *Facts on Cancer Incidence UK*. Fact-sheet 1.1. Cancer Research Campaign.

Clifton, B. (1992). Health promotion goes AWOL. *Nursing Standard*, 24 February, 7(23), 49.

Clifton, B. (1993). Overpowering empowerment. *Nursing Standard*, 21 April, 7(31), 45.

Cook, R. (1993). Health promotion in an inner city area. *Nursing Standard*, 2 June, 7(37), 25–28.

Craig, H. M. and Edwards, J. E. (1983). Adaptation to chronic illness: an eclectic model for nurses. *Journal of Advanced Nursing*, 8(5), 397–409.

Day, M. (1994). Smoke alarm. *Nursing Times*, 9 March, 90(10), 16.

Dean, K. (1986) Lay care in illness. *Social Science and Medicine*, 22(2), 275–284.

DeFriese, G. H., Woomert, A., Guild, P. A., Steckler, A. B. and Konrad, T. R. (1989). From activated patient to pacified activist: a study of the self-care movement in the United States. *Social Science and Medicine*, 29(2), 195–204.

Dellasega, C. (1990). Self-care for the elderly diabetic. *Journal of Gerontological Nursing*, 16(1), 16–20.

Department of Health (1992). *The Health of the Nation: A Strategy for Health in England*. HMSO, London.

Ditto, P. H., Jemmott, J. B. and Darley, J. M. (1988). Appraising the threat of illness: A mental representational approach. *Health Psychology*, 7(2), 183–201.

Eben, J. D., Gashti, N. N., Nation, M. J., Marriner-Tomey, A. and Nordmeyer, S. B. (1989) Dorothea E. Orem self-care deficit theory of nursing. In Marriner-Tomey, A. (ed.) *Nursing Theorists and Their Work*, 2nd edn, pp. 118–129. C. V. Mosby, St Louis.

Eisenthal, S. and Lazare, A. (1976). Evaluation of the initial interview in a walk-in clinic: the patient's perspective on a 'negotiated approach'. *Journal of Nervous and Mental Disease*, 162, 169–176.

Eveleigh, M. (1993). Health promotion in 1993. *Practice Nursing*, 6–19 April, 8–10.

Gammon, J. (1991). Coping with cancer: the role of self-care. *Nursing Practice*, 4(3), 11–15.

Gantz, S. B. (1990) Self-care: perspectives from six disciplines. *Holistic Nursing Practice*, 4(2), 1–12.

Gibb, E. and Lucas, B. (1993). Portakabin care. *Nursing Standard*, 19 May, 7(35), 18–19.

Girdano, D. A. and Dusek, D. E. (1988). *Changing Health Behaviour*. Gorsuch Scarisbrick, Scottsdale, AZ.

Ham, C. (1992). *Health Policy in Britain: the Politics and Organisation of the NHS*, 3rd edn. Macmillan, Basingstoke.

Ham, D. (1993). Orem's model of self care. *Practice Nursing*, 2–15 March, 24–25.

Hatch, S. and Kickbush, I. (eds) (1983). *Self-help and Health in Europe*. WHO, Regional Office for Europe, Copenhagen.

Haug, M. R., Akiyama, H., Tryban, G., Sonoda, K. and Wykle, M. (1991). Self care: Japan and the U.S. compared. *Social Science and Medicine*, 33(9), 1011–1022.

Haynes, R. B. (1976). A critical review of the determinants of patient compliance with therapeutic regimens. In Sackett, D. L. and Haynes, R. B. (eds) *Compliance with Medical Regimens*, pp. 26–39. Johns Hopkins University Press, Baltimore.

Heidt, P. (1981). Effect of therapeutic touch on anxiety level of hospitalised patients. *Nursing Research*, 30, 32–37.

Hollingsworth, S., Walton, S. and Hallawell, R. (1994). Student perceptions of total quality. *Nursing Standard*, 2 March, 8(23), 34–35.

House of Commons (1942). *Social Insurance and Allied Services*. Report by Sir William Beveridge. HMSO, London.

Jordanova, L. J. (1980). Natural facts: a historical perspective on science and sexuality. In MacCormack, C. and Strathen, M. (eds) *Nature, Culture and Gender: A Critique*, pp. 42–69. Cambridge University Press.

Jowett, S. (1992) A health model for community nursing. *Nursing Standard*, 11 March, 6(25), 33–35.

Kappeli, S. (1986). Nurses management of patient's self-care. Occasional paper, *Nursing Times*, 82(11), 40–43.

Kickbush, I. (1989). Self-care in health promotion. *Social Science and Medicine*, 29(2), 125–130.

Krasnick, A. (1986). Moving towards self-care: a Danish experiment. *Impact of Science on Society*, 143, 255–262.

Kronenfeld, J. (1979). Self care as a panacea for the ills of the health care system: an assessment. *Social Science and Medicine*, 13A, 263–267.

Kyle, B. A. S. and Pitzer, S. (1990). A self-care approach to today's challenges. *Nursing Management*, 21(3), 37–39.

Lacy, A. L. (1988). Health beliefs and health behaviour in elderly, chronically ill males. Rush University College of Nursing, DNSc, Chicago.

Laffan, G. (1993). A new holistic science. *Nursing Standard*, 13 January, 7(17), 44–45.

LeGrand, J. (1982). *The Strategy of Equality*. Allen & Unwin, London.

Levin, L. (1981) Self-care: toward fundamental changes in national strategies. *International Journal of Health Education*, 24, 4.

Lorenzo, P. and Drick, C. A. (1990). Self-care identity formation: a nursing education perspective. *Holistic Nursing Practice*, 4(2), 79–86.

MacCormack, C. P. (1980). Nature, culture and gender: a critique. In MacCormack, C. P. and Strathen M. (eds) *Nature, Culture and Gender: A Critique*. Cambridge University Press.

McKee, P. A., Costelli, W. P. and McNamara, P. M. (1971). The natural history of congestive heart failure: the Framingham study. *New England Journal of Medicine*. 285, 1441–1446.

McMahon, R. (1991). Therapeutic nursing: theory, issues and practice. In McMahon, R. and Pearson, A. (eds) *Nursing as Therapy*. Chapman & Hall, London.

Marks, M. (1993). Palliative care. RCN Nursing Update, unit 002. *Nursing Standard*, 29 September, 8(2).

Martin, J. (1993). Lying to patients: can it ever be justified? *Nursing Standard*, 20 January, 7(18), 29–31.

Masterson, A. (1993). Tomlinson: a social perspective (part 1). *Nursing Standard*, 19 May, 7(35), 38–40.

Michael, M. M. and Sewall, K. S. (1980) Use of adolescent peer group to increase the self-care agency of adolescent alcohol abusers. *Nursing Clinics of North America*, 15(1), 157–176.

Moore, E. J. (1990). Using self-efficacy in teaching self-care to the elderly. *Holistic Nursing Practice*, 4(2), 22–29.

Muetzel, P. (1988). Therapeutic nursing. In Pearson, A. (ed.) *Primary Nursing: Nursing in the Burford and Oxford Nursing Development Units*. Croom Helm, London.

Mulli, V. (1980). Implementing the self care concept in the acute care setting. *Nursing Clinics of North America*, 15(1), 177–190.

Musci, E. C. and Dodd, M. J. (1990). Predicting self-care with patients and family members' affective states and family functioning. *Oncology Nursing Forum*, 17(3), 394–400.

Nowakowski, L. (1980) Health promotion/self care programs for the community. *Topics in Clinical Nursing*, 2(2), 21–27.

O'Connor, M. A. (1987). Health/illness in healing/caring – a feminist perspective. In Orr, J. (ed.) *Women's Health in the Community*. John Wiley, Chichester.

Orem, D. (1991). *Nursing Concepts of Practice*, 4th edn. Mosby-Year Book, St Louis.

Ottawa Charter for Health Promotion (1986). *Health Promotion*, 1, iii–v.

Peplau, H. E. (1969). Professional closeness. *Nursing Forum*, 8(4), 342–360.

Porter, R. (1984). Do we really need doctors? *New Society*, 9 August, 87–89.

Richardson, A. (1991). Theories of self-care: their relevance to chemotherapy-induced nausea and vomiting. *Journal of Advanced Nursing*, 16, 671–676.

Roberts, S. J. and Krouse, H. J. (1988). Enhancing self-care through active negotiation. *The Nurse Practitioner*, 13(8), 44, 47, 50–52.

Roberts, S. J. and Krouse, H. J. (1990). Negotiation as a strategy to empower self-care. *Holistic Nursing Practice*, 4(2), 30–36.

Rowe, A. and Miles, M. (1994). Coping strategy. *Nursing Times*, 9 March, 90(10), 32–34.

Runyan, J. W. (1975). The Memphis Chronic Disease Program: comparisons in outcome and the nurse's expanded role. *American Journal of Medicine*, 231, 264–267.

Sanderson, H. and Carter, A. (1994). Healing hands. *Nursing Times*, 16 March, 90(11), 46–48.

Sayre-Adams, J. (1994) Therapeutic touch: a nursing function. *Nursing Standard*, 19 January, 8(17), 25–28.

Scambler, A., Scambler, G. and Craig, D. (1981). Kinship and friendship networks and women's demand for primary care. *Journal of the Royal College of General Practitioners*, 26, 746–750.

Scambler, G. (1986). Illness behaviour. In Patrick, D. L. and Scambler, G. (eds) *Sociology as Applied to Medicine*. Baillière Tindall, London.

Seedhouse, D. (1988). *Ethics. The Heart of Health Care*. John Wiley, Chichester.

Sorofman, B., Tripp-Reimer, T., Lauer, G. M. and Martin, M. E. (1990). Symptom self-care. *Holistic Nursing Practice*, 4(2), 45–55.

Tannahill, A. (1985). What is health promotion? *Health Education Journal*, 44(4), 167.

Townsend, P. and Davidson, N. (1988) *Inequalities in Health*. Penguin, London.

Turner, T. (1994). Prescription for fitness. *Nursing Times*, 6 April, 90(14), 14–15.

Williams Utz, S. (1990). Motivating self-care: a nursing approach. *Holistic Nursing Practice*, 4(2), 13–21.

Further reading

Allan, J. D. (1990). Focusing on living, not dying: a naturalistic study of self-care among seropositive gay men. *Holistic Nursing Practice*, 4(2), 56–63. This research shows the positive benefits of self-care in increasing empowerment and improving coping strategies in a chronic life-threatening illness.

Bentzen, N., Christiansen, T. and Pedersen, K. M. (1989). Self-care within a model for demand for medical care. *Social Science and Medicine*, 29(2), 185–193. The concept of self-care is seen as part of a continuum in the provision of care. Health diaries and a mathematical model are used to study self-care and the economics of self-care.

Bowling, A. (1992). Setting priorities in health: the Oregon experiment (Part 1). *Nursing Standard*, 3 June, 6(37), 29–32. Bowling, A. (1992). Setting priorities in health: the Oregon experiment (Part 2). *Nursing Standard*, 10 June, 6(38), 28–30. These two articles examine consumer (i.e. patient) participation in needs assessment, leading to the prioritisation of health services. This took place in Oregon in the USA. The situation is then related to the NHS.

Clifton, B. (1993). Freedom up in smoke. *Nursing Standard*, 26 May, 7(36), 46. This article examines the paternalistic attitude of health professionals towards smoking. It is useful for self-reflection on attitudes to 'unhealthy' behaviours.

Conn, V. S. (1990). Joint self-care by older adults. *Rehabilitation Nursing*, 15(4), 182–186. Research, examining self-care activities for joint problems, in a group of independently living older adults.

Coons, S. J. (1990). The pharmacist's role in promoting and supporting self-care. *Holistic Nursing Practice*, 4(2), 37–44. This article is about the role of the community pharmacist in the USA, but it is becoming increasingly relevant to the UK as individuals are being encouraged to use more OTC preparations via the media.

Friend, B. (1992), Self-service. *Nursing Times*, 28 October, 88(44), 26–28. Self-care for those individuals with a severe chronic illness who would usually be cared for in hospital, e.g. receiving total parenteral nutrition.

Gibson, C. H. (1991). A concept analysis of empowerment. *Journal of Advanced Nursing*, 16, 354–361. A useful article explaining the concept of empowerment and its problems and benefits from a nursing perspective.

Hanucharurnkui, S. and Vinya-Nguag, P. (1991). Effects of promoting patients' participation in self-care on postoperative recovery and satisfaction with care. *Nursing Science Quarterly*, 4(1), 14–20. An interesting research paper showing the benefits of self-care in promoting a quicker and less stressful recovery following surgery.

Holzemer, W. L. (1992). Linking primary health care and self-care through case management. *International Nursing Review*, 39(3), 83–89. This article parallels Orem's theory of self-care with a health-promoting strategy in primary health care, i.e. individuals, families and communities can be encouraged to take responsibility for their health in the future.

McLean, J. and Pietroni, P. (1990). Self care – who does best? *Social Science and Medicine*, 30(5), 591–596. Research, examining the benefits of self-care for stress and anxiety management, in general practice.

Rourke, A. M. (1991). Self-care: chore or challenge? *Journal of Advanced Nursing*, 16, 233–241. This article examines Orem's self-care deficit theory of nursing, and the challenges that it presents to the traditional paternalism that exists in the 'medical model' style of nursing.

Segall, A. and Goldstein, J. (1989). Exploring the correlates of self-provided health-care behaviour. *Social Science and Medicine*, 29(2), 153–161. Research, in Canada, examining the self-care behaviours of a cross-section of the population of Winnipeg. The article also investigates the possibility of any correlation between certain health beliefs and attitudes and the practice of self-care.

Ward-Griffin, C. and Bramwell, L. (1990). The congruence of elderly client and nurse perceptions of the clients' self-care agency. *Journal of Advanced Nursing*, 15, 1070–1077. This research has potential implications for the provision of health care at a community level. It examines the differences (and similarities) between nurses' and older clients' perceptions of the ability of the clients to provide self-care.

Winkler, R., Underwood, P., Fatovich, B., James, R. and Gray, D. (1989). A clinical trial of a self-care approach to the management of chronic headache in general practice. *Social Science and Medicine*, 29(2), 213–219. Research showing the effectiveness of self-care in the management of headache in general practice.

9

PROMOTING LEARNING: A HELPING RELATIONSHIP

Sue Hinchliff

Introduction – the practitioner as teacher

Reflective point

Before starting to read this chapter, pause for a moment and think about the extent to which your job involves teaching and consider the following questions: is teaching written into your job description as a major component of your role? Do you see yourself as a teacher? When are you teaching? When do those around you see you as teaching?

The extent to which you teach in your present post will obviously depend on your clinical area and the role you are fulfilling. Clearly, if you are specialising in the care of patients with stomas, then your job will entail almost non-stop teaching of patients, relatives and colleagues. Equally, if you work in the community as a nurse, midwife or health visitor, you will be teaching colleagues on placement, as well as patients in their homes and their carers or relatives, about a range of topics. As a practitioner in the hospital environment, you will be working with patients in preparing them to manage their own health-care needs, ready for discharge to the community.

Not all teaching, though, is as explicit as these examples suggest. You are teaching as an exemplar for much of the time you are on duty, commu-nicating to those around you your values, attitudes and expectations, as well as your knowledge and skills.

Reflective point

Consider your last span of duty and write down all the opportunities you took to teach explicitly. Now write down what else might have been learned from your conduct, bearing, actions and words during that period.

Patients and colleagues may only perceive you as teaching when you give them cues that you expect them to be learning from you, for example, when teaching how to manage stress levels or wound care. They may have expectations that teaching is going on when they are asked to watch or listen to you ... usually whilst sitting down, and are able to write down what they have been taught, or are given a hand-out.

When you carry out nursing actions such as:

- settling a patient for the night and making his pillows comfortable
- maintaining a patient's dignity whilst she is being examined
- spending time to help a patient to plan an appropriate menu choice
- discussing with a carer how she might manage her husband's mood swings

you are teaching by acting as a role model. You are modelling caring behaviours, the value that you attach to ensuring the patient meets his nutritional needs within his own food preferences and the way in which you value individual needs. All these are teaching opportunities that can be explored and developed. It must be remembered, though, that not all teaching by example is so positive. When you forget to say goodnight to a patient for whom you have been caring, or talk with a colleague rather than your patient, whilst carrying out an aspect of care, you are teaching that you are not really caring for, or valuing the individual in the fullest sense.

Whether or not teaching features in your job description, there is an expectation of you as a registered practitioner that you will teach. *The Code of Professional Conduct* (UKCC, 1992) makes implicit rather than explicit reference to this. It states:

> As a registered nurse, midwife or health visitor, you are personally accountable for your practice and, in the exercise of your professional accountability must:
>
> 1. act always in such a manner as to promote and safeguard the interests and well-being of patients and clients;...
> 5. work in an open and cooperative manner with patients, clients and their families, foster their independence and recognise and respect their involvement in the planning and delivery of care;
> 6. work in a collaborative and co-operative manner with health-care professionals and others involved in providing care, and recognise and respect their particular contributions within the care team.

Whilst the teaching commitment is not spelled out, it could be argued that it is inherent in meeting all of those responsibilities.

The English National Board in its *Framework for Continuing Professional Education for Nurses, Midwives and Health Visitors* (1991) is more direct. It includes amongst its suggested learning outcomes for the ten key characteristics that practitioners must be able to demonstrate the ability to:

- discuss and teach clients, carers and team members concepts of health promotion, health education, prevention and health protection
- understand and apply the principles and practice of health promotion in the practitioner's work setting
- facilitate clients' responsibility and choice for healthy living
- apply the principles of teaching, supervision, facilitating and assessing; select appropriate methods to meet specific situations

- act as a role model in the practice area, encouraging staff in teaching, supervising, facilitating and assessing
- create and sustain a supportive teaching and learning environment in their own practice setting.

This chapter sets out to analyse the process of teaching and learning principally as it relates to patients or clients, examining and reflecting on what learning is, what influences whether it occurs and how best it can be facilitated. There will be a focus on the stages of:

1. assessment of both the learner and the environment in which teaching will take place
2. planning to use appropriate methods and resources
3. intervention, building on effective teacher–learner relationships, breaking down barriers to communication, and enhancing teaching skills;
4. evaluating teaching, learning and supervision.

Learning in practice

Most educational psychologists would agree that learning can be defined as a relatively permanent change in behaviour, that occurs as a result of experience. Gagne (1985) would add that this change takes place over a period of time and is not the result simply of growth or maturation.

This definition implies that:

- if the change is relatively permanent, memory is involved and conditions must exist that are not likely to extinguish the learning
- the change in behaviour results in different knowledge, attitudes or skills on the part of the learner after learning has occurred
- experience ... interaction with the environment ... is a key determinant of learning.

So can learning occur without a teacher? Think for a moment about the ways in which a baby learns to explore his or her world safely or learns to use a spoon, or how a person learns to save text on a word-processor. Clearly the presence of a teacher is not a necessary condition for learning to occur. However, teaching strategies, when successful, ensure that effective experiences are provided by which the student can learn more quickly than by trial and error.

Teaching, then, can be seen as a way of managing the learning environment; it refers to an activity which facilitates or enables learning to take place; it involves setting up the conditions in which learning is most likely to take place and developing the right sorts of helping relationships that will promote learning. All this represents a shift away from the didactic approach that some clients may be used to.

It is not the purpose of this chapter to provide a lesson in educational psychology, and explain in detail how learning occurs. That would involve discussing at some length cognitive, social and behavioural approaches to learning, exploring short- and long-term memory, individual differences in perception, attitudes, motivation and skills. For this background try to read the first three chapters of Quinn (1988) listed in the Further Reading section.

What the chapter will do, though, is to give you some pointers for ensuring that the environment in which you work is conducive to learning; offer you some strategies for facilitating learning and help you to use them effectively.

Factors that influence learning

It was during the 1980s that the bulk of the substantive research into the learning climate in nursing took place. This research clearly relates to the ways in which nurses learn within the hospital, but the results are transferable both to patient/ client learning situations and to the community setting. The main research studies are those of Fretwell (1980, 1982), Marson (1982), Ogier (1982) and Orton (1981); all of which continue to be worthy of further study.

What can we learn from this work that will enable us to plan effective conditions for learning?

Factors that facilitate learning include

- A sharing, collaborative relationship, in which teacher and learner are equally involved, with shared values and beliefs (Marson, 1990)
- an awareness of and consideration for the learner's physical and emotional needs and differences (Orton, 1981; Ogier, 1982)
- an approachable manner on the part of the teacher (Ogier, 1982), with mutual respect, trust and support in identifying both learner strengths and weaknesses (Marson, 1990)
- good teamwork, with a lack of hierarchy and an ethos of negotiation (Fretwell, 1982)

- good communication network within the workplace, with information freely available (Fretwell, 1982)
- encouraging a spirit of enquiry (Fretwell, 1982), which includes openness to new ideas and risk-taking (Marson, 1990)
- acceptance of the right to make mistakes and toleration of levels of performance which fall short of perfection (Marson, 1990)
- evidence of a planned teaching programme (Orton, 1981) with clear learning outcomes
- an enjoyable learning environment (Marson, 1990)
- the teacher having had some training (Fretwell, 1982)
- good staffing levels and a feasible workload (Fretwell, 1982).

Factors that inhibit learning include

- Environments where there is an emphasis simply on getting the work done and an orientation towards task achievement (Fretwell, 1982)
- routinisation of work, leading to automatic performance (Fretwell, 1982)
- teaching being given low priority (Orton, 1981).

Principles of facilitating learning

Brookfield (1986) cites six principles of effective practice in facilitating learning which you may find helpful in preparing to teach patients and clients.

The decision to learn is the learner's

People may engage in learning for a variety of reasons, for example, for self-gratification, to acquire new skills or to find out more about something that interests them. Whatever the motivation, so long as it derives from the learner, learning is likely to be more effective. Teachers need to remember, however, that learners can equally decide **not** to participate in learning. If you have ever tried to hold a discussion with a group of learners who have decided to 'switch off' you will know how powerful and necessary cooperation can be. In order to retain this cooperation the teaching offered has to match the learners' needs.

Teacher and learner must respect each other

Teaching implies a partnership. Any behaviour that denigrates either participant will hinder learning.

Sarcasm, embarrassing the other, or any form of abuse is, in Brookfield's words, 'disastrous'. This does not mean that any teaching encounter has to be gratuitously familiar, nor does it preclude challenging the other's opinion, but a culture should be fostered in which such challenges can be offered in a spirit of mutual trust.

Teaching is a collaborative process

Teacher and learner need to work together to assess needs, work out objectives, plan how to achieve them and to evaluate whether they have been reached.

Activity is central to the learning process

'Activity' does not necessarily mean the need to be up and doing, it may refer to mental or emotional work. It does, though, imply a dynamic process – and note that it is a process – if you like, a journey – rather than a product or an endpoint. The process involves exploration, action, reflection and interpretation, and is cyclical.

Learning involves critical reflection

Teachers should help learners to cultivate a 'healthy scepticism' towards what they hear and what they read. Assumptions should be challenged, contexts examined and alternative views sought. Knowledge should not be assimilated uncritically, without probing both its source and its context.

Facilitation should cultivate self-directed, empowered learners

The learner should have control over the learning process, and this should have relevance to them as an individual. They should have the freedom to determine and express their own needs throughout the learning experience.

Reflective point
Take a few moments to re-examine the findings of the nurse researchers relating to factors which facilitate learning in the workplace and match them to Brookfield's six principles.

You should be able to see that Brookfield's points about how learning in adults can be brought about more effectively have a close correspondence with the researchers' findings on the ward learning climate.

Having examined some of the conditions necessary for learning to occur we are now in a position to move on to look at what is involved in the assessment stage of learning.

Assessment

We are using the term 'assessment' here in the sense of it being the first stage in any systematic approach to teaching, in exactly the same way that it is used in relation to the nursing process. It is not being used to mean 'evaluating results' or 'determining the level of performance' after teaching has taken place; these are both issues that will be addressed in the section on evaluation.

Before any decisions about what to teach or how to teach it can be made it is essential to carry out an assessment of:

- the learner
- the learning environment
- the knowledge/skills required of the teacher.

Your teaching – and the extent to which the learner learns – will only be as good as your assessment.

Assessment of the learner

It is essential, in any teaching situation, if it is to be planned to meet individual needs effectively, to find out as much about the learner as possible. Your list may include some of the following points:

Reflective point
Stop for a moment and make some notes about the sort of information you would need about the learner if you were to be able to plan content, strategies, and meet resource needs, etc., for an individualised teaching session – in this case, with a client. (It may help you to imagine a specific client with particular learning needs.)

- his or her present state of knowledge and need for further teaching
- state of motivation

- ability to learn
- readiness to learn
- preferred learning style
- dexterity
- use of language
- physical and psychological state.

You may have thought of other points but we will focus on these:

Find out 'where the learner is' and determine learning needs

Whatever the teaching situation, it is essential to find out what the learner already knows in order to be able to build on this in planning your teaching. Never assume prior knowledge on the learner's part. If you miss out this step you may end up pitching your teaching below the learner's present level of knowledge and thus risk patronising him or her; equally you may pitch your teaching above the learner's level of comprehension and so risk him or her switching off because there is no hope of understanding what is being taught.

So how do you find out 'where the learner is'?

You may be able to assess this from directly observing the person carry out an activity, where skills are in question. Remember, though, that what appears to be competent skill performance may not be matched by an equally good knowledge-base. Additionally, skill performance may be affected by observation, for example, the very act of watching someone carry out a procedure could make him highly nervous and therefore fumbling; alternatively, watching could make him take much greater care over how the skill is performed.

You may be able to tell from the sorts of questions asked by the learner, or from responses to questions you pose in conversation; these may give you an idea of the person's level of self-awareness and something about their insights, strengths and weaknesses.

Non-verbal behaviour may supply you with clues, for example, whether the person appears puzzled, confident or has low self-esteem.

Try to find out from written medical and/or nursing records what the person has been told previously – although this does not tell you what they now remember, nor what they actually understood at the time. Conversations with partners or parents may give you some idea of understanding and any potential confusions.

However you assess it, it is good practice in teaching to start off any session with, if not a recap, then at least a conscious attempt to be aware of, and acknowledge, the learner's existing knowledge-base. This may be considerably easier when teaching another professional than when teaching a client. It is usually possible to be able to predict, with a reasonable degree of accuracy, what it might be reasonable to expect a nurse to know or be able to do, at a certain stage of training and experience. Indeed, we are normally familiar with the intended learning outcomes of periods of clinical experience or education, and these can be used to inform our predictions. Remember, though, that they are only predictions and all learners are individuals and respond to both teaching and experience differently.

Assess the learner's motivation

Motives are hypothetical constructs which are used to explain behaviour (Stipek, 1988). Thus, we may explain the behaviour of the athlete who trains rigorously to win a race as being driven, or motivated by, the need to compete or the need to improve on his or her personal best performance. Motivation provides the drive towards a goal, and theories of motivation attempt to explain **why** people act in a certain way.

Reflective point

Think for a moment about some of the things that motivate you in your behaviour throughout the day. What makes you undertake certain actions? For example, why are you reading this chapter?

You may do some things because you fear sanctions if you fail to do them ... if you consistently fail to report for duty at the allotted time you may be disciplined.

Other things may be done in order to please someone or to gain their approval ... you may go out of your way to give a colleague a lift home because you like him or her. Equally, it could be that you do this because you think it would help you get a good reference or you want to ask her a favour!

You may be reading this chapter because you are about to undertake a course in teaching and assessing and you want to get ahead of everyone else in your preparation, or you may be reading it out of interest or in order to stretch your existing skills and knowledge. Whatever the reason, you are likely to be motivated by the need to achieve. This is affected by both the desire to succeed and the fear of failure.

You may put in extra hours at work because you simply enjoy your job and derive a lot of personal intrinsic satisfaction from performing it well. Alternatively, you may be aware of an increasing number of redundancies in your NHS Trust or organisation recently, and want to insure your own position by drawing your diligence to the attention of your manager.

In some areas of your life you may lack motivation. If your partner fails to notice when you make a special effort to cook dinner, you may with justification resort to cooking mundane meals or use convenience foods.

Over this century psychologists have attempted to explain behaviour using theories of motivation. It must be clear to you, from the above activity, that there are a number of motivating forces that shape behaviour, and a knowledge of these is useful in planning teaching strategies.

You may be familiar with Maslow's theory (Maslow, 1987) which has been used quite extensively, and sometimes uncritically, in nursing. [For a critique of Maslow's methodology see Clark (1990).] Maslow focused on the healthy individual's potential for personal growth and self-fulfilment and his theory of motivation is based on a pyramid or hierarchy of human needs. Maslow postulated that only when lower level needs were met could a person become capable of working towards meeting higher level needs (Fig. 9.1).

Maslow differentiated between behaviour shaped by deficiencies (for example, lack of sleep, food or water causes people to adopt behaviour designed to remedy the lack), tending to occur at the four lower levels of the hierarchy, and that impelled by growth, occurring at the apex. In this latter category he put the desire to seek out new experiences, leading to self-fulfilment; this he saw as being possible only when deficiency needs had been met.

In planning teaching, therefore, it makes some sense to ensure that the lower levels of needs in Maslow's hierarchy are met before embarking on teaching aimed at meeting higher level needs. For example, it is no use planning a session focused on

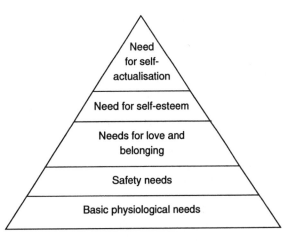

Fig. 9.1. *Maslow's hierarchy of needs (from Maslow, 1987).*

helping a nurse to enhance her skills in breaking bad news to clients if she is tired, hungry and just due to go off duty!

Motivation may depend on the expectations of those around you. If someone expects you to perform well, then it's likely that you will put in a greater effort. Conversely, if someone gives you every impression that they do not expect you to succeed, then you are less likely to. This notion was tested originally in the classroom by Rosenthal and Jacobson (1968) in the USA, who explored the idea of a self-fulfilling prophecy in education. Teachers were told that certain children (who were, in fact, selected at random) were brighter than the rest. After several months, during which all the children were given repeated intelligence tests, these children performed significantly better than previously, ascribed to the fact that their teachers' expectations of them as bright positively affected their achievement. It is worth bearing this work in mind to prevent yourself falling into the trap of accepting uncritically another's assessment of a client's abilities and responding accordingly.

For a helpful exposition on the affects of expectations (of either the teacher or the learner) on learning see Chapter 11, Communicating Expectations, in Stipek (1988).

A lack of motivation may derive from the feeling that one is unable to influence the course of events, that one has no control over the circumstances of one's life. This sense of being disempowered has been described as 'learned helplessness' by Seligman and Maier (1967). They subjected dogs to mild electric shocks which were unavoidable, that is, nothing the dogs did could prevent the shocks being delivered. The dogs soon became passive, even when later placed in a situation where they could have avoided the shocks. Similar behaviour can be observed in some schoolchildren who believe that despite what they do they will fail.

It does not take much imagination to envisage situations in health care where clients experience learned helplessness. Clearly if teaching is to be effective this becomes more feasible where the learner feels he or she has some control over the situation, and teaching strategies can be used which increase this sense of ownership and control.

Find out about the learner's ability and readiness to learn

Assessment of any learner must include an assessment of his or her existing abilities in order to be able to pitch teaching at the right level. Obviously this should not be taken to mean that you need to administer a full-scale intelligence test to your learner, but there are several pitfalls that you need to beware. Do not assume that the client who is articulate in general conversation is necessarily *au fait* with medical terminology or possesses manual dexterity; nor assume that the client whose command of the spoken language is not so good is not capable of absorbing health teaching when it is phrased simply and broken down into small steps. It must be remembered, though, that for some clients, using a link-worker to interpret for you may be the only sure way of communicating effectively. The only rule here is that each learner deserves to be assessed individually.

Separate from ability is the concept of the person's readiness to learn. This implies that the learner has reached a level of maturity and has acquired enough experience to be able to benefit from the particular piece of teaching. Implicit within this is the fact that the teaching has to be relevant to the learner's 'need to know'. Redman (1976) identifies two aspects of readiness to learn in relation to teaching patients and clients. Firstly the patient or client has to be ready emotionally for the learning, and secondly s/he has to be ready in terms of experiences, abilities, attitudes and skills. Linked with this you need to reflect on a client's cultural predisposition to learn.

> **Reflective point**
> Think of an example from your own area of practice where this concept is relevant in helping to determine the right time or way to teach a client something.

For example, suppose you are working with a patient who has recently had a stoma formed. Before you begin to teach the patient how to manage the stoma herself, you need to be sure that she is able to look at the stoma, and is beginning to come to terms emotionally with the change in her body-image. If she has not reached this stage of readiness she will not be able to cope with you teaching her how to change her colostomy bag.

In patients a significant factor which may affect readiness to learn may be their illness. Uncertainty and anxiety about their diagnosis, or about the outcome of a known diagnosis can be disabling in terms of ability to take in new information. Coming to terms with the knowledge of a poor prognosis or with the diagnosis of a chronic disease takes time. Coping strategies, such as the use of denial as a defence mechanism, can block learning.

A particularly difficult example might be judging the readiness to accept teaching aimed at helping someone to stop smoking. Here the readiness to learn is complicated by the physiological needs engendered by the confirmed smoker's addiction to nicotine, and the benefits the smoker perceives he receives from smoking. This serves to illustrate that motivation and readiness to learn are interlinked and are by no means simple when applied to individuals.

Assess learning styles

People are usually aware of the way in which they prefer to learn. You will sometimes hear people describe themselves as 'plodders', or as someone who learns best 'by doing'; some people know that they grasp something better if they can see it as a whole, rather than as a series of steps. Clearly it is helpful to have this information in order to plan teaching strategies to suit the individual.

Much of the research that has been done on cognitive styles, the ways in which individuals prefer to learn, has been done with children or college students. However, a great deal of what has been learned is transferable to the health-care arena.

The work of Dunn and Dunn (1978) provides a

useful framework for planning teaching based on individual client preferences. They identified four areas where people differ in their needs:

1. **environment**: learners differ in their preferences for silence or background noise; bright or dim lighting, comfort and design of furniture, and ambient temperature
2. **motivation and mood**: some people are intrinsically motivated, whilst others may need to be motivated by the teacher; some give up if they do not learn easily, others are more dogged; some learn best when they can see a discernible structure to what they are taught; certain individuals learn best when they feel responsible for their own learning
3. **one-to-one versus group teaching**: learners differ in their preferences for learning in isolation (rather as you are doing in interacting with this text), one-to-one with the teacher, in twos, in larger groups or using a variety of approaches
4. **physical differences**: most people have some idea whether they learn best by listening, seeing, touching or doing, or by using a combination of these approaches; similarly, people usually have a good idea whether they are larks – learning best early in the day, or owls – preferring to study late into the night.

Some of you may be familiar with the work of Honey and Mumford (1990) on categorising and using learning styles. They devised a Learning Diagnostic Questionnaire which allows the learner to assess the extent to which he or she is an activist, reflector, theorist and pragmatist and to capitalise on opportunities for learning.

They see learning as a cycle in which one has an experience (activist), reviews the experience (reflector), reaches a conclusion based on this (theorist), and plans the next step (pragmatist). People vary, though, in their interest and capacity to learn from the four stages of the cycle.

- **Activists** tend to enter fully and with enthusiasm into the challenge of new experiences, often acting first and considering the consequences later. They are open-minded, willing to 'try anything once', thriving on finding solutions to new problems, but finding less attractive the stages of implementing solutions and consolidation.
- **Reflectors**, on the other hand, like to spend some time considering the consequences and

different perspectives before reaching any sort of conclusion. They tend to be thoughtful and may not be at the forefront of meetings, preferring to observe.

- **Theorists** like to be able to reach a rational conclusion in a logical, analytical and objective manner. They tend to prize certainty above divergence, creative and lateral thinking.
- **Pragmatists** are keen to try out ideas to see if they work in practice. They tend to be practical, down-to-earth people who like 'to get on with it'.

Whilst these categories can be helpful, it is important to remember that Honey and Mumford saw all four styles entering into effective learning, and that whilst a person may have a tendency to act in one way rather than another, he or she can be helped to develop other capabilities. So, for example, the person who tends to prefer action can be helped to become more reflective.

Reflective point

Try to get hold of a copy of The Opportunist Learner *and work through some of Honey and Mumford's exercises; diagnose how you could maximise your own learning opportunities. Before you do this, use Dunn and Dunn's framework to decide the best way of undertaking this, i.e. where? when? who with?, etc.*

Finding out something about the way in which a client learns best can be time well spent before you plan any piece of teaching.

Identify any health factors that can affect learning

Reflective point

Picture a patient in a hospital ward and list some of the factors that may impede his or her learning process. You may find it helpful to think back to the conditions you identified as being necessary to your own learning.

The ward is seldom an ideal environment for learning. It may be noisy and patients are all too aware that they can be overheard. They may be frightened of missing seeing the doctor or visitors and there are frequent distractions. They may have had little sleep, may be hungry or quite possibly be in pain. Some patients may have impaired sight, hearing or touch. Additionally, patients in hospital may frequently experience feelings of anxiety. Tobias (1980) found that anxiety interferes with the ways in which we attend to information, mentally organise it, retain it, apply it and use it.

If you want your teaching to be effective, then you need to consider minimising all these impediments to learning by choosing your time and place carefully, and making sure your client is as relaxed and comfortable as possible, both physically and psychologically, and can both see and hear you easily.

Activity
Select a client for whom you are currently caring, who will shortly need to be taught about an aspect of health care. Using the above information, plan to spend some time with him or her to assess learning needs prior to the teaching session. This activity is one which we will follow through to the end of this chapter.

Assessment of the environment for teaching

When we talk about the environment for teaching we need to think not just about physical conditions but also about the atmosphere in which the teaching will take place.

Activity
Review the section on the factors which influence learning, in particular the work of the nurse researchers on the ward learning climate. Now carry out an educational audit of your own workplace and assess the extent to which it could be considered to be conducive to learning. If you identify any areas which need improvement, discuss with your colleagues how this could be done and devise an action plan with a realistic time-scale for achieving objectives.

The assessment you have carried out on your chosen client's learning style will tell you something about how physical conditions might best be

arranged. For example, if the person has impaired hearing on one side this will determine where you place your chair; if he seems to be very tired and has difficulty in retaining information, then you may need to time your session after he has had a rest and for a time when you can be fairly sure you will not be interrupted. If he seems highly anxious about an aspect of care unrelated to your planned teaching, it may be counter-productive to do anything about this until his particular anxieties are relieved. He may indicate that he would prefer to learn in the company of his partner, or he may feel the need for absolute privacy.

Remember that sights, smells and sounds in the clinical environment that may be 'normal' and familiar to you may be acutely disturbing to your client, to such an extent that learning may be affected. Although it is not always possible to remove such impediments completely, try to be alert to clients' sensitivities.

It is helpful, for future reference, to document your assessment of the client's learning needs and any needs for adaptation of the environment and these can be incorporated into your teaching plan.

For a discussion on the use of an audit tool applied to the clinical learning environment see the work of Spouse (1990) in the Further Reading section at the end of the chapter. Spouse developed a list of criteria and a questionnaire to assess the suitability of the workplace in terms of meeting students' learning needs, and suggests that the results can be used to negotiate improved working conditions.

The knowledge/skills required of the teacher

It is important to take some time to assess what the teaching is likely to demand of you as a teacher before launching into it. It is never enough simply to feel comfortable with the knowledge you hope to impart to the client. As a teacher you need a considerable reserve of knowledge and skills in order to feel confident in answering any potential queries your client may raise.

It is recognised by teachers that you never really 'know' something until you come to teach it. For example, you may feel fairly secure in your knowledge of blood-groups. Stop for a moment now, though, and think how you would explain to a junior colleague why someone who is Group O Rhesus positive is regarded as a 'universal donor'. If you can do this with no difficulty, congratulations! However, most people would begin to flounder without spending some time revising their knowledge and rehearsing the logic of their explanations.

Note that I am not saying that you should be able to teach without preparation. On the contrary, I am advocating taking some time, firstly to assess your present state of knowledge and competence, and secondly to develop and enhance this by further reading and preparation. This will ensure that you are in the best position to answer questions and that you approach the session with confidence.

Assessing your own degree of knowledge and competence, prior to teaching, may present an interesting challenge. Polyani (1966) explored the notion of 'tacit knowledge', where practitioners, under certain circumstances 'know more than they can tell'. This is akin to Schon's (1987) 'knowing-in-action', where expert practitioners use knowledge derived from experience to reach new, and often creative solutions to the sort of complex, frequently messy problems with which clients present. In preparing to teach it is often technical, rational knowledge that is sought, rather than the knowledge that is embedded in practice. Powell (1991) argues that, as practitioners, we should attach more value to this latter kind of knowledge.

For an interesting study on how this sort of knowledge can be taught to other practitioners, see the work of Davies (1993). Davies studied a cohort of first-year undergraduate nursing students who were encouraged to observe role models in the clinical situation, as a means of discovering the knowledge embedded in practice. She found that, by following expert role-models, the students were able to uncover more of the artistic aspects of practice, rather than scientific elements, issues to do with caring and showing concern. They began to be able to make judgements about what constituted 'good' and 'bad' practice.

Reflective point

Focus on the proposed teaching session you identified above. Spend some time deliberating on the knowledge and skills you will need to carry out this teaching effectively. How confident do you feel in your existing knowledge-base? How much 'spare' knowledge do you possess, over and above that which you will need to teach your client? What will you need to do to remedy any knowledge/skills deficit? Draw up an action plan for this now.

You may find it an illuminating exercise to differentiate between what Schon described as the technical, rational knowledge that you need for your particular piece of teaching, and the knowledge that derives from your experience. The former can be found in research studies and texts, and hence is accessible to novices as well as to experts; the latter lies in the province of specialist and advanced practitioners, and results from critical reflection in and on practice.

Planning

The inclusion of a section here on planning assumes that all teaching that occurs in the clinical environment is planned. It has to be said at the outset, that however desirable this may be in theory, in practice some teaching, of necessity, could be called 'crisis teaching'. White and Ewan (1991) describe the clinical environment as 'unpredictable, volatile, dynamic, close and personal', and as such it can be 'a powerful centre for learning' (p. 3). This lends to any teaching situation a degree of uncertainty, with the potential for a crisis or problem emerging at any point.

To describe teaching as 'planned' indicates that the teacher has control over the process. This is clearly so in the case of a distance learning package, or a videotaped teaching session; however, the degree of control lessens as one moves from lecture, through seminar, discussion, tutorial to one-to-one teaching in the clinical area, where teaching itself can be 'dynamic, close and personal'.

This continuum obviously presents an increasing challenge to the teacher; the more control one has over the process of teaching, the less threatening and taxing it is likely to be. With decreased control, the more necessary it is to feel confident in rising to whatever challenges the situation may present. It is for this reason that teachers who are less experienced often feel more comfortable using teaching strategies over which they have greater control.

Planning strategies for teaching

If learning refers to the relatively permanent change in behaviour described at the beginning of this chapter, then teaching has to be planned to make that change as efficient, effective and comfortable as possible.

Reflective point

Think about your proposed teaching session with your client. Look at the factors you came up with in the activity on assessing this client's learning needs. What help does this give you in planning how to structure the session? What sort of language to use? The level at which to pitch the teaching? What method you might choose? What resources you might select to enhance learning? You will find it helpful, first of all, to identify exactly what you are hoping to achieve in your teaching.

What are you trying to achieve?

The aim of the session is quite clearly specific to each individual's learning needs and his or her existing state of knowledge. It needs to be identified clearly and agreed between teacher and learner before the teaching can be planned.

For example, are you building on existing knowledge or starting from scratch? Does the client need to revise previous learning, or has s/he learned erroneously in the past and perhaps needs to correct misunderstandings? Obviously you will only be able to reach a decision on any of these points if your assessment has been comprehensive.

Identifying intended learning outcomes

Once an aim (i.e. an overall goal) for the session has been defined and agreed you are in a position to work out the intended learning outcomes, that is, what it is you want the learner to be able to do *en route* to achieving the aim. Specifying these steps allows you to break down content into manageable chunks. It is important for the learner to experience success at each of these sub-goals, since this reinforces his or her sense of self-esteem and motivation. It is also important for you to share these intended learning outcomes with your client. Identifying intended learning outcomes is a key component of the evaluation of teaching and learning, where you measure the extent to which these outcomes have been met.

Scheduling your teaching

It is helpful at this stage to begin to think about

timing. How much time have you got at your disposal to teach the client? Is this ideal? Will you need to break down the session into shorter periods, each focusing on one particular theme and its relevant intended learning outcomes? If so, it may be useful to give your client a written plan of what you are both hoping to accomplish for each session.

Selecting a suitable method and resources

This will depend entirely on each intended learning outcome in relation to the specific client. The method chosen is likely to have implications for the place where teaching will occur and how this setting might most appropriately be arranged.

For example, if you need to teach something that is practical and requires a degree of manual dexterity, then a demonstration is likely to be appropriate. You may need to use diagrams, models, equipment or mock-ups. You may carry out the demonstration yourself, you may prefer to use a videotape or you may wish to bring in a clinical specialist to support your teaching. You will certainly have to build time into your schedule for supervised practice.

In order to make this process clearer, let us consider the example of teaching Mrs Sinclair, who is 62 and recently diagnosed as having non-insulin dependent diabetes mellitus, how to care for herself in order to keep her blood glucose at an acceptable level, whilst maintaining her normal life-style and avoiding the complications of diabetes.

Your assessment will have told you something about how well motivated Mrs Sinclair is, how able she might be to grasp what you need to teach her, whether she would prefer to learn alongside her husband, what her previous knowledge of diabetes is, and any misconceptions she might have, her level of anxiety with regard to her diagnosis, her degree of manual dexterity, details of her normal lifestyle (in particular information about her diet, alcohol intake and exercise levels) and so on.

You can discuss the general aim, given above, with Mrs Sinclair and find out if she has any other specific learning needs. You need to work out how much time is likely to be necessary in order to achieve your overall aim. To do this, you need to spend some time working out what Mrs Sinclair's intended learning outcomes might be.

You might decide to structure your sessions on the following themes.

1. What is diabetes? Different types of diabetes and how they can be treated, with a focus on Mrs Sinclair's own clinical features, diagnosis and management

Here the intended outcome is to give Mrs Sinclair the tools with which she can discuss her diabetes with health professionals and others in her life and understand what they are asking of or explaining to her, without misconceptions.

The language and sentence structure used should be simple, no matter how intelligent you might assess her to be, without recourse to jargon, unexplained medical terms or abbreviations. Note that it is not the intention to avoid all technical terms. It is important for the patient to have a facility with relevant terms in order for her to achieve independence, understand other members of the health-care team or written material about her condition and to be a partner in future communications.

Never attempt to teach too much at one session. Learners will frequently remember that which is taught first, when they are freshest, and that which is taught last, which has the least chance of being 'overwritten'. If too much is offered between these two points, then it is likely not to be retained, unless it is of particular personal importance (Ley and Spelman, 1965).

It is important to allow frequent pauses to allow Mrs Sinclair to assimilate the information and to consolidate her learning. Some learners need space to rehearse what has been taught, going over it in their minds to ensure understanding.

You may need to repeat information which she has not understood. Since to teach something clearly relies on it being presented in a logical sequence, it is important that each step is comprehended, in order for the learner to build on it in learning the next step. Ideally, therefore, you need to assess learning throughout the session, rather than just at the end. If Mrs Sinclair has failed to understand a crucial piece of information near the beginning of the teaching, then the rest of the session is likely to have been wasted.

Remember that the average span of attention for anybody is in the region of 20 minutes. This is likely to be shorter for someone who is anxious, who has disturbed homeostasis, is in pain, very young or very old. This does not mean that no teaching session can be longer than 20 minutes, merely that you need to be aware of the need to provide breaks, summaries or a change of activity at frequent intervals.

It is almost invariably helpful to end each session with a written summary of what you have taught. This might take the form of a printed leaflet, a summary which you have prepared or notes made by the client at the end of the session under your guidance. Whatever sort of hand-out you offer your client, it is vital that it is readable. Material written using short sentences and simple words is likely to be clearer and does not have to compromise accuracy or credibility (Ley, 1989).

Generally it is not a good idea to ask the client to make notes as you go along, as she may be so intent on doing this that she fails to take in what you are saying, or to query points she does not understand. Simply asking the client to summarise orally what she has understood from the session gives you a valuable opportunity to assess and evaluate her learning, and to correct misapprehensions where they have arisen.

You are likely to need to set aside about an hour – uninterrupted – for this. Learning is an active process and distractions should be avoided. You may need to draw diagrams, to write down definitions or spell medical terms for her, so be prepared with any equipment you might need.

2. How blood glucose levels are normally maintained and how this mechanism is altered in diabetes, with a focus on Mrs Sinclair's assessment of her own blood glucose level and potential glycosuria

At the end of this session Mrs Sinclair should be able to state what the range of normal is for her blood glucose level and how she would monitor and record it. She should recognise the importance of correctly testing her urine for glucose and recording the results and she should be aware of what action to take to manage any deviations from normal. (These would be her intended learning outcomes.)

Depending on Mrs Sinclair's ability to grasp new information (which may in turn depend on her level of concentration, anxiety, tiredness, blood glucose level, etc.) you may decide to split this session into two, one focusing on blood glucose levels, the other focusing on urine testing.

Each session could then be further broken down

into even smaller steps. For instance, in a teaching session on urine testing, intended learning outcomes might relate to:

*   recognising the reagent strips needed to perform this test
*   identifying whether these are out-of-date or damaged in any way
*   knowing how to obtain more when supplies are low
*   correctly obtaining a specimen of urine of the right amount and freshness
*   using the reagent correctly
*   reading the results accurately
*   interpreting the significance of the results and knowing what action (if any) is appropriate
*   recording this correctly.

Other themes which you would need to develop into intended learning outcomes might focus on:

*   the relationship between diet and blood glucose levels, and how diet can be used to stabilise blood glucose, with reference to Mrs Sinclair's normal preferences
*   the role of exercise in the management of diabetes and its incorporation into Mrs Sinclair's lifestyle
*   the recognition of skin, foot, eye, circulatory or cardiac problems related to the development of complications of diabetes and how Mrs Sinclair might recognise these in herself.

Note that each theme sets out to increase Mrs Sinclair's knowledge in direct relation to herself. Unless information is seen as meaningful to the individual it will not readily be learned.

It is not the place of this chapter to go into each of these themes in detail, but you should be able to see from the worked examples how a teaching session can be planned to have a structure and sequence which will facilitate learning.

Like the stage of assessment, planning is key to the success of any teaching. It is worth spending some time examining the research relating to giving clients information, before moving on to consider implementing the plan. Ley (1988) found that patients are often dissatisfied with the amount of information given; they do not always understand what they are told; they do not consistently follow instructions they are given, nor do they remember what they are told. It has to be said that Ley's research relates mainly to patient–doctor communications, but there are lessons to be learned here for all health professionals.

Reflective point

Bearing in mind what has been discussed so far in this chapter, identify some possible reasons for these findings.

You may have thought of:

*   patients being frightened to question what the doctor/teacher says
*   too much information being given at once
*   information being poorly structured or too complex
*   presenting information (telling) rather than teaching it
*   failure to assess the patient's learning needs adequately
*   failure to be specific and make learning meaningful for the client
*   insufficient time being allocated to the teaching session
*   failure to put the patient at ease, or relieve pain or anxiety
*   insufficient space being allocated for questioning, rehearsal and repetition
*   insufficient supervised practice when a skill is to be learned

There are a range of other potential reasons why a client may not take in what he or she is taught that are specific to the client in question. Most of them do, though, relate to failures on the part of the teacher, rather than any ineptitude on the part of the client!

Activity

Go back to the teaching session you propose to hold with your chosen client. In the first reflective point in this section of the chapter you began to identify what you are trying to achieve in your teaching. This needs to be negotiated with your client. Next:

*   *consider the total period of time you will need in order to achieve your agreed aim*
*   *divide what is to be taught into themes, with an appropriate time-span for each*
*   *make sure that these are sequenced logically*
*   *specify intended learning outcomes for each theme*
*   *identify what you will need to teach to bring about each learning outcome*
*   *decide what teaching resources you will need.*

You should now have produced, through the suggested activities and reflections, a plan for teaching your chosen client.

Intervention

Having assessed your learner's needs and planned your teaching accordingly you are now in a position to deliver the teaching. Before you do this, though, it is important to spend some time looking at the learner–teacher relationship, communication skills and potential barriers to communication and the implications for the teacher.

Learner–teacher relationships

It goes without saying that the best teaching should be learner-centred. This does not always happen, of course, and it may be the context in which teaching takes place that prevents this sort of approach. For example, it would be difficult to be learner-centred when teaching physiology to 80 students in a lecture theatre. However, for all of the occasions when you will be teaching clients it should be your aim. What does it mean, though, to be learner-centred in your approach?

First of all, it implies building your teaching on an understanding of how people learn, and since most of your clients will be adults, you need to know something about the assumptions that can be made about how adults learn. Knowles (1980) used the term androgogy to refer to the study of the ways in which adults learn (as opposed to pedagogy, which is used to refer to the teaching and learning of children at school).

Knowles made four assumptions about the needs of adult learners.

1. Although in some situations they may become more dependent, **adults show a tendency to be self-directed in their learning.** That is, they are independent, autonomous beings, able to determine their own needs and act to fulfil these and to construct their own reality.

If you take a moment to consider this statement, though, you will begin to see that this is not invariably the case. Socialisation in childhood, cultural and ethnic differences, disempowerment through political or economic circumstances, emotional immaturity, illness or decreasing abilities through ill-health or in extreme old age may all serve to cause an individual to be less than self-directed. Equally, it would be wrong to assume that many children are **not** self-directed.

Adults may need help in becoming more self-directed. Self-direction implies knowing how and where to go to meet learning needs; it also implies possession of skills in analysis and critical enquiry, and these need to be facilitated. The degree to which one is able, as a learner, to be self-directed may have a considerable effect on one's self-concept. The sort of teaching, then, which fosters self-direction, can have a positive influence on the learner's personal growth and self-awareness.

2. **Adults have a wealth of experience which they bring to a learning situation and these experiences affect how they perceive their world.** This is, unarguably, the case. The clients whom you are teaching are not blank slates; they bring to you a rich resource on which to base teaching and learning. Such learning is referred to as experiential learning. If learners are to be encouraged to build on their prior experience, then they may need to be taught skills in reflecting critically upon it.

Kolb and Fry (1975) described an experiential learning cycle (see Fig. 9.2), which seeks to explain how a person undergoes a concrete experience (stage 1), then looks back on the experience, reflecting on it and examining observations made at the time and subsequently (stage 2), then forms abstract concepts and generalisations as a result of the first two stages (stage 3), then tests out these ideas in new situations (stage 4). These new experimental situations then act as new concrete experiences and so the experiential learning cycle starts again.

Reflective point

What sorts of skills are required of the learner if he or she is to learn from experience in this way?

You might have come to the conclusion that:

- first of all the learner has to be receptive to new experiences
- then s/he has to be able to reflect on them in a fairly objective way. Kolb and Fry point out that learning is often more effective if this stage takes place in a group, where reflections can be challenged and examined. It is self-evident, though, that such group work needs to be handled with care and sensitivity if its objectives are to be

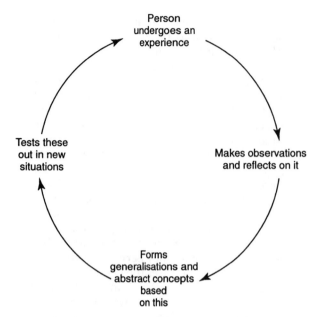

Person
undergoes an
experience

Makes observations
and reflects on it

Forms
generalisations and
abstract concepts
based
on this

Tests these
out in new
situations

Fig. 9.2. *An experiential learning cycle (after Kolb and Fry, 1975).*

achieved, and it is essential that a spirit of trust is engendered from the outset

- the learner then has to be able to generalise and draw conclusions from this, in order to come up with new ways of acting to apply to future situations. At this stage the learner commonly has to learn new information to increase his or her knowledge-base
- the last stage, that of experimentation, may demand a degree of courage on the part of the learner, and a willingness to try a fresh approach and evaluate it.

The sorts of teaching strategies which promote the use of experience are likely to be more successful with adults, for example, group-work, discussion, debate and problem-solving.

Whilst, in general, adults derive personal satisfaction from feeling that their experience has value, it should be remembered that at times, past experiences may hinder current learning, and it may be painful to revisit and critically reflect upon some experiences and this discomfort should be recognised and acknowledged.

3. **Adults become aware of learning needs as they arise out of the circumstances and problems of their lives**. The implication of this is that teach-

ing should relate to the adult's personal circumstances and needs: that is, they will learn best that which is useful to them within their own context and which they need in order to function. This might cause you to examine what you are teaching. Does it really relate to the learner's needs or to your need to teach it? What will the learners be able to do with it if you do teach it? Can they apply it to meet their needs? Indeed, are they ready to learn it?

This statement should cause you to ask, though, do people always know what it is that they need to know?

4. **Adults tend to relate learning to their performance needs, that is, their need to develop competency**. Whilst, at first these last two assumptions seem to be seductively sensible, there is a danger here that if they are accepted at face value, they could lead to an instrumental, narrow and reductionist approach to teaching and learning, which neglects learning for personal growth and as a way of extending oneself.

Androgogy is, without doubt, a useful and in many ways an attractive way of looking at adult learning, which focuses on a belief about the ways that a teacher should be treating the learner. It is not, though, without its critics; for a helpful critique see *Androgogy: Alternative Interpretations and Applications* in Brookfield (1986).

Reflective point

Spend a few moments considering your response to Knowles' assumptions about the ways in which adults learn. To what extent are these notions taken into account in the teacher–client encounters in your own clinical area? Do you now need to amend your teaching plan in any way to take on board androgogical approaches?

Let us go back to the need to be learner-centred which we discussed earlier. We started off by saying that we need to know something about how learners learn. Once we have gained this knowledge we then need to recognise the individuality of every single person whom we teach. For each person's needs will be different. This serves to emphasise, yet again, how crucial the stage of assessment is to the process of successful learning and teaching.

Communication skills

Good communication skills are clearly essential elements in the repertoire of teaching skills. We have described teaching (or promoting learning) as 'a helping relationship' in the title of this chapter, and so far we have identified a number of ways in which the teacher is acting 'to help' the client, by:

- collaborating and sharing
- accepting and encouraging
- empowering and supporting
- modelling caring attitudes
- showing respect for the worth of the client
- discussing feelings
- helping to reflect on experience
- helping to make decisions
- changing knowledge, attitudes and skills.

It is interesting, looking at the above list, that it is not until we get to the last point – changing knowledge, attitudes and skills – that we come to a helping behaviour that would quite categorically come under the heading of 'teaching'. Most of the rest would simply be considered elements of good interpersonal relationship skills, skills that would be common in caring social interactions.

Bridge and Macleod Clark (1981) suggest that there is a continuum of communication needs on the part of clients, ranging from the need for simple social interaction, through information, advice, reassurance, discussion of diagnosis, treatment and prognosis, discussion of feelings to counselling. They suggest that whilst practically all clients need social interaction and information of some kind, both of which can take place at a relatively superficial level, not all will need counselling, an activity which requires considerable preparation and skill in its exercise, together with a deeper nurse–client relationship.

If you look at the above list of helping behaviours again, you will notice that not all of the actions need to be entirely (if at all) verbal. Non-verbal communication plays a powerful role in the development of a helping relationship when aiming to promote learning. Knapp (1978) posits that non-verbal communications convey 65 percent of the message. That being so, we cannot afford to neglect developing our awareness of the messages we convey to our clients, through eye gaze, body language, touch, silence and listening behaviours.

Therapeutic communication and teaching within nursing

In effect, then, much of what we might want to achieve under the heading of teaching the patient or client could be regarded as 'facilitating learning' a term preferred by Carl Rogers (1983), which implies setting up the best conditions for learning to occur, using a partnership approach.

Vaughan (1991) cites Peplau's (1952) view that nursing is a developmental process in which a 'professional closeness' is forged between nurse and client. In this relationship (which demands experience on the part of the professional) the nurse 'is able to manage her own behaviour in such a way as to help a client to develop and learn through a personal health crisis. ... With professional closeness one of the major functions of nursing can be seen as the creation of environments in which clients can feel safe and learn more about themselves which can be of both short and long term benefit to them. This does not, however, negate the fact that in each new nursing situation the nurse will also learn something new which can be added to her total repertoire of knowledge for future practice.' (Vaughan, 1991, pp. 91–92.)

In examining the concept of the nurse being in a partnership relationship with the client, Brearley (1990) suggests that this may extend from 'complete passivity to full activity' on the part of the client. Interactions may occur at any point on this continuum depending on client preference, type of health problem in question and the client's ability to participate. Once the client's stance is determined, the nurse has to take up a complementary position. Clearly, there may need to be some negotiation of stances between client and professional, where, for example, the professional feels that the client's position is too passive.

What is necessary in order for communication to become therapeutic? The Latin root of the verb 'to communicate' includes the meanings 'to share' and 'to participate'; 'therapeutic' refers to 'contributing to treatment'. Murray and Zentner (1989, pp. 52–55) cite examples where they see nursing interactions as forming part of therapeutic communication:

- facilitating a relationship based on collaboration and cooperation
- empowering the client to have a firm sense of 'self'
- accepting ... being non-judgemental and following the client's train of thought

- using thoughtful silence to encourage the client to talk
- using open-ended questions
- using exploration to help the client to clarify understanding and to describe how he or she is feeling
- sharing with the client how you perceive him or her to be feeling and verbalising what you think is implied, making sure that you reach an understanding which is mutually agreed
- helping clients to see events in context and perspective
- bringing the client back to reality when you feel s/he is straying
- restating the client's ideas to ensure perceptions are accurate
- reflecting back what the client has said to elicit further elaboration/clarification
- helping the client to evaluate the point which s/he has reached
- encouraging the client to develop an action plan.

Reflective point

Take some time now to reflect on what might act as barriers to this sort of beneficial communication, that sets out to facilitate growth in the client.

By carrying out an effective assessment of the client, before attempting any therapeutic communication (which includes teaching), the practitioner hopes to avoid potential barriers, such as:

- using inappropriate language (including body language), or jargon
- failing to acknowledge cultural/ethnic/class/gender differences and needs
- basing teaching/health promotion on your values rather than those of the client
- forgetting when the client has impaired sight, hearing or memory, pain, anxiety or is distracted
- offering false reassurance
- mis-timing or offering inappropriate interventions
- being judgemental/ threatening.

To summarise then: in order to be an effective communicator the practitioner needs to develop a repertoire of skills that can never be complete. Clearly people do not come to nursing with these skills already developed. The skills continually evolve and are refined throughout years of preparation and cultivation, through training, role-model-

ling, mentoring, preceptorship, supervision, reading, experience and reflection. Professional and personal maturation and growth are prerequisites, and these demand of the practitioner a readiness to learn from both clients and all that experience can teach. Such learning must be based on honesty and humility. There is no room for complacency or any sense that the skills are complete and that learning is over.

Evaluation

[Note that in this chapter 'evaluation' is used to refer to the measurement of performance (of either teaching or learning), whereas 'assessment' is used to refer to measurement of need for teaching or learning to occur. In other texts the terms may be used interchangeably.]

Evaluation (of what the learner has learnt and how the teacher has taught) forms the last part of a systematic approach to teaching, before the cycle starts again, since any deficits diagnosed at evaluation require further corrective assessment, planning and intervention. It is likely that, whether or not the teacher builds evaluation into the process, both teacher and taught will come to some sort of judgement. This may be more or less explicit, sometimes amounting simply to an unexpressed feeling of satisfaction (or otherwise) with what went on. We have all come away from doing some teaching, at one time or another, and felt that somehow 'it wasn't quite right', or even worse, that it went disastrously wrong. Clearly, this sort of intuitive feeling about our performance is an insufficient basis on which to build improvements to future practice.

If evaluation (which can occur both during and after the exercise of teaching and learning) is to be objective, rather than being based merely on subjective feelings of how well it went, it must be based on some preset criteria of success. These criteria, you will recall, are set at the planning stage, when 'intended learning outcomes' are set. Look back now at the section on identifying intended learning outcomes and remind yourself of how intended learning outcomes relate to the aim of a piece of teaching.

Formative and summative evaluation

You may have heard these terms applied to the evaluation of professional learning. Formative evaluation refers to measuring continuously what the process of learning is like. It is a diagnostic type of measurement, which allows for alterations and adjustments to be made in order to meet learning objectives or outcomes. Formative evaluation may take place in sessions with mentors, preceptors and supervisors, or in situations of 'professional closeness' with clients. These relationships are by definition formative, that is, they contribute to 'shaping' learning.

Summative evaluation occurs at the end of the learning exercise and this measures the product of the teaching , that is, exactly how much learning occurred. An examination is a form of summative evaluation.

What should be evaluated?

Coutts and Hardy (1985) suggest that the same criteria on which standards are constructed are used in evaluation, namely, structure, process and outcomes.

Using this framework, evaluating structure causes you to focus on the context in which the teaching/learning occurred; the resources, human and inanimate; the environment; timing, and the degree to which participants expressed satisfaction.

Examining process allows both partners to evaluate what went on in the teaching, the nature of the relationship, the strategies employed, the effectiveness of communication skills, in fact, consideration of all the influences which were brought to bear on how learning took place.

Outcome criteria explore the results of the teaching encounter. If the purpose of the teaching has been properly identified, by way of delineating an aim and meaningful desired outcomes of learning, then this stage consists of measuring what actually happened against the intended standards. It may be, of course, that it is found at this stage that the intended learning outcomes were inappropriate in their scope or feasibility.

How can we evaluate learning and teaching?

Evaluation is essentially a stage of data collection, interpretation and recording of results, similar to that of assessment. Data collection needs to be readily carried out, with speed and ease, and asking questions orally of the client is frequently the most effective method. Questioning allows the

practitioner to check understanding and retention.

From time to time it may be appropriate to use written questions to evaluate a client's grasp of what you have taught. For some people this may remove from the situation any anxiety associated with the feeling of being 'put on a spot', which may accompany oral questioning. For others it may carry associations of examinations and testing, and so may provoke anxiety. Only adequate client assessment can tell you which method is likely to be most useful for each individual client.

You may find it helpful to provide the client with a written checklist of the intended learning outcomes and ask him or her to rate the extent to which s/he feels that you have mutually achieved what you set out to do.

If you have been teaching a practical skill to your client, then supervision of client practice is an appropriate method of evaluation.

It should be remembered that evaluation provides the teacher with an opportunity to give the learner feedback on what has been achieved. Positive feedback, where you are confirming for the client that learning has occurred, is always pleasant both to give and to receive. However, learning may not have taken place effectively, and it is equally important, if less pleasant, to give the learner this knowledge. Only when you have given the client detailed feedback on his or her performance, with emphasis on identified strengths and how these can be built upon in the future, can s/he use feedback as a developmental tool, providing the foundation for future improvements and success. Allowing the client to see that you are working towards this in collaboration, and in a step-wise fashion facilitates a sense of confidence, increased motivation and progress in both teacher and learner.

It is not only the learner who needs feedback in order to develop. For the teacher to be able to extend skills in the future s/he also needs information about the effectiveness of strategies used and structured support in the teaching role. Clinical supervision is suggested as a way forward towards the continual development of primary, specialist and advanced practice and personal and educational growth; this may take the form of one-to-one, peer or group supervision. The supervisory relationship is also a helping one, and is based on sensitivity, trust, willingness to learn and intellectual rigour (Butterworth and Faugier, 1992).

Activity

After you have completed the piece of teaching which you have been planning throughout this chapter, evaluate what your client has learnt and give him or her appropriate feedback.

What have you learned about your own teaching and how it could be improved? Plan to build on this exercise in the next teaching that you do. Spend some time reflecting on this and note down what you feel are your teaching strengths. Also note down any areas where you think you need to improve your skills.

As the next step in your personal and professional development, try to read the text by Tony Butterworth and Jean Faugier on clinical supervision in the Further Reading section and reflect on how you might access this sort of support in your own area of practice. A supervisor who has good teaching skills would be most help to you in the light of the last activity.

Conclusion

With the trend towards a shorter in-patient stay, and with potentially decreasing contact between professional nurses and clients, it is vital that the nurse develops and uses his or her role as an educator to its fullest, wherever the client is. It is also crucial to this helping relationship that the client sees the nurse as his or her most appropriate partner.

Casteldine's (1991) examination of the advanced nurse practitioner cites communication as one of the necessary core competencies. Communication can take place without teaching expressly occurring, but teaching cannot occur without some form of communication. If we accept the argument that teaching a client is a form of helping relationship, then possession to a high level of a range of communication skills is key to this relationship. The acquisition of such skills should form a continuing thread throughout the professional practice of a nurse.

Throughout nurse training and in the initial stages of primary practice the profession has accepted the notion of mentorship and preceptorship as tools for developing practice. In order to make learning a life-long professional activity clinical supervision is advocated as a means of giving practitioners the support they need in developing their teaching and helping role.

References

Brearley, S. (1990). *Patient Participation: The Literature.* Scutari Press, London.

Bridge, W. and Macleod Clark, J. (eds) (1981). *Communication in Nursing Care.* John Wiley, Chichester.

Brookfield, S. (1986). *Understanding and Facilitating Adult Learning: A Comprehensive Analysis of Principles and Effective Practices.* Open University Press, Milton Keynes.

Butterworth, T. and Faugier, J. (eds) (1992). *Clinical Supervision and Mentorship in Nursing.* Chapman & Hall, London.

Casteldine, G. (1991). The advanced nurse practitioner (part 2). *Nursing Standard,* 24 July, 5(44), 33–35.

Clark, E. (1990). *Developmental Psychology,* Part 2, *The Developing Person,* Distance Learning Centre, South Bank University, London.

Coutts, L. and Hardy, L. (1985). *Teaching for Health: The Nurse as Health Educator.* Churchill Livingstone, Edinburgh.

Davies, E. (1993). Clinical role modelling; uncovering hidden knowledge. *Journal of Advanced Nursing,* 18, 627–636.

Dunn, R. and Dunn, K. (1978). *Teaching Students Through Their Individual Learning Styles: A Practical Approach.* Reston Publishing, Reston, VA.

ENB (1991). *Framework for Continuing Education for Nurses, Midwives and Health Visitors, Guide to Implementation.* English National Board for Nursing, Midwifery and Health Visiting.

Fretwell, J. (1980). An enquiry into the ward learning environment. *Nursing Times,* occasional paper, 76(16), 69–75.

Fretwell, J. (1982). *Ward Teaching and Learning: Sister and the Learning Environment.* Royal College of Nursing, London.

Gagne, R. (1985). *The Conditions of Learning and Theory of Instruction,* 4th edn. Holt, Rinehart and Winston, New York.

Honey, P. and Mumford, A. (1990). *The Opportunist Learner: A Learner's Guide to Using Learning Opportunities.* Published and distributed by Peter Honey, Ardingly House, 10 Linden Avenue, Maidenhead, Berks.

Knapp, M. (1978). *Nonverbal Communication in Human Interaction,* 2nd edn. Holt, Rinehart & Winston, New York.

Knowles, M. (1980). *The Modern Practice of Adult Education: From Pedagogy to Androgogy,* 2nd edn. Follett, Chicago.

Kolb, D. and Fry, R. (1975). Towards an applied theory of experiential learning. In Cooper, C. (ed.) *The Theories of Group Processes.* Lilley, London.

Ley, P. (1988). *Communicating with Patients.* Croom Helm, London.

Ley, P. (1989). Improving patients' understanding, recall, satisfaction and compliance. In Broome, A. (ed.) *Health Psychology: Processes & Applications*. Chapman & Hall, London.

Ley, P. and Spelman, M. (1965). Communications in an out-patients setting. *British Journal of Social and Clinical Psychology*, 4, 114–116.

Marson, S. (1982). Ward sister – teacher or facilitator? An investigation into behavioural characteristics of effective ward teachers. *Journal of Advanced Nursing*, 7(4), 347–357.

Marson, S. (1990). Creating a climate for learning. *Nursing Times*, 25 April, 86(17), 53–55.

Maslow, A. (1987). *Motivation and Personality*, 3rd. edn. Harper & Row, New York.

Murray, R. and Zentner, J. (1989). *Nursing Concepts for Health Promotion*. Prentice-Hall, Hemel Hempstead.

Ogier, M.(1982). *An Ideal sister? A Study of the Leadership Style and Verbal Interactions of Ward Sisters with Nurse Learners in General Hospitals*. Royal College of Nursing Research Series, Scutari Press, London.

Orton, H. (1981). *Ward Learning Climate: A Study of the Role of the Ward Sister in Relation to Student Nurse Learning on the Ward*. Royal College of Nursing Research Series, Scutari Press, London.

Peplau, H. (1952). *Interpersonal Relations in Nursing*. Putnam, New York. Cited in Vaughan, B. (1991). Patient education in therapeutic nursing. In McMahon, R. and Pearson (eds) A. *Nursing as Therapy*, Chapman & Hall, London.

Polyani, N. (1967). *The Tacit Dimension*. Doubleday, New York.

Powell, J. (1991). Reflection and the evaluation of experience: prerequisites for therapeutic practice. In McMahon, R. and Pearson, A. (eds) *Nursing as Therapy*. Chapman & Hall, London.

Redman, B. (1976). *The Process of Patient Teaching in Nursing*. C. V. Mosby, St Louis, MO.

Rogers, C. (1983). *Freedom to Learn for the Eighties*. Merrill, Ohio.

Rosenthal, R. and Jacobson, L. (1968). *Pygmalion in the Classroom*. Holt, Rinehart & Winston, New York.

Schon, D. (1987). *Educating the Reflective Practitioner*. Temple Smith, London.

Seligman, M. and Maier, S. (1967). Failure to escape traumatic shock. *Journal of Experimental Psychology*, 74, 1–9.

Stipek, D. (1988). *Motivation to Learn: From Theory to Practice*. Prentice-Hall, Englewood Cliffs, NJ.

Tobias, S. (1980). Anxiety and instruction. In Sarason, I. (ed.) *Test Anxiety: Theory, Research and Applications*. Erlbaum, Hillsdale, NJ.

UKCC (1992). *Code of Professional Conduct for the Nurse, Midwife and Health Visitor*, 3rd edn. United Kingdom Central Council for Nursing, Midwifery and Health Visiting.

Vaughan, B. (1991). Patient education in therapeutic nursing. In McMahon, R. and Pearson, A. (eds) *Nursing as Therapy*. Chapman & Hall, London.

White, R. and Ewan, C. (1991). *Clinical Teaching in Nursing*. Chapman & Hall, London.

Further reading

Butterworth, T. and Faugier, J. (eds) (1992). *Clinical Supervision and Mentorship in Nursing*. Chapman & Hall, London. Do try to read this important text, which sets out to apply supervision to a range of clinical environments. Supervision is increasingly being seen as a key tool for professional development.

Coutts, L. and Hardy, L. (1985). *Teaching for Health: The Nurse as Health Educator*. Churchill Livingstone, Edinburgh. A very useful book with a focus on improving nursing care.

Hinchliff, S. (ed.) (1992) *The Practitioner as Teacher*. Scutari Press, London. A practical, interactive text, with a focus on experiential and reflective learning, aimed at helping all nurse practitioners develop their teaching role.

Kenworthy, N. and Nicklin, P. (1989). *Teaching and Assessing in Nursing Practice: An Experiential Approach*. Scutari Press, London. A useful resource for those acting as a mentor to student nurses.

Powell, J. (1991). Reflection and the evaluation of experience: prerequisites for therapeutic practice. In McMahon, R. and Pearson, A. (eds) *Nursing as Therapy*. Chapman & Hall, London. An excellent chapter which examines the part played by both reflection and knowledge derived from experience in making a positive difference to a client's health status.

Quinn, F. (1988). *The Principles and Practice of Nurse Education*, 2nd edn. Chapman & Hall, London. This text provides a sound background in learning and teaching theory ... a useful reference.

Spouse, J. (1990). *An Ethos for Learning*. Scutari Press, London. A research study focusing on the development of suitable learning opportunities in the workplace, for student nurses.

Stipek, D. (1988). *Motivation to Learn: From Theory to Practice*. Prentice-Hall, Englewood Cliffs, NJ. Chapter 11, Communicating Expectations, is particularly useful in helping to explain how both teachers' and learners' expectations can affect learning, either positively or negatively.

Tanner, G. (1989). A need to know. *Nursing Times*, 2 August, 85(31), 54–56. An examination of the notion of readiness to learn as it relates to patients.

White, R. and Ewan, C. (1991). *Clinical Teaching in Nursing*, Chapman & Hall, London. Equally applicable to a hospital or community setting, this comprehensive text explores the strategies that can be used to facilitate clinical teaching.

10

STRATEGIES FOR ORGANISING CARE

Gerald S. Bowman and David R. Thompson

General introduction

The organisation and management of health-care services is sophisticated and complex. In the current climate of market-led health care no single occupational group can lay claim to understanding the full impact of health services on its consumers, whether they be individuals, families, health organisations or society as a whole. True multidisciplinary work is necessary for excellence in practice, and it is, therefore, important for nurses to have a clear appreciation of their role. This role should be a strong one built around a core of knowledge and skills acquired and developed over many years. This chapter aims to offer an insight into the role played by nurses in an effective health-care system and an introduction to a range of issues and strategies for organising care that ultimately results in its effective and efficient delivery of care.

Issues covered include a historical perspective giving an insight into how nursing was managed and the reasons for the transitional processes of today. The problems of nurse leadership are discussed. Factors that impinge on the work environment and influence practice, and methods currently used to measure nursing activity are explained. The ways in which nurses' work methods can be organised is described; so too are the problems associated with change in the workplace.

Historical introduction

In western society care organised and delivered outside of the family began with the Christian church. Christian teaching exhorted concern for the welfare of those who were sick. Care was seen as a vocation based on Christ's command that neighbourly love was as binding as the love of God (Calder, 1974), and personal service and ministering to the sick were emphasised. A major effect of this principle was the establishment of infirmaries that were built within Christian communities. 'Visiting' the sick was also undertaken. The Church officiated over the appointment of the visitors, who included virgins, widows, deacons and deaconesses. Some worked from their homes, others lived in monasteries. Monastic rules commanded that those who were sick should be considered above all things (Austin, 1957).

During the crusades of the 10th century AD, orders such as that of St John of Jerusalem emerged as a response to the needs of those who were wounded or exposed to exotic infectious diseases. In these institutions the Knight Hospitallers and serving brothers ministered to those who were sick.

The Nightingale era

Organised care, as it is understood today, is generally believed to have first been made possible through the efforts and dramatic success of Florence Nightingale at Scutari, during the Crimean War. Following a vigorous campaign for army sanitary reform, she significantly improved the morale of the army and dramatically reduced the mortality of wounded troops. She returned from the Crimea determined to do something to improve the quality of nursing. In response to her success, and after much political lobbying with her powerful and influential connections, she established the Nightingale School of Nursing at St Thomas's Hospital in 1860. Nightingale's philosophy of care had three objectives: 'to help the patient to become well; to help the patient die comfortably; and to keep the individual well' (White, 1978, p. 215). Duties were physically demanding for the trainees, who were Christian ladies with an educational background that was akin to home maintenance skills, being inculcated with the virtues of cleanliness, order, quietness and gentleness (Maggs, 1982).

Services for visiting the sick poor and destitute in their homes were initiated by Anglican nursing orders, who developed the regimen of punctuality, cleanliness and obedience to matron's orders, coupled with skills in directing domestic staff, observing and controlling patients, applying dressings and administering enemas and other treatments. These orders were often established under the supervision of a clergyman. Perhaps the best-known philanthropist who did most to initiate and organise home care was William Rathbone, considered to be the founder of modern district nursing. His compassion for those who were poor and suffering encouraged him in 1859 to employ a nurse to relieve suffering and to teach the rules of health and comfort (Hardy, 1981). The value of the work was such that, supported by Nightingale, he opened a nurse training school at Liverpool Royal Infirmary.

In the mid-19th century nursing rapidly developed as a male-dominated service. The men were not nurses, but were clerics, medical practitioners and philanthropists who were assuming control of a workforce comprised mainly of women, trained and able to manage their own affairs. Nurses of the calibre of Florence Nightingale and Ethel Bedford-Fenwick were opposed to such controls. Miss Nightingale, who was against a central examination for, and the registration of, nurses, and Mrs Bedford-Fenwick, an ardent supporter of women's rights and the leader of the movement for the registration of nurses, strengthened the matron's role, so that in nursing matters the matron reigned supreme. This created many tensions and political problems within institutions at that time because of the inferior position of women in society. However, the system of matrons organising nursing was to become the means of controlling and developing nursing for over a century.

The matrons

The matrons appointed from the era of Nightingale were reformers. They were trained nurses who had a mission to change the ill-disciplined nursing workforce into a well-organised profession whose members received 'in-house' training. The matrons wrested power from medical and clerical hands by challenging the legitimacy of nurses having to account to non-nurses. They were responsible for the nursing service, including nurse training, the domestic service and, sometimes, the catering service. The matrons strengthened their position when Bedford-Fenwick founded the Matrons' Council in 1894. The aim of this body was to establish the principle of a register of nurses. It was felt that the registration of nurses would firmly place power and control of the profession in the hands of nursing. It was not until 1919 that this aim was achieved.

The matron system proved successful because, at its inception, it had adapted to the needs of patients, society and a female workforce that demanded a legitimate role in the wider society.

The ultimate demise of the matron system occurred because it was unable to adapt to changes occurring in medical science and technology, especially following the explosion of medical knowledge after the Second World War. Also, women were gaining access to a wide range of other occupations, such as teaching.

By the 1960s it was clear that the matron system had to change. There were a variety of reasons, the main ones being that young women no longer wished to enter an occupation that still operated as a strongly authoritarian and hierarchical system based on military and religious principles, and that the system produced a high wastage of trainee and qualified staff.

Education

Until relatively recently, nursing was seen as a vocation, with the emphasis placed on training; there was a general resistance to higher education. Following the Registration of Nurses Act in 1919 it took some years to set up training schools and the means of monitoring them by the new nurses' professional body, the General Nursing Council for England and Wales. By the late 1930s it was clear that nurse training needed some amendments. Since the early 1940s reports had recommended changes in nurses' education, the type of institution that might deliver it and who should contribute to that education [Royal College of Nursing (RCN), 1943, 1964; Ministry of Health (MoH), 1947; DHSS, 1972]. The general consensus of these reports was that nursing education should be independent of hospitals and health service management, there should be fewer nurse education establishments, nurses should be *bona fide* students during their education and courses should be linked to degrees.

As early as 1947 nurses were given the opportunity to improve their education but they rejected it. Nurses were still wedded to their now anachronistic systems to such a degree that real change was almost impossible. In 1979 the General Nursing Council (which set and monitored educational and professional standards) was replaced by the more autonomous United Kingdom Central Council for Nursing, Midwifery and Health Visiting (UKCC). Not until the 1980s, with a strong reforming government that demanded change across all the social institutions, did real reform in nurse education take place. These reforms are in effect an amalgam of many features of the post-Second World War reports. The benefits of the reforms may take many years to be realised.

Management

The Salmon Report (Committee on Senior Nursing Staff Structure; MoH, 1966) described the confusion in the matron system (in community and midwifery services, the superintendent was equivalent to the matron). The title 'matron' was used indiscriminately and was not necessarily linked to responsibility. Lines of communication were unclear and roles were vague. Often, 'assistant' matrons had a non-nursing role, such as being in charge of the nurses' home or the linen service.

The Salmon Report recommended a line management structure, in which status was meant to be related to the quality of decisions taken (clinical decisions were not seen as being as high in quality as administrative or managerial decisions). Three levels of management for the nursing service were determined:

1. first level (concerned with the role of staff and charge nurse grades)
2. middle level (concerned with the role of nursing and senior nursing officer grades)
3. top level (concerned with the role of principal and chief nursing officer grades).

This delineated a comparatively straightforward structure that offered career progression for nurses, although it excluded provision for the development of clinical careers.

As a response to the Salmon Report, the Mayston Committee was set up to establish whether 'Salmon' could be applied to community nursing and midwifery services (DHSS, 1969). A Salmon-style structure was recommended that was based on population size and geography. The line structure recommended for hospitals was also accepted for community nurses and midwives.

Health services were managed in a line structure that stretched from the DHSS through the regional health authority to the district health authority.

National Health Service (NHS) trusts

Hospitals and community services are now managed in clearly defined units.

Trusts are independent units; they are self-governed and have a chairman, chief executive and board of directors and are empowered to make decisions concerning services and development. There is some external control in that they have to provide core services agreed with purchasers in order to earn their revenue. Purchasers of services include general practitioners (GPs) who hold their own funds, district health authorities who may purchase some speciality services (e.g. cardiac surgery) and private patients who may choose to be treated by a trust because of its facilities and expertise. NHS trusts have to agree with a purchaser the costs of services they provide; they have the authority to borrow money and, if necessary, dispose of assets to develop or maintain services.

The development of trust status for units has caused much controversy. Those against these reforms argue that the emphasis is on cost-cutting exercises making care cheaper but less effective and isolated from other services. Oversupply of some services with undersupply of others is also considered likely to occur. Advocates of the changes believe that health services will be fitter, more competitive, give more consumer choice and be more flexible.

Current developments

The dynamic and disruptive consequence of these changes show signs of shifting the health service out of its cosy corner of security into the wider competitive society with all the uncertainties that accompany commercial life. Whether benefits will be realised is not yet possible to determine. What is clear is that there can be no return to the unsatisfactory systems of the past. From a nursing perspective it is likely that four major changes will determine the shape and fitness of nursing to flourish in the future:

- nursing leadership
- nursing education
- nursing practice, and
- nursing research and development.

Nursing leadership

The push in the 1980s by a radical government for a more efficient and accountable health service resulted in the creation of significant management changes, emanating from the publication of the *NHS Management Enquiry*, chaired by Sir Roy Griffiths (DHSS, 1983). There is no longer a single management structure for the whole service. Local needs dictate local circumstances, but the universal philosophy is that organisational and fiscal management is separate from professional leadership. This means that nurses occupying senior positions are there because of their management skills rather than their nursing expertise and it is unlikely that nursing structures will extend beyond the level offering direct services to specific groups of patients.

Nursing education

Project 2000 (UKCC, 1987), the result of the many recommendations to reform nurse education, provides students with a nursing education at an academic institution free from hospital control. The purpose is to produce 'knowledgeable doers'. Those in favour of the reforms believe that competent professionals will emerge who are more flexible and adaptable. Those opposed to the reforms believe that the final product will be a deskilled workforce. What is clear is that nurses who have spent three years in a higher education establishment, and have had most of their practice supervised, will not view nursing in the same way as their forebears. The successful completion of a Project 2000 education will result in the award of a diploma (in health education or nursing) as well as registration as a nurse (there are also some undergraduate nursing degrees based on the framework of Project 2000, i.e. a common foundation programme followed by a branch programme). The academic credits obtained on completion of the course can be linked into other appropriate courses leading to a degree after a further year of study or into the post-registration and practice scheme to gain sufficient credits for a degree.

The post-registration education and practice project (PREPP) (UKCC, 1993) proposals are intended to build on existing developments in nurse education and practice and to effect changes once Project 2000 is fully implemented. The proposals are:

1. conditions concerning eligibility to practise
2. a period of support under the guidance of a preceptor for newly registered practitioners
3. the requirement that all practitioners maintain a 'personal professional portfolio', undertake a statutory minimum of five study days every three years and complete a statutory return to practise course after a break of five years or more
4. the concept of and preparation for advanced practice.

This total professional development programme will be offered in a flexible form and will not be less than equivalent to a first degree. The importance of this is not only the obvious benefit of creating a more confident and committed nursing/midwifery workforce but the potential to set benchmarks for promotion within the service.

From 1995 nurses registering will be advised what requirements they need to fulfil before re-registering in 1998. By April 2001, nurses will have to meet PREPP requirements in order to re-register.

Nursing practice

As the general population has become healthier, and longevity is a reality for more people, the health needs of society have changed. Individuals are surviving acute illness episodes and, as a consequence, are often left with chronic residual health problems. A major challenge for nurses is to enable patients to adjust to their changes in health state. Nurses have responded in a patchy way to this challenge. Importantly, there has been a rediscovery of nursing as a therapy which in itself supports and aids recovery. The nurse–patient relationship is being examined more closely and ways of enhancing it, e.g. through primary nursing, are now being explored in many centres. Patients' views and experiences are increasingly accepted as significant and considered as a basis from which care can be agreed. Thus, apart from the accepted biological knowledge and motor skills a nurse requires, there is now a demand for well-developed human and social skills. Further, nurses need to be able to assess, systematically and competently, the patients needs to facilitate care. Tutored competence in the following skills is required by nurses:

- interview skills: to be effective in acquiring information
- health education knowledge: to effectively inform the patient
- counselling skills: to be effective in facilitating change in the patient
- stress management techniques: to reduce emotional damage from patient involvement
- research awareness: to use, appropriately, new knowledge in practice.

Nursing development units (NDUs) are the result of an initiative that was first described in Oxford during the early 1980s (Pearson *et al.*, 1992). The notion that health care and recovery from illness is more than medical diagnosis and treatment has been explored since the Nightingale era. The huge expansion in medical science and technology has dominated health care and inhibited the development of nursing. Today, individual responses to health care are accepted as an important variable in adaptation and recovery following illness and disability. The relative success of the Oxford nursing development units (Pearson *et al.*, 1992) in meeting patients' needs, and the subjective evidence of a speedier and better recovery, have led to their introduction in a range of nursing specialities. Proponents of the initiative see NDUs as another example of nursing's capacity to respond to the needs of people and of the ability of nurses to pioneer new ideas (Evans and Griffiths, 1994).

NDUs aim to monitor and critically evaluate their own practice, to develop and test assessment tools and to disseminate findings to the profession. Clear leadership with an appropriate philosophy is thought essential if these units are to achieve such objectives. Those involved in this initiative believe it has an important place in the organisation and development of nursing. For example, Vaughan and Gough (1993) state 'What makes them special is their constant innovation and continuing critical evaluation and dissemination of their work' (p. 28).

A recent report (Shaw and Bosenquet, 1993) recommends the consideration of NDUs by any health-care organisation that is seeking to provide high-quality care. They believe that NDUs provide a way of developing nurses and practices when resources are finite.

There are understandable criticisms of this practice-based initiative, such as these units appearing élitist; that it is unjust for one ward, out of many in a hospital, to be a designated development unit with the additional resources this status brings. Arguably such developments should be occurring throughout an institution.

Nursing research and development (R&D)

Research in nursing is to a large extent likely to be determined by the major developments in the NHS, particularly the NHS R&D programme. The three main aims of the NHS R&D programme are:

- to base decision-making at all levels in the health service on reliable information based on research
- to provide the NHS with a capacity to identify problems that may be appropriate for research
- to improve the relations between the health service and the science base; this includes the biological and physical sciences, the social and behavioural sciences, economics, as well as engineering and biotechnology.

The taskforce on the strategy for research in nursing, midwifery and health visiting (DoH, 1993) set within the context of developments in the management of the NHS; health policies (*The Health of the Nation*, DoH, 1992); health service research (*Research for Health*, the NHS R&D Strategy); nurse education (UKCC, 1987) and more generally within nursing (*A Strategy for Nursing*, DoH, 1989), made four major recommendations:

- the integration of nursing issues and researchers within the new organisational structures for R&D in the NHS
- targeted investment in research education and training for nurses
- the identification of an enhanced range of sources and types of funding for research in nursing
- an improvement in the dissemination and implementation of R&D in nursing.

These recommendations are currently being addressed. Research in nursing is most likely to focus on nursing practices, nursing services and service delivery. A fundamental research task is to evaluate the effectiveness, including costs, of clinical procedures, practices and interventions. Investigation of the effectiveness and efficiency of clinical interventions is essential in order to establish outcome measures. Further research is needed in other areas of nursing, including workforce characteristics, the management of nurses and the process and outcomes of education and training. The scope for developing nursing research is huge and is likely to involve the use of a range of methodologies.

The gap between research and practice is well recognised and is due to a variety of factors, including many nurses having a poor understanding of the research process, resulting in a number of nursing research studies which are poorly designed or conducted. It is unrealistic to expect all nurses to design and conduct independent research, but they should be able to participate in research projects and to examine the research literature when producing clinical guidelines and protocols.

The need for research training, funding and career development in nursing in general is well recognised by the recent taskforce. However, it will be some time before structure and support mechanisms for nursing widely exist in the UK.

The future for research in nursing is challenging and exciting. It will involve nurses acknowledging the importance of research, recognising their own strengths and weaknesses in understanding and conducting research, welcoming the opportunity to share ideas and work with others, embracing a range of methodologies, and accepting that research in nursing needs to be seen in the wider context of health services research.

The health service culture

Culture refers to the pattern of development in a group's system of knowledge, ideology, values, laws and day-to-day rituals (Morgan, 1990). Organisations have their own cultural life which may be quite different from that of wider society, and places of work influence culture today as much, if not more, than the church or home.

Health care was traditionally rooted in religious culture. Within hospitals, in particular, the vestiges of religious Victorian culture are still evident. Nurses wear uniforms which are a mix of those worn by parlour maids and nuns. Relationships between nurses and doctors tend to mirror the Victorian household, with the doctor as the father figure and the 'sister' as manager of the household. The patients position within this is as the passive child. In effect, the health service has mirrored the traditional, élitist class-based system that has been so damaging to Britain in the modern world. The changes taking place within the health service provide the opportunity for these unfortunate relationships to evolve into more mature and adult ones that demonstrate respect for all involved.

Reflective point

Nurses need to consider who determines the direction of nursing in everyday practice. You might reflect on what you have seen or experienced during an allocation. How was the registered nurses' work structured and how much autonomy for practice did the nurses display?

Within your scope of experience, are registered nurses setting their own professional agenda, or is it set for them? For example, do registered nurses need to refer to medical staff before determining nursing care? Do registered nurses use their assessments effectively to solve a range of patient problems, or is assessment viewed as a chore?

Do registered nurses mainly pursue medical, management or nursing objectives, and do you think the balance is right?

As a registered nurse, what would you want to achieve for patients under your care? Does this differ from what you have seen in practice so far?

The current changes in the organisation of nursing has produced a range of work methods operating and offers opportunities to compare practices. Workplaces that are unresponsive to recent philosophies, exhorting methods of independent practice, are likely to operate central decision making (the most senior nurse on duty making the care decisions). In other workplaces, the registered nurse may have a clear patient group for whom care decision making will be determined by these patients and her. These will be the extremes of practice.

Leadership

Management or leadership?

Occupations concerned with human service need to appreciate the difference between management and leadership. Many people in society work in organisations whose main objective is to produce or sell goods in order to make a profit. The individual knows the organisation's aims and generally accepts the management arrangements which facilitates the business. Occupations that have a direct influence on and control of peoples' lives make decisions of a personal, moral and ethical nature that may have profound personal consequences. Such decisions should be informed by the latest research knowledge and information. The health service consists of many professional groups that require leadership to set standards. The management of estates, resources and personnel is no different in the health service than it is for any other organisation. Leadership as a means of organisational goal attainment is important to occupations such as nursing because of issues of accountability. Registered nurses, for example, are not only accountable to the organisation in which they work, but also to their patients, society in general and to their statutory body, the UKCC. This accountability is implicit in the various acts of parliament.

Burns (1978) states that leaders lead people while managers control things. Management is fundamentally about the task or how things are operated. The main concern of management literature is the creation of conditions that make people more effective in achieving the organisation's goals. Factors such as motivation, reward and punishment tend to be concentrated on as means of enhancing productivity.

The view that management and leadership are different does not infer that managers are not concerned with people or that the role of manager and leader cannot be present in the same individual. Management is, in effect, how power and influence are utilised. Managers tend to be concerned with attaining short-term goals and developing routines. This controlling of events is an act of power. Leadership is not about the use of power but a process of influence over others by enhancing their voluntary compliance (Bryman, 1985). Leaders, as members of a group, have to demonstrate that they are effective in their role. Once accepted by the group as credible, the leader can then become innovative. Change is brought about by leaders when they influence the thinking of individuals through a vision of what is desirable, possible and necessary (Zeleznik, 1981). Florence Nightingale is a good example of a 'visionary' leader who reformed through influence. Ethel Bedford-Fenwick sought to control and limit access to nursing and can be considered an early managing force in nursing.

The nursing dilemma

The distinction between management and leadership is important to nursing. Nursing has tended to be over-managed and under-led. There are too few initiatives for recognising potential leaders and developing them for the future.

Following the introduction of the Griffiths Report (DHSS, 1983) and the NHS reforms, medicine has a perception of itself as providing leadership within the NHS (White, 1993). If nurses are not given the freedom to develop their own contribution to patient care, short-term medical outcomes will become the aim of health care. Initiatives within nursing, such as Project 2000, PREPP, nursing development units and research, have the potential to create a more dynamic and assertive occupation with therapeutic value, but without effective leadership operating at a clinical level these initiatives may well be lost.

In a recent discussion document on nursing leadership, Rafferty (1993) expresses concern about the lack of nurse leaders in decision-making positions in health-care units. She outlines the possible routes for nurses to achieve leadership positions within the reformed health service. These routes include attaining specific qualifications, such as a master's degree in business administration (MBA), being mentored and being 'fast tracked' (accelerated promotion for able individuals). These routes may be designed to get nurses to the top, but this does not necessarily mean that once these nurses arrive there that they will represent nurses and nursing. What is essential is effective leadership at the clinical level. Ultimately this is more likely to result in significant contributions to patient care, such that policy-makers will feel compelled to include nurses in their deliberations.

Leadership abilities

Early leadership research (pre-1940) concerned itself mainly with trying to establish the traits (inbuilt characteristics) that leaders possessed (Bryman, 1989). Since that time the issue of traits as indicators of leadership potential has lost favour, first to style (what leaders do), and then to contingency (behaving as the situation demands). More recently, transactional (reciprocal influence between leader and led) and transformational (leaders with visions) leadership have assumed dominance (Bryman, 1989).

An organisation needs to be able to recognise leaders from within its membership. There are many characteristics associated with leadership personalities, for example, Bray *et al.* (1974) list 25 of them, including the possession of intelligence, imagination and resilience, an ability to communicate, assess objectively and make good decisions, and a desire to please others, enjoy work and want personal progress.

Leadership styles

The idea that the leadership style will directly influence issues such as job satisfaction, role clarity and group performance is in doubt. It is just as likely that these issues will influence the group and the leader. In everyday life, relationships between management and workforce do seem to range between three general styles of relationship. It is not uncommon for a dominant style to be present with shifts into other styles occasionally taking place.

The autocratic leader is mainly concerned about the task in hand. Decisions are made and others are expected comply; there is little attempt to acknowledge the views of those who have to carry out the tasks or to consider the effects of the decisions on them. Inflexible organisations tend to

operate in this way; the work is usually highly structured and those who enforce the structures are viewed positively by the senior members of the organisation. Thus, in some organisations there may be rewards for individuals who behave in an autocratic way towards those they supervise.

The democratic style of leadership is in stark contrast to the autocratic style. There is consideration for the opinions of those who have to carry out the tasks. Individuals and groups are involved in decision-making processes concerning their work. The valuing of people, their knowledge, experience and skills is central to this style. Through such participation it is thought that staff are likely to feel valued and responsible for their work.

The *laissez-faire* style of leadership is characterised by the low consideration of processes and group decision making. Initiative is left to the individual who is given no direction and who has complete freedom; this produces an uncoordinated group with no boundaries. In organisations (or parts of organisations) that depend on creativity at an operational level this may be the only way to achieve the desired outcome.

Two factors are thought to be necessary for effective leadership: consideration of colleagues, and the initiating structure (to give people clear precise roles). Also, four leadership dimensions are thought to be significant:

- support – which gives individual staff a sense of worth
- interaction facilitation to produce satisfying relationships in the group
- goal emphasis – unpressured stimulation and enthusiasm
- work facilitation – providing the means to accomplish the goal (Bryman, 1985).

Leadership is a complex issue, however, some simpler concepts have emerged in attempting to clarify this difficult subject. Hersey and Blanchard (1982), for example, described leadership as either task-oriented (authoritarian), concerned with the pursuit of goals, or the relationship-stressing approach (democratic), concerned with strengthening and maintaining the group. After studying leadership in depth, Likert (1979) considered that the issue should be based on the simple principle of supportive relationships.

The history of nursing has been typified by autocratic relationships. Autocratic control always creates informal leadership structures (leadership outside of the formal organisation). In nursing and health care generally, autocratic relationships are damaging for the patient, the nurse and the organisation. The problem facing nursing now is how to find competent leaders.

The need for leadership

It is common for nurses to be managed from an impersonal central administration. Nurses are consciously attempting to base their work on research evidence to improve practice. When individuals have well-developed knowledge and skills it is natural that they will want to express them in their work as the opportunities arise. No longer is it feasible for non-nurses to claim a level of knowledge and experience that matches that of an educated, experienced, practising nurse.

Within nurses' work there is little latitude for mistakes, and the consequences may be severe for patients and nurses, particularly now that nurses have a code of conduct which is quite specific about professional responsibility. As nursing is a highly stressful occupation, finding ways of supporting staff and reducing stress is a major challenge to nurse leaders (Stewart, 1990). This means that leadership should be close to patient care and competent in nursing. Supportive relationships between the nurse and the nurse leader at ward level and above would help provide this need.

The qualifications and abilities of nurses are many and diverse. Nurses are predominantly women and their careers can be frequently interrupted for family reasons; part-time work is often desired. These factors influence the support resources required, such as crèches, and the character of in-service (continuing) education. To develop knowledgeable and skillful nurses there is a need for more appropriate continuing education. Good in-service education may be more cost-effective than sending staff on a series of study days, it also utilises the talents of available staff. Basic education and training seldom fully equip nurses, particularly those who are newly registered, for the role expected of them in practice. In particular, the development of interview techniques, assessment skills, assertiveness training, counselling and stress management are subjects that are essential to a nurse's armoury if he or she is to provide an effective service.

Ultimately, the issue of quality in nursing care is a question of how well nurses are equipped to perform their central role.

Background for leadership

Predicting who is likely leadership material is problematic. Many of the tests claiming to determine leadership qualities actually measure supervisory or management ability (Bryman, 1985). Nurses have a history of being highly compliant, and individuals who are intelligent and question practices are likely to become frustrated by the system and leave (Birch, 1979). There needs to be a system in nursing that recognises and rewards personal development and achievement in order to promote a culture from which leaders will emerge.

The recent major reforms in the NHS, including *Caring for People* (DHSS, 1989) and *The Health of the Nation* (DoH, 1992), have led to changes in nursing, for example, *A Strategy for Nursing* (DoH, 1989) and more recently *A Vision for the Future* (NHS Management Executive, 1993). This latter document gives 12 targets, with time limits, for all nursing units to achieve. It addresses issues related to five main areas of nursing activity and responsibility: quality, outcomes and audit; accountability for practice; clinical and professional leadership; clinical research and supervision; purchasing and commissioning; and education and personal development. All nursing units have to demonstrate that they are meeting these objectives. *A Vision for the Future* clearly sets the agenda for the development and role of nursing in the changed health service, and nursing leadership is obliged to focus on these key issues.

> ### Reflective point
> It will be useful if you can identify how leadership is operated in your place of work and the influence it has on those who are led.
>
> What is your impression of the senior nurses you have met?
>
> From this reflection you may be conscious of either a negative, neutral or positive image of the senior nurse. What factors led to your perceptions? The style of leadership may have been influential: how leaders make decisions and encourage others to act can, if attractively presented, be positively viewed by staff regardless of leadership style (the benevolent dictator). Did the way you were motivated by the senior nurse influence your opinion? Did the or she ever discuss care problems with staff, praise them or become involved with patient or staff problems?

Did you feel recognised and included or ignored and excluded when in the presence of the senior nurse? Did you ever see him or her? Points like these may give you some clues as to how you formed your opinion.

Factors influencing nurses' work environment

Motivation at work

Much of the literature on work motivation has emerged from theories and research associated with industrial production. Some of the experiences of industry can readily be applied to the health service. The essential difference is that the focus of the health service is vulnerable, sick and disabled people, and staff have a moral and ethical duty to utilise their knowledge and skills in a way acceptable to the patient.

In the performance of work where tasks are carried out, several factors influence an individual's motivation (Cooper, 1973):

1. the environment, type, pace and variety of work, and the volume of people with whom the employer interacts
2. giving people choice and discretion when task problems need solving
3. being able to contribute to constructive changes that effect the total task, and being given feedback regarding final decisions and
4. goal characteristics that are clear, realistic and not too difficult.

Nurse training has been described as a conditioning process rather than an educational experience (Bowman and Thompson, 1989). Behavioural approaches to work motivation can be used to influence performance at work. The conditioning approach of the behaviourists is founded on three main principles: that the focus of attention is on observable behaviour; that behaviour is learnt; and that the strength or weakness of a behaviour depends on the consequences of that behaviour. The consequences are the end product of the technique known as operant conditioning (Robertson and Smith, 1985). There are four main types of consequences: positive reinforcement, aimed at increasing the frequency of a given behaviour; negative reinforcement, aimed at the removal of unpleasant stimuli that may prevent the learning of behaviour that is desired; punishment, in which unpleasant experiences associated with specific behaviour will reduce the likelihood of unwanted behaviour being repeated; and extinction of a behaviour, when there are no consequences or feedback occurring as a result of the behaviour. It is not unusual for nurses to experience two of the four consequences in the work situation: positive reinforcement and punishment.

The process theory (Robertson and Smith, 1985) examines the psychological processes that facilitate motivation. The main thrust of this approach is that people are goal-directed and the higher the value the individual puts on the goal the greater will be his or her motivation, for example, nurses who put a high value on 'practice' may be motivated to stay within clinical practice. Realism in the setting of goals is of great importance: goals that are too easy or too difficult can, in themselves, be demotivating. Productivity of people at work can indicate how well motivated individuals and groups are. Hernandez *et al.* (1988) looked at nursing by relating organisational factors to productivity. Their analysis indicated the strong positive factors that enhanced productivity and included the climate within the organisation, the supervisory support and involvement, how peers supported one another and how group members interacted and that by using job enrichment methods (e.g. primary nursing) nurses work was more productive.

In nursing the consideration of work motivation should include the effects of such strategies on patients. Punishment of the nurse may cause him or her to feel anger and resentment which may, unwittingly, be transferred to the patient and have adverse repercussions on the quality of relationships and work. The use of concepts that establish human need and development may be more valuable in motivating nurses. These are known as hygiene theories. Maslow (1970) proposed a theory of needs in a hierarchy that offers five levels of human achievement and motivation:

- physiological needs
- a need for safety
- a social need or feeling of belonging
- a need for esteem and

- a self-actualisation need, that is, the need to realise one's potential.

The lower needs, physiological and safety, become less important if the higher needs can be realised. This notion of different levels of personal needs can be applied to both the patient and the nurse in the workplace. Patients are more likely to be concerned with the lower needs of physiological survival, safety and belonging, especially in the acute phase of an illness. Later, they may use the illness experience as a positive development in themselves having coped effectively with a difficult and demanding experience. The nurse, however, may be more concerned with the higher needs, including the sense of belonging and need for esteem to self-actualisation. Another of the hygiene theories of work motivation is offered by Hertzberg (1968), who proposed two factors of importance in the work environment: the satisfiers or motivators that come from elements within the work (intrinsic factors), such as the challenge or meaning of the work, which are considered to be of a higher need; and the dissatisfiers (extrinsic factors), such as management styles, pay and conditions, which are considered to be of a lower need. The removal of dissatisfaction from the lower need (e.g. give a pay rise) does not in itself create satisfaction, it merely removes a dissatisfaction.

Leaders can influence motivation (Oldham, 1976). Motivating leaders exhibit more positive reward behaviour and less punishing behaviour, are more inclined to design feedback systems (letting people know how they are performing at work), and are more participative.

Work control

Every organisation has key aims, these are often published as 'mission statements' indicating to staff what the organisation believes in. Organisational aims set the scene for the behaviour and standards of those who work within it. Work in large organisations, such as hospital and community units, is of a complex nature, and depends on the contribution of different groups of people. This places controls on the freedom of the individual nurse, doctor and others to operate in precisely the way they may wish. The concept of 'control' for the individual will be influenced by the nature of the work and the variety and number of other staff involved. For example, a district nurse may have

more control over the organisation of his or her daily work activity than a nurse in a surgical day-case ward.

Most people want to exercise control over their own lives. Humans are described by Lazarus (1985) as seeking to control events and understand them by being active, manipulative, searching and evaluative. He suggests that any lack of control leads to stress. How much latitude an individual is given at work will depend on his or her knowledge, skills and areas of responsibility and accountability. Nurses are primarily responsible and accountable for assessing the needs of the patient, devising a plan for care, ensuring care is carried out according to the plan and evaluating the effects of care. The nurse should possess not only the skills and knowledge to do this, but should also have the resources and freedom to fulfil this primary role. However, in many situations the work of others takes precedence (like the doctor demanding a nurse's time and attention), thus displacing this prime function of the nurse and putting nurses in situations in which they have little or no control. Indeed it is not uncommon for nurses to state that they are 'too busy' to undertake patient assessment and evaluation because of other pressures. This is where nursing leadership has the potential to clarify and determine the nurse's contribution and direction.

The need for control is strong within individuals. An individual's desire to act declines in situations he or she has failed to control. This can lead to helplessness and a reluctance in the person to face change (Aronsson, 1989). Nurses and nursing have suffered from a lack of control, which, in turn, may have contributed to the poor leadership and inability of nursing effectively to invoke changes in work practice. Bowman *et al.* (1990) suggest that when registered nurses' work is organised in a way that gives them more control over patient care (e.g. primary nursing), more status and independence is experienced by the nurse. Also, when individuals have more flexibility in scheduling their work they experience fewer psychological stress symptoms (Pierce and Newstrom, 1983).

Nurses need to be clear about their span of control because others also have legitimate areas of control that can impinge upon them. An understanding of this can prevent conflict arising and will enable the nurse to cope more effectively.

Discipline

Organisations can base their success on the discipline of their members. The need for rules in society to maintain order and equity are appreciated as rational by most people. The way discipline is applied to individuals within an organisation often depends on the decision-making process and the roles of individuals and groups. Rules and policies impose limitations and determine the degree of freedom individuals and groups may have. For discipline to be effective it has to be seen to be fair and just.

Discipline can be discussed as a means of exercising control over groups of people, as in a school or the army, or it can be used to describe a mental or moral process that establishes rules of personal behaviour.

In society generally, it can be seen that the professional is given more freedom to exercise and control his or her own judgement. This is on the understanding that they have had the moral learning that enables them to operate with fewer controls, this requires self-discipline. Within organisations, workers who have well-developed motor skills tend to have fewer opportunities for decision making. For example, the architect will make decisions about the design of a building and the materials used. For the plans to be accomplished successfully, the builder needs to conform to the architect's plans. Most systems of organising nursing care are based on the tradesman model because of the basis on which decisions are made. For example, many nurses depend on a medical diagnosis before they feel able to intervene in making patient care decisions. More recent approaches to the organisation of nursing, where the nurse is making decisions based on the patient's physical, emotional and social problems, do not require any other perspective to initiate nursing care. These changes indicate that nurses are able to operate with the freedoms enjoyed by other professions, but they also need to develop the self-discipline that must accompany this freedom. This is probably best illustrated by Kinston (1987), who used his levels of work measure in various nursing organisations and found that registered nurses operating the more traditional work methods were classified at level 1 (prescribed output: where tasks are concrete and completed one at a time), the tradesman level. Registered nurses who worked within an organisation that operated primary nursing were classified at level 2 (situational response: several tasks are handled simultaneously and priorities determined by the operator), or at the professional level of working.

The hierarchical nature of work in many care settings often imposes tight controls on the registered nurse's decision making. Many nursing organisations offer little opportunity for nurses to utilise their knowledge and skills to help individual patients. Most nursing care methods use group discipline as a means of achieving standards in patient care; that is constantly making each other aware of any mistakes made or deficiencies in practice. Sometimes it is difficult to avoid such arrangements with the many changes in pace and volume of work that can occur over a short time. The issue of nurses' responsibility, authority and accountability can be confusing when work responsibilities are shared, and it may be impossible in practice to determine who is accountable for what.

The road to professionalism, with nurses operating in a system where there are fewer controls on decision making and behaviour, may be attractive but it is not an easy option. Not all nurses are prepared for or desire such a role. Changes in education for nurses, such as Project 2000 and PREPP, will provide some of the support necessary to shift to systems that require confidence to operate more independently. If nursing is to become more autonomous, then open leadership (where staff are free to express their opinions without recriminations) is needed to give the decision-making nurse the confidence to consult colleagues about patient care (Bouman and Landeweerd, 1993). If the right type of support and development of staff is not in place there is a real danger that the rush for independent practice will not achieve the success it deserves.

Social support

The influence social support has on an individual's successful adaptation and coping is the subject of much research. Although there are still gaps in understanding how social support affects individuals there is no doubt that its study will provide useful information concerning human relations. Social support is the interaction of four components in human relations: emotional concern; instrumental aid; information exchange; and appraisal

(House, 1986). In 1976 the World Health Organization (WHO) recognised four general situations that were important to psychological stress: uprooting, where individuals may be deprived of support and a sense of belonging; dehumanisation of societies and institutions, the impersonal and mechanistic provision of services with over-reliance on technology; psychological side-effects of the spread of innovation, where technology isolates individuals or changes relationships; and psychosocial factors as constraints on environmental and health programmes and activities, e.g. differences in aims and aspirations of doctors, nurses and managers.

Social support in the work situation is thought to be dependent on three key relationships; the support given within the home (problems at home are frequently carried into work and can influence performance), the support from colleagues and the support from immediate supervisors (Dignam and West, 1988). Generally, good support in the work situation can reduce the effects of stress. Effective support can influence perceived job stress and strain to the point of having a mental health effect (La Rocco *et al.*, 1980). Also, nursing leaders who show social consideration have a positive effect on nurses' responses to their job, while those who are production-orientated provoke a variety of health problems in their staff, including general health problems, anxiety, depression and irritability (Bouman and Landeweerd, 1993). Nurses seem to be more satisfied when leaders operate a combination of these styles.

The mixed style is one that is currently operating in the health service. There is an emphasis on efficiency and productivity and at the same time attempts are being made to produce a more egalitarian workforce with the emphasis on multidisciplinary teamwork. Nurses will be unable to contribute effectively to these 'teams' without a supportive leadership that gives them the confidence to so do. Practical measures for structures that will be socially supportive might include: leaders above the level of charge nurse who have a responsibility for a number of wards/departments and personal contact with all registered nurses and clinical credibility; an educational programme that will enable nurses to contribute to professional teams and patient care (in line with PREPP); and work that is designed to give the registered nurse a clear indication of their accountability, responsibility and authority in relation to patient care.

Regardless of the implementation of support strategies, some individuals may display intrinsic behaviour which reduces their opportunity for receiving social support. For example, individuals may avoid their work seniors, not avail themselves of available educational opportunities and or not accept responsibility, accountability and authority.

The nurse–doctor relationship

The relationship between nurses and doctors is generally reported to be poor (Game and Pringle, 1983; Katzman and Roberts, 1988). Yet in order to have an effective patient care and treatment service there is a need for close collaboration between the two occupations where each offers their services in an atmosphere of mutual trust and understanding. Unfortunately, the relationship tends to be based on power and the traditional gender roles of men and women, and it is not unusual for both doctors and nurses to deny that there is anything intrinsically wrong with this relationship. In reality, problems have existed since the inception of nursing, with medicine wanting to control nursing activity and development.

Nightingale expressed concern about the lectures that were given to trainee nurses by doctors because of the danger that nurses might become 'medical men'. She felt that the content of the medical staff's lectures was not appropriate to nursing, and she was suspicious of the 'medical model'; her ambition was to have educated women teach the 'handicraft of nursing' (Baly, 1986). Such was the domination of nursing by medicine that many of Nightingale's theories of nursing remained undeveloped. Nursing theory did not emerge again for 100 years until nurses such as Henderson and Orlando in the 1950s in the United States began the present movement of nursing theory development.

Game and Pringle (1983) depict the abnormal sex-role relationships in the health arena as related to Victorian figures that are paternalistic and maternalistic in nature. Such relationships are abnormal, according to Stein (1967) who feels that attitudes towards these 'games' need to change. He viewed the relationship between doctors and nurses as a transactional neurosis (abnormal interaction). This view is supported by more recent investigation. Katzman and Roberts (1988) found that the views of nurses on patient care issues were subordinated to the decision making of physicians; this subordination was interpreted as the traditional male–female roles as played within the traditional family. Katzman and Roberts (1988) argue that this relationship severely hampers nurses' ability to set their own boundaries, as their inferior position lacks any power in the workplace. One assessment found that the medical influence on nurse education and the hiring of 'good' nurses by doctors encouraged a sex-role stereotype of the nurse because their view of a 'good' nurse was an attractive, compliant female (Keddy *et al.*, 1986).

Many nurses feel angry at the way they are treated by doctors and in some situations nurses are reported to be drawing up their battle lines (Gray, 1987). In Britain almost half the nurses responding to a survey were not happy with relations between themselves and doctors (Heenan, 1991).

However, some medical staff do not sympathise with nurses' claims that they are being treated as second class. They do not necessarily agree with the analysis of the problems associated with traditional nursing. Stanley (1983) argues that it is normal for one group to be dominant and another to be submissive, subject to challenges and competition. He also expresses the view that nurses have chosen to be submissive and defer to doctors.

These power relationships clearly need to change. Nurses need to acknowledge the issue of responsibility, accountability and authority as a means to encourage the expression of views: Dimond (1987) argues that nurses cannot continue to hide behind medical coats as legal accountability has to be faced.

Not all doctor–nurse relationships are poor or perverse; good relationships are possibly as common. Porter (1991) found that in the absence of the consultant the nurse's contribution to clinical decision making was considerable and senior nurses were less deferential to medical staff when involved in decision making. Some believe that less rigid role demarcation is needed, with more shared roles and shared education (e.g. Brooking, 1991). The rational view is that as health decision making and research becomes more collaborative the power relationships are more likely to be broken down.

Personnel

In health-care organisations judgements have to be made about the number and type of staff required to provide an effective and efficient service. Each department has to justify the costs they incur on staff, and nursing is no exception. Nursing has a problem, however, in accurately estimating the number and skill mix of staff needed for a given population of patients. The nature of nurses' relationships with patients is determined by patients' needs; physical needs being easier to measure and understand than psycho-social needs. The effective utilisation of registered nurses is important to the delivery of a high-quality service. Issues such as how much of a registered nurse's time should be spent on administrative/clerical duties, and how much time is realistic to allow any nurse to be with patients, pose difficulties in terms of precision. Skill mix levels (the number of registered, trained and untrained personnel) in a department are problematic issues that nurses must address. The best evidence to-date indicates that wards with higher ratios of staff employed at grade 'D' (registered nurses) and above provide higher quality of care with better outcomes and are more cost-effective than wards who carry a larger proportion of unqualified staff (Carr-Hill *et al.*, 1992).

A rule-of-thumb method of calculating nursing staff requirements is by nurse–patient ratios. This method determines the number of nurses by specialty to bed. Intensive care units have a higher ratio of staff per bed than other specialties, and paediatric wards have a higher ratio of nurses per bed than general wards. Small wards are offered a percentage increase to give sufficient staff to facilitate 24-hour cover. In the community, nurses are calculated based upon population size. In the equation additional staff are calculated for each student nurse, approved leave and sickness. Today other less simplistic methods of calculating staff are available.

Nursing workload or patient dependency measures are viewed as a more scientific and rational approach to finding the right mix of staff for a particular clinical setting. The objective of workload/dependency studies is to assess the demand for nursing time, to ascertain how staff may be deployed and to provide a level of quality in care acceptable to user and provider.

Workload/dependency measures can be quite sophisticated in assessing, with reasonable accuracy, the amount of nursing time needed in a clinical area. However, there is still the problem of identifying every activity that occurs between the nurse and patient; some patients will demand more time during well-defined procedures than others; the time for effective education and adaptation will vary between patients. As systems become more sophisticated allowances for such differences can be calculated, when the frequency of these variables are known. The problem with estimating manpower requirements by workload/dependency measures is that they currently address the quantitative aspects of care but are unable to be accurate about the qualitative aspects of nurses' work. What workload measures try to do is determine the number of nursing hours required to provide a prescribed level of care. The factors taken into account include the time to carry out the care, the individual's need for care, the quality or standard of care expected and the level of skill or skill mix required to deliver the care.

Work study methods are often chosen as a means of sampling nursing work activity. Work is observed that is either patient related, and has a direct or indirect input to the patient, or non-patient related. Modification of this approach is necessary, depending on the type of environment and services being offered (e.g. intensive care units have higher patient dependency than a general ward and allowance has to be made for this).

Other non-work study methods have been developed that centre more upon the nurse's perception of the patient's needs. These are considered by some to be as reliable as those that employ a quantitative approach. Schroeder *et al.* (1984) found that simple workload measures were just as accurate in the information gained as detailed, more expensive measures. Development of this approach continues.

Outcomes

In principle, the correct balance of personnel should result in the correct outcome for the patient. Shortage of staff, for example, can lead to complications for the patient. Upon discharge patients should have an understanding of their health status and strategies for coping; their level of understanding and coping will be influenced by nurses. Patients will also have feelings, impressions and personal evidence of how they were treated by staff. They will know whether they physically feel better, no different or worse than they did prior to any health-care intervention.

Nurses have not yet determined outcome measures that have universal acceptance. Outcomes that can be directly observed may be more easily measured, for example the incidence of pressure sores and wound infection, and the severity of pain. Other outcome measures include educational factors, such as patients' understanding of their condition and the processes associated with their care. Changes in psychological factors, such as levels of anxiety and depression, following health care might also be used as an outcome. The most common method of measuring outcome in nursing is through patient satisfaction surveys. These may indicate strengths and weaknesses within a nursing service and the available resources but might not address more important personal issues. The development of outcome measures is currently a high priority for nursing.

Audit

For many nurses the use of auditing methods in determining the quality of care may not seem appropriate. It could be argued that a key component of nursing is the helping relationship with patients and it is the subtleties within this relationship that culminate in care outcomes. Nurses, however, must accept their responsibility to account for the care given. The lack of tools to measure nursing care is a reflection of the priorities of the past.

Nursing audit is primarily achieved by effectively assessing care needs and evaluating outcomes. There are three ways in which care quality can be audited. Where patients may be at risk of complications, for example, wound infections and pressure sores, a **prospective** assessment may indicate the need for preventative interventions. These preventative interventions can then be assessed as they occur or at a later date. The assessment of a patient's care and recording of outcomes while the patient is still receiving care is called a **concurrent** audit. A **retrospective** audit examines the effects of care once interventions cease. The real purpose of any audit is to collect as much factual information as possible to facilitate better planning and development of a service.

A report by the Audit Commission (1991) illustrates how this approach offers useful information. The report found that only 15 percent of the wards studied practised primary nursing and 40 percent allocated nurses different patients from shift to shift. Also, it was found that if nursing time spent on clerical and housekeeping duties was reduced to 8 percent, a saving of £40 million would be made. Some wards continued to be run by routine, and care planning and documentation was generally poor across all wards. The nurses on the 'best' wards spent 20 percent of their time planning, evaluating and documenting care, and the report claimed that this activity saved nursing time by eliminating unnecessary routines. Such audit reports provide information that is advantageous to patients, nurses and the health service.

Quality assurance

Nurses are accountable for the quality of care they deliver. Although there has been a concerted effort to improve the quality of care and services to patients, no-one has yet established a clear meaning of the term. By examining literature related to 'quality' in nursing care that spanned 30 years, Attree (1993) found confusion about what was meant by quality and what should be measured. Theory development and research are needed to clarify this concept as it applies within different contexts. When discussing quality assurance in nursing one is usually talking about the best example, or standard, that can realistically be achieved with some certainty. Good standards of care can only be assessed when the care is planned systematically around the individual patient.

For nurses to be clear about the standards they and their colleagues aspire to, it is usual for a nursing directorate to agree a philosophy. This will help determine the nursing activity, the expertise required by staff and the direction of any education and training programmes.

Nurses working in clinical practice are usually involved in the setting or writing of standards. Standards are set by considering the structure (this indicates a minimum level of expectation in terms of environment, organisation, expertise and resources), the process (what the nurse actually does and its implementation) and the outcome (the expected response of the patient to planned care) according to Donabedian (1966). There are seven steps to writing standards (Dunne, 1991): selecting the area for which the standard is to be written; stating the objectives the nurse wishes to achieve; specifying the type of nursing action necessary to achieve the objectives; where appropriate, giving a time scale for each action; writing it up in a logical sequence; reviewing the written standard to eliminate anything that cannot be evaluated; and testing the new standard for feasibility.

A good quality assurance programme that is clear about the nursing contribution sets achievable nursing standards, matches skills and knowledge to the work, educates staff to achieve quality of care and monitors performance through appraisal and audit methods.

To be effective, quality assurance and auditing systems need to be highly structured and require investment. For full effect the positive cooperation of staff is essential. They will need to participate in the setting up of systems and be aware of benefits that can accrue to their practice. Good quality assurance and auditing programmes should demonstrate positive and measurable benefits for patients which reflect dynamic and innovative practices. Dissemination and discussion of findings is essential if the information obtained is to be effective.

Resource management

Nurses are now responsible for the effective use of those resources that impinge on the quality of service to the patient. Wilson (1991) states that there are four key elements to resource management: improving the quality of care; involving in the management process all those professional groups whose decisions have a direct commitment of resources to care and treatment of patients; improving information; and effectively controlling available resources.

Competent assessment of patients' needs is essential in enabling information from all healthcare professionals to be combined (case mix data) and stored in one file. Such information should make it possible to track patients' treatment and progress throughout their hospital stay. Information gathered in this way can enable costs to be determined more accurately. Other benefits include a reduction in the use of manual information systems that might be more time consuming.

The main elements of a nurse management information system are: care planning; workload measures; rostering; and patient case mix cost details. The benefit of this type of system for nursing is the more efficient use of staff and equipment. Other issues, such as the way the patient's day is organised, more flexible duty planning over a 24-hour period and matching patient admissions to the available staff on duty, can also be addressed (Wilson, 1991).

Job design and skill mix

Most nurses are unclear of, or unable to articulate, their contribution to health care. This has left nursing open to criticism and nurses are frequently challenged about what it is they do, whether they are effective and what role they should take. The reality is that there is insufficient evidence to put forward compelling arguments supporting a unique contribution from the nurse. A few studies, such as that of Carr-Hill *et al.* (1992), provide an indication of the benefits of using more rather than fewer registered nurses. There is no doubt that registered nurses are frequently used inappropriately, and many part-time registered nurses do not assume the same degree of responsibility at work as do their full-time colleagues. In some situations the role of the 'bank' registered nurse may not be any different from that of the trained health-care assistant.

The intention to embrace holistic care principles is currently paramount. To achieve the best for patients and to have regard for costs nurses must ask themselves whether their education and training is being used fully to benefit practice. For example, how necessary is it for a registered nurse to be involved in the bathing of patients? Involvement in this type of activity may well be necessary to take the opportunity to assess the patient, to use the time to educate the patient or to strengthen the relationship, but as a motor skill it does not require a registered nurse. What should the registered nurse actually be doing whilst working? Questions such as this are crucial and they need to be addressed through job design and skill-mix exercises. The emphasis on work methods like primary nursing have begun to address these issues by defining the professional relationship between the patient and registered nurse; Bowman *et al.* (1991) have described this relationship as a companionship attachment because of the desire of the patient to be in the company of someone who understands the problems facing the patient and the system in which the patient is 'travelling'.

Job design is concerned with observing and recording peoples' work activity and analysing it to improve efficiency, involvement, job satisfaction and, where possible, to reduce costs. Nurses need to know how such objectives can be achieved.

Probably the first method of studying job design was the **time and motion** study. The basic principle behind this was to time specific activities with a stopwatch, the main purpose being to identify and eliminate wasteful time. In human services, action may not be the most important part of a process, thus time and motion have limited uses. The **methods improvement** approach is dependent on drawing in all available data surrounding a process, such as the environment, type of work carried out, staff and other resources, policies and cost, to improve goal achievement. Flow charts show how a function is achieved from beginning to end; materials and the person performing the function can be tracked. **Job simplification** aims to remove difficult, time-consuming parts of the work to give individuals more time for other work. Another person may be employed to cope exclusively with the discarded task. A consequence of this may be a reduction in the variety of work with a subsequent reduction in job satisfaction. To increase variety in work **job rotation** can be used; staff exchange shifts or roles on a regular, planned basis. A negative effect of this is lack of continuity. The **job enrichment** approach is concerned with expanding a role to develop or utilise a wide range of skills and abilities, while at the same time offering staff more control over their work. This is the approach of nurses who recommend individualised care planned and delivered by individual nurses.

All the above approaches will in some way affect work motivation, satisfaction, absenteeism and turnover. The work circumstances of staff, their expectations, level of development and support will have an influence on how effective any of these approaches might be. Many good intentions for developing work have been lost because those leading the change have not judged or prepared for these issues effectively.

Skill mix is concerned with obtaining the right balance of the various grades of nurses within a particular care setting for optimum efficiency. The skill mix debate has come about for many reasons, including the increasing ageing population, the reduced number of school leavers, the shortage of staff in 'high-tech' areas, the changes in nursing strategies and education, the introduction of resource management, increased competition in health care, quality of care issues and the clinical regrading exercise. The most important grade in the skill-mix debate is that of the registered nurse. How best can their education, training and skills be utilised? Should the job be focused on being a nurse, doctor's assistant, ward supervisor or a combination of these? The view of Eric Caines, who was the NHS personnel director, is that nurses (and other professionals) should be more flexible in work practices; also he believes that professional demarcation lines need to be eliminated with staff acquiring a wider range of skills to meet patients' immediate health-care needs. He envisages that over time there will be fewer people who could be defined as nurses in the narrow way it is today (Naish, 1992).

Regardless of developments the key role of the nurse is that of the professional who assesses patient care needs. Once the role of the registered nurse is clarified, the roles of the charge nurse, trained health-care assistant and so forth will be easier to determine. The central role of the registered nurse within any care setting, whether hospital or community, should be focused on helping and teaching patients and their families how to cope and adapt. The volume of time spent on these activities will depend on factors such as the ratio of patients to a registered nurse, the frequency of assessment and evaluation, and the communications with other professionals.

A major concern for nurses regarding skill-mix exercises is that they are driven by a desire to save money. It is also argued that the measures used are crude, mechanistic and insensitive to the subtle aspects of nursing. A further criticism is that there are no apparent attempts to evaluate objectively the qualitative impact of care on patients after changes in skill mix have been carried out (Buchan, 1993). While in principle skill mix appears a perfectly rational process, what is actually required are more sensitive measures that capture the real essence of nursing work and not just a few simple procedures.

Reflective point

What decisions and activities do you think a registered nurse should be involved with during a 37.5-hour week? It may be helpful to analyse a week's activity of your own.

Determine the volume of time you would spend in direct and indirect (preparing for patient interventions, writing notes) patient care and ward/department management.

Nurses' work organisation methods

The Code of Professional Conduct for Nurses Midwives and Health Visitors states that each registered nurse, midwife and health visitor shall act, at all times, in such a manner as to:

- safeguard and promote the interests of individual patients and clients
- serve the interests of society
- justify public trust and confidence and
- uphold and enhance the good standing and reputation of the professions (UKCC, 1992).

The code, given to all registered nurses, goes on to list 16 ways in which nurses are accountable for their practice.

When considering nurses' work organisation methods the position of the registered nurse in relation to the code of conduct needs to be examined. Difficulties may arise in an organisation where decision making is centralised, and the registered nurse's ability to fulfil his or her patient care responsibilities may be compromised. The public is encouraged to demand higher standards of care (e.g. *The Patient's Charter*). It is therefore important to utilise fully the skills and knowledge of registered nurses. To be effective in the health-care system, nurses need to be clear about what expertise they have to offer and how it can be best utilised. An independent, objective view of nursing was provided by Kinston (1987) from the Brunel Institute of Organisation and Social Studies. He found that nurses were confused about the actual kind of nursing to be done, and that there were too many layers of management, inappropriate expectations of staff and insufficient integration of nursing with medical and support services. A more confused system would be difficult to contrive. A shift from such a position takes many years to achieve and requires a strategy such as that proposed by the chief nursing officer (DoH, 1989; NHS Management Executive, 1993) gradually to strengthen nursing. It is not uncommon for patients to feel that they are there to do as they are told and to fit in with health-care organisations. The organisation should respond to the patient – not vice versa. By examining the various ways nursing can be organised it may be possible to determine which methods enable nurses to fulfil effectively their legal and moral obligations to patients.

The definition and classification of work organisation methods is fraught with difficulties. Many of the methods have emerged from practice with little or no testing of their effects on patient care quality or staff satisfaction. The literature on nurses' work methods is sparse, anecdotal and rarely research based. The notable exception is that pertaining to primary nursing. The confusion is such that nurses describe the same work methods in a variety of ways. The brief descriptions that follow serve to indicate the approaches taken to organise nurses for care delivery.

Main features of nurses' work methods

Task (functional) nursing

When organising nursing care through a task system the patient has to relinquish responsibility (Menzies, 1960) and become a passive work object in order to fulfil the prescribed role (Fretwell, 1980). The nurse uses a medical model to conceptualise the patient's problem. The consequence of this is that nursing care is targeted at combating the patient's 'disease'. Task orientation gives a fragmented impression of the patient and a lack of continuity in the delivery of care (Marks-Maran, 1978; Fretwell, 1980; Chavasse, 1981). Work is allocated by listing tasks on a daily or shift basis, the advantage being that these can be completed during a span of duty (Chavasse, 1981). Nurses are responsible for the individual tasks they carry out, the tasks themselves assuming priority over the patient (Chavasse, 1981). Block prescription of care for categories of patients occurs which leads to a hierarchy of tasks. The more complex task is given to the more highly trained or more senior nurse and the prescribing of care becomes a one way process with no opportunity for patients to ask questions or contribute (Fretwell, 1980). Relationships are avoided, there is no allowance for emotional support, close observations are less likely and important clinical changes often go unnoticed (Marks-Maran, 1978). The ward routine follows a predetermined and rigid course making day-to-day work planning simple and easy (Chavasse, 1981).

Progressive patient care

In progressive patient care patients are assigned according to their level of dependency to a geographical area of a ward/unit, where a team of nurses delivers the care. Usually the ward is divided into four discrete groups of patients (Sjoberg *et al.*, 1971), e.g. intensive care, high care, average care and minimal care. The patient's condition and dependency is reviewed daily and the patient is placed in the area judged most appropriate to their needs. Responsibility for patient care is decentralised to the person in charge of the team. The composition of staff in each team is organised according to the skill mix required. Thus, the intensive care team would have a high complement of registered nurses and the minimal care team would have fewer registered nurses.

Patient allocation (case method)

Allocation of patients to nurses usually occurs in one of two ways: most commonly on a shift basis (Pearson, 1988), far less commonly on the basis of a weekly span of duty (Marks-Maran, 1978). The patient need not necessarily be allocated to a registered nurse (Chavasse, 1981) but this nurse will be responsible for the delivery of total care while on duty. The nurse will plan care for the period of duty which decentralises management and creates a more participative style (Heslin, 1987) with ongoing care planning by those nurses directly involved with care. In this way the senior nurse's role is supervisory although it may involve care planning and responsibility for patient outcome.

Team nursing

The purpose of team nursing is to maximise the use of available nursing skills making them more readily available to patients (Shukla, 1982). The registered nurse is supported by a team of junior nurses. Usually, wards are divided into two teams, although there may be more than two. Each team is led by an experienced registered nurse, whose role it is to create a good team with a strong group identity (Shukla, 1982; Pearson, 1988). According to Shukla (1982), the team leader's role is fourfold:

- to plan nursing care through participative planning strategies
- to delegate specific tasks and/or patients to team members

- to provide part of the professional care and
- to supervise, coordinate, and evaluate the care provided by team members.

The team leader may use a patient allocation method or task approach to organising care (Marks-Maran, 1978). The emphasis in team nursing is to increase each group member's participation in the management of care thus creating group identity.

The patient is cared for by fewer nurses and may be involved in the planning of care, which may improve nurse–patient relations (Reed, 1988). The hierarchy within this system is traditional with the team leader responsible and accountable to the senior nurse, the team assuming collective responsibility for its actions. Such participative management may increase job satisfaction and motivation in the nurse (Pearson, 1988).

Primary nursing

The basic tenet of this method is that the registered nurse has

> total responsibility for a patient while he receives nursing services from a particular department or agency ... within the context of this relationship the patient knows that one (registered) nurse is in charge of his care while the patient is in this particular area ... the system is recognised as one where an individual nurse has responsibility both for giving care and for making decisions and where acceptance of responsibility is both visible and well understood (Manthey, 1988, p. 645).

In primary nursing each patient is assigned to a registered nurse on admission to hospital. The registered nurse is responsible and accountable for the welfare of the patient throughout his or her hospital stay (Pearson, 1988). This change in relationship between the registered nurse and the patient should facilitate a strong bond or attachment between the patient and nurse (Gillies, 1982). Each registered nurse has responsibility for between one to eight patients (Hegyvary, 1982; Follett, 1982; Gillies, 1982; Shukla, 1982) which gives the nurse maximum accountability during her time on duty.

The registered nurse has a clear patient workload and full responsibility for the delivery of care. She has autonomy, responsibility and accountability for the coordination of services to the patient. The primary nurse's main responsibilities, according to Shukla (1982), are for assessing, planning and coordinating care throughout the patient's stay in hospital and for formulating the provision of direct services to the patient and family at all times.

An associate nurse is a less experienced registered nurse who works with the primary nurse helping to carry out agreed care. The associate nurse may also make changes to the patient's care plan during the absence of the primary nurse (Shukla, 1982; Pearson, 1988). The ward senior nurse's role changes to that of a clinical leader who acts as consultant and advisor to primary nurses and as a teaching resource to all staff in the unit; this changes the traditional hierarchical relationships to peer relationships (Bowman and Thompson, 1989). Ideally, the primary nurse is released from most administrative duties and the ward routine, which is organised around the patient, should be less rigid.

Effects of work methods on patient care and the nurse

As primary nursing has received most attention in both opinion and research literature, direct comparisons of different work methods are exceedingly difficult. The study of nurses' work and its consequences is at an early stage, and any interpretation should be tempered with caution as the many variables are not yet understood.

Work design may prove to have more of an impact on the nurse than is currently accepted. Broadbent (1985) argues that job design may well have an important effect on the way that individuals perceive their work. The common view is that an individual's personality is often the cause when work is viewed negatively. Broadbent believes that his, and other studies, indicate that it is the work itself which may have an effect on the individual's psychological health. For example, paced production causes anxiety in most people; social isolation at work induces depression and a lack of support can provoke depression and a reduction in job satisfaction. Despite industrial origins, such information can be understood from a nursing perspective. Experienced nurses will recall feelings of anxiety on occasions when the pace of work increases due to a rapid influx of admissions or increased workload. They will also be able to recall the detrimental effects of unsupportive senior colleagues.

The effects of work and its organisation on nurses has received scant attention. The available literature tends to utilise primary nursing as a model practice and comparisons between this method and others (usually team nursing) are made. A further problem is that the research available has consistently failed to determine the difference between the various work methods, compounding the difficulty of interpretation.

The cost effectiveness and quality of different work methods has received some attention, although studies have been almost exclusively confined to hospitals. Generally the findings indicate that primary nursing can be shown to improve productivity (Marram, 1976; Hernandez et al., 1988; Bond et al., 1991) with no increase in costs (Marram, 1976; Betz, 1986; Chavigny and Lewis, 1984; Wilson and Dawson, 1989). Primary nursing, when compared to other forms of nursing, at worst makes no difference to patient satisfaction and care quality (Chavigny and Lewis, 1984; MacGuire, 1991) and at best improvements are shown (Sellick et al., 1983; Reed, 1988; Wilson and Dawson, 1989; Bond et al., 1991). Patient assignment systems have shown improvement in nurses' understanding of patients' problems as well as creating more positive attitudes towards patients (Athlin and Norberg, 1987). However, the lack of operational definitions and the variety of research instruments used makes the various findings equivocal.

Similar findings are apparent when addressing staff satisfaction. Most of the available research literature indicates greater satisfaction in those nurses practising primary nursing compared to other work methods (Carlsen and Malley, 1981; Sellick et al., 1983; Perella and Hentinen, 1989), though some studies have found no difference (Chavigny and Lewis, 1984; Armitage et al., 1991) or less satisfaction (Giovanetti, 1986). The lack of standard instruments and procedures in assessing nurses' satisfaction makes interpretation difficult. It may be the case that in many of the studies primary nursing systems were still developing. Sometimes a new change provokes enthusiasm and generates interest in staff initially. If measures are taken on the effects of the change during this initial enthusiasm then unreliable results will be obtained, this is called a 'Hawthorne' effect.

Stress associated with different nursing work methods has not received so much attention as work satisfaction. The available studies indicate that nurses whose work is designed to give them more autonomy and control will experience less stress from their work (McGrath et al., 1989; Bouman and Landeweerd, 1992; Escriba-Aguir et al., 1993).

Identifying nursing work methods

The problems associated with inappropriate work methods, that resulted in poor relationships for patients and nurses, were first described graphically by Menzies (1960). The authoritarian social structure and work processes that existed at that time were judged to be harmful to both nurse and patient. Difficulties for nurses were related to their perception of the patient being subjugated by the medical perspective. In essence, the medical model breaks the patient down into a series of functions. In such a model, dysfunction is corrected by medical interventions, and in such an environment nurses have no control over their relationships with patients or events associated with patients; work is broken down into a series of tasks that the patient and nurse have to fit in with.

Nursing theories that emerged (mainly from the United States) following the Second World War, expressed views on health and care that acknowledged the experience and knowledge of both the patient and the nurse. These theories have developed in practice to such an extent that the nurse is now able to make care decisions without the need for constant checking with medical staff. The nurse can offer a unique service to the patient that is in itself beneficial and therapeutic. This enables the nurse to play a full role in the health-care team. The acceptance of the patient as a sentient, knowing individual who has a right to choose whether to be involved in the care decision process is only problematic for those who view the patient as a series of biological processes. Such contrasts in views of health work can only be explained by describing them. What is needed is a method of breaking nurses' work down into its various components so that a more objective assessment of what is operating in practice can be made.

Descriptions of nurses' work methods are unreliable because it is probable that staff in different work environments, who describe their work in the same way, will have areas of their work organised differently. There is a tendency for nurses to see work methods as packages, when in reality there may only be minor differences in work practice between nurses who claim to be operating a primary nursing system and those operating a team system. This packaging of work methods has led authors and researchers to try and describe work methods in isolation. MacGuire (1989a, b), for example, described ten principles of primary nursing, how they may be operationally defined and how to assess whether these principles are operational in wards where elderly people are cared for. The assessment is complex to use and will only inform the user of the extent to which primary nursing is practiced. Others have examined particular characteristics as if they are unique to primary nursing. For example, Watts and O'Leary (1980) described primary nursing as the five 'A's:

- accountability
- advocacy
- assertiveness
- authority
- autonomy

and the five 'C's:

- collaboration
- continuity
- communication
- commitment
- coordination.

Clearly these components are not unique to any one form of nurses' work organisation. What may be different is the way they are operationalised. Thomas and Bond (1990) attempted to distinguish between primary, team and task nursing. Their questionnaire addressed six aspects (grouping of nurses and length of allocation to specific patients; allocation of nursing work; organisation of the duty rota; nursing accountability for patient care; responsibility for writing patients' nursing notes; and liaison with medical/paramedical staff) of nurses' work but was ultimately unable to discriminate between the three work methods in their sample.

It is possible to utilise industrial models to determine how nurses may be working. Bouman and Landeweerd (1992) used Hackman and Oldham's (1976) jobs characteristic model to differentiate nurses' practice when studying social support, coping and work satisfaction. This model looks at core job dimensions such as skill variety, task identity, task significance, autonomy and feedback. How these are organised should have an effect on the individual at work. Such universal

work models may be helpful in understanding the general characteristics of a working situation.

Kinston (1987) stated that registered nurses can organise their work in three ways:

- by being involved with routine tasks and responding to situational changes, involving themselves with all aspects of care
- by handling most of the patient care but having an assistant to help them with routine work
- by prescribing care. All routine work being carried out by others under the registered nurse's management.

Components of all work methods can be placed into three major organisational modes of work:

- primary nursing, in which a registered nurse is the main person who interacts with the patient and has the best opportunity for a consistent relationship with the patient
- team nursing, in which several of the available staff interact with the patient and have an equal opportunity for developing a relationship with the patient
- task nursing, in which all staff interact with the patient and have an equal opportunity for developing a relationship with the patient.

Bowman *et al.* (1991) suggested that all nursing work contains the same components, it is how they are operationalised that determines the prevailing work method. They proposed a system that classifies nurses' work methods as either primary, team or task nursing, depending on how specific components of the registered nurse's work are organised. The classification system indicates the type of relationship achieved in practice between the registered nurse and patient. Thirteen components central to all nurses' work, regardless of specialty, are assessed as to how they operate (Bowman *et al.*, 1991, 1993). The 13 items are:

1. The basis of the patient's assessment.
2. The assessment and evaluation of the patient.
3. The degree of managerial control.
4. The accountability for patient care.
5. The responsibility for patient care.
6. The authority for patient care.
7. The senior ward nurse's role in decision making.
8. The method of communication between professional groups.
9. The method of allocating patients to nurses.
10. The leadership style operating on the ward.

11. Responsibility for communication with relatives.
12. The patient's awareness of who has responsibility for care.
13. The patient's involvement with decision making.

Patients are interviewed regarding items 12 and 13, those chosen for this will come from the patient population for whom the registered nurse considers him- or herself to be responsible. A total score is achieved from all 13 items: the higher the score the greater the opportunity of a close relationship between the patient and the registered nurse. A high score equates with primary nursing, a moderate score with team nursing and a low score with task nursing. Each work method can be arbitrarily categorised as strong, moderate or weak to indicate more precisely the score.

The benefits of this system are that it is relatively simple to use (assessment will take up to one hour), it addresses the main components of a registered nurse's work and it can be used to determine the organisational work method. Such a classification system may be used:

- as a monitoring instrument to diagnose practices when changing to primary nursing or the named nurse principle
- to determine the work method for research purposes
- for managers to determine the effects of different work methods on productivity, quality and satisfaction with care.

Reflective point

Patients clearly benefit from nursing care. Nurses should be able to articulate how they help and contribute to care, health maintenance and recovery in a way that other health professionals do not.

Determine how you offer the patient a unique service and use your knowledge and skills. Consider how this might complement the services others give.

This exercise is not easy but should make you clearer about the decisions you are allowed to make as a nurse and how such decisions shape your role. It may also make you think about issues of accountability and responsibility. In all health-care situations some areas of work are shared; you should be quite clear about what is shared and who has the authority to initiate such work!

The need to change nursing practice

In order for services to be effective they should be responsive to changes in health-care needs or priorities, medical science, technology, research and demands from society. The traditions within nursing have created an occupation that finds it difficult to adapt effectively to change.

There is a clear demand for systems that offer individualised care organised and accounted for by named registered nurses. Patients permit care to be given by others because they accept that they are unable to care for themselves. The patient is vulnerable and will accept almost any intervention. While some patients may want others to assume responsibility for decisions that affect their health and welfare, because they may feel unwell, have difficulty in understanding the technology or wish to take a passive role (Biley, 1992), most want to retain some degree of control over decisions that affect their lives (Dennis, 1987). To understand the patient's view nurses need to accept patients' experiences as a basis for decision making (Bowman et al., 1992) or differences in perception of need between patients and nurses will occur (Webster et al., 1988; Farrell, 1991).

Nurses often feel ill-prepared for their role (Moores et al., 1982; Lathlean, 1987). Systems of work that put nurses in a role with little latitude are destined to create insecurity and result in the avoidance of responsibility and accountability. Those nurses who work in systems that offer support in taking accountability, responsibility and authority are more satisfied with their work, suffer less stress and are more productive. Decision making is also improved and becomes more appropriate to patient care (Kinston, 1987).

Resistance to change

Real change in social institutions is always difficult and protracted. Coercive approaches to change generally achieve little of significance and can damage human relations. Watson (1970) gives an account of those factors that inhibit change. These are likely to reflect some of the problems that one may experience when involved with change:

- Resistance in social systems: individuals tend to function through habit, generally shaped around the 'norms' of social systems designed to keep behaviour in check (conforming to norms). Change in one part of an organisation cannot take place without repercussions elsewhere (there must be systemic and cultural coherence associated with the change). Where economic costs may be too great or the prestige of individuals might be affected (an expression of vested interest) and when there is disturbance of taboos or rituals in people's work (the sacrosanct), then resistance will occur. Most change tends to come from outside the organisation and as a consequence is viewed with suspicion (rejection of outsiders).
- Resistance in personality: when work circumstances are pressured and individuals find the work too demanding innovation may not be welcomed (wishing to maintain the *status quo*). There is a tendency for people to respond to situations in ways to which they are accustomed (old habits die hard). The experience of an individual who has coped successfully with a previous situation may encourage them to persist with coping in the same way to other stresses (this is called primacy). There is also a tendency to respond to new suggestions from a position of established attitudes (selective perception and retention) and conformity to previously influenced behaviour (dependence). There is also a desire within individuals to maintain standards that have been handed down (super-ego) and a strong desire to condemn and repress impulses that do not correspond to known social order or routines (self-distrust). Finally, there is a desire for the contentment and security of the past (fear of insecurity and regression).

It is, however, not altogether unhealthy or wrong to resist change. The need to establish adaptative and coping strategies during resistant periods is important to prevent individuals from being overwhelmed. If a major change is to be effective it should be desired by the majority of those affected. Reality for the individual is affected when there is a threat of change. Values, competence, autonomy and self-esteem may all be undermined. There is an obligation by those who plan change to minimise the effects of any change on others' lives. Plans for change that are kept secret from those affected indicate suspicious motives on the part of the planners (Klein, 1976).

Stable groups are not receptive to change. Suggestions for change are thus more likely to emerge from external sources. If it is desirable to keep a group together then sustained efforts to present the change in different ways can help the change fit the group and help to maintain the *status quo*. According to Klein (1976), there are three reasons why defensive positions to change are a healthy response:

- it may be that there are unanticipated consequences affecting the system under change that constitute a real threat
- changes may also undermine the integrity of the system
- change agents may fail to appreciate the values of the system undergoing change.

The most successful change processes are likely to be those in which individuals and groups have the opportunity to take possession of new information and have the necessary support to give them the confidence to make changes themselves. In doing this individuals control the pace of change and are more likely to develop positive attitudes (Bowman *et al.*, 1983), creating a climate that will equip future members with appropriate attitudes (Bowman *et al.*, 1986).

Cultural change

The change from traditional methods of nursing to primary nursing is not a simple mechanistic shift in work arrangements. It is, in effect, a culture change that is influenced by a nursing philosophy. Organisational cultures influence the undertaking of change. Dyer (1984) proposes a seven-point plan to manage culture change successfully:

1. Conduct a culture audit: identify cultural beliefs and values; note differences between what people say and what they do.
2. Assess culture and need for change: cultural change is often needed if the prevailing culture pattern is not solving problems. There is a need to establish whether prevailing values, beliefs and behaviour are appropriate to changing conditions.
3. Assess cultural risk: the proposed change may cut across current cultural values.
4. Unfreeze the cultural pattern: this proposes that only major events like leadership change, basic strategy or structural change and technical innovation will 'unfreeze' a cultural system.

246 Gerald S. Bowman and David R. Thompson

These changes destabilise the culture making it amenable to change.

5. Elicit support from the cultural élite: ensure support from senior management.
6. Select the intervention strategy: decide how to introduce the change and how to encourage staff to adopt new values and introduce education/training towards the proposed change.
7. Monitor and evaluate: cultural change takes time to bring about. Monitoring could be achieved by using measurements that indicate changes in behaviour or practice.

This follows the action research model of introducing change and is favoured by many nurses who advocate systematic controlled change. It may be of particular value in geographically defined areas, such as wards where people interact almost continuously. In community settings, where nurses may be more isolated, other approaches may be appropriate.

The most important element of the introduction of planned change is the handling of human conflicts, doubts and insecurities. The change agent needs a knowledge of human psychology and organisational behaviour. Understanding the technology (nursing theories and systems) is comparatively easy. A brief account of three more strategies for coping with change (Bennis et al., 1976) is given below.

Empirical–rational strategy

This strategy is based on the assumption that humans are rational and will do what is in their own interest. The liberal principle behind this strategy is that human systems will progress if they are equipped with the knowledge to help them to change. The first step is to commission research in areas where knowledge is lacking, as the knowledge grows it is then disseminated through general education. Once the knowledge is available the challenge is to introduce and apply it in practice. Questioning the fitness of those in charge of practice to lead the change is the next stage. Removing those not accepted as fit and replacing them with selected personnel who are judged as able is considered a rational procedure. It is implicit in this strategy that information will continuously be used to analyse the effects of change. Within human systems practical, applied research is seen as a means of identifying problems and then solving

them. The empirical–rational strategy is not without an imaginative or creative dimension; a utopian vision of the future is encouraged, provided it is rationally convincing and preferably related to values associated with human sciences. The clarification of language within a system to facilitate good understanding and relationships is thought to be of importance.

One can see this strategy being applied on a national basis, in the changes occurring within nursing such as A Strategy for Nursing, Project 2000, PREPP and the desire for research.

Normative–re-educative strategy

The assumption for this strategy is that humans are active in responding to and finding out about their environment.

Successful re-education is dependent on the individual being active in the process. The idea of self-discovery and awareness led to the development of an action research strategy. The normative–re-educative strategy is concerned with knowledge acquisition, but the main purpose is to change attitudes, values, relationships and social norms using collaboration as a means of change. A central consideration of this strategy is to improve the problem-solving capabilities of a system. This is achieved by adapting internal and external orientation to reality. Reality for nurses has often been confused. Their value system and knowledge base has not always been congruent with their role. Work methods associated with competent care assessment and more autonomous practice enables nursing knowledge to be externally expressed and the values of care to be enacted. Fostering growth and development of individuals is seen as essential for motivation to achieve higher needs. The equipping of nurses with well developed human skills can accomplish this. Strategies like this need positive support. Individuals want to know, through example, that the organisation values, respects and rewards those who make the effort.

Power–coercive strategy

The assumption here is that power is implicit in all human activity. How power is applied and created during change is the basis of this strategy. The emphasis lies in the use of political and economic sanctions as a means of encouraging change. Nonviolent strategies, as used by Mahatma Gandhi and Martin Luther King, are examples of coercive action to bring about political and social change. The use of parliamentary lobbying or attachment to political institutions is another means of achieving change through legislative power. The use of power élites within organisations and in society generally may be a means by which ideas get supported and ultimately economical and organisational backing.

The strategies briefly discussed here are not mutually exclusive. Most serious change processes will have elements of different theoretical strategies. It is likely that one particular approach will form the central thrust as the means of initiating and facilitating change. The method used should be chosen for its appropriateness to the change situation. Change should be viewed as an exciting challenge but real lasting change is rarely accompanied by overnight success and seldom goes to plan. Some staff will also be left behind as the change speeds up, this will be indicated by unequal skill and knowledge acquisition. In the early stages of change few people cope effectively. The problem with most organisations is that individuals (who usually initiate the change) are offered little support to cope (Callan, 1993). Both individual and organisational-level strategies should be available to help staff cope.

Reflective point

Within your experience of practice can you identify a workgroup whose behaviour and attitudes are maladapted? What do you think might need changing? How would you begin to change the group? Recall the influence of different personalities in the group and how they might help or hinder the change process.

Groups of people tend to share values and beliefs which may prevent them from making appropriate adaptations in their work. It is useful to establish where most resistance to change is coming from within the group, is it from the leadership or at a lower level? Examining the leaders attitudes and relationships may offer most insight into the problems.

Conclusion

Nursing is a complex activity. It is primarily an art that is increasingly based on scientific knowledge. Thus, the philosophical basis that drives practise demands regular, close scrutiny. Organisational strategies and management practices need to take into account the current position of nursing philosophy and knowledge in order to effect the best care. The effective organisation and management of resources is crucial if full use of staffs' talents is to be achieved. Historically, weaknesses in nursing systems were a product of leadership that could not adapt. Competent leaders who have the ability to facilitate a positive and clear nursing role in a changing health-care system are essential. Emphasis has been placed on clinical leadership because it is at this level that the volume and grade of staff operating within a clinical setting will be agreed and the shape and content of nurses' work determined.

It could be argued that nursing is at a crossroads. Current changes evolving in the the NHS will affect all groups. Nurses can choose to be passive and allow others to determine the type and range of activity they are to be engaged in, or they have the opportunity to prescribe and develop a valuable role. This chapter has discussed those topics believed to be essential for nurses to address. Consideration of the relationship between the registered nurse and the patient is central when contemplating change within nursing practice.

References

Armitage, P., Champney-Smith, J. and Andrews, K. (1991). Primary nursing and the role of the nurse preceptor in changing long term mental health care: an evaluation. *Journal of Advanced Nursing*, 16, 413–422.

Aronson, G. (1989). Dimensions of control as related to work organisations, stress, and health. *International Journal of Health Services*, 19, 459–468.

Athlin, E. and Norberg, A. (1987). Caregivers attitudes to and interpretation of the behaviours of severely demented patients during feeding in a patient assignment care system. *International Journal of Nursing Studies*, 24, 145–153.

Attree, M. (1993). An analysis of the concept 'quality' as it relates to contemporary nursing care. *International Journal of Nursing Studies,* 30, 355–369.

Audit Commission (1991). *The Virtue of Patients: Making Best Use of Ward Nursing Resources.* HMSO, London.

Austin, A. L. (1957). *History of Nursing Source Book.* Putnam, New York.

Baker, D. E. (1978). Attitudes of nurses to the care of the elderly. *Nursing Research,* 28, 208–212.

Baly, M. (1986). *Nursing and Social Change.* Heinemann, London.

Bennis, W. G., Benne, K. D., Chin, R. and Corey, K. E. (eds) (1976). *The Planning of Change.* Holt, Rinehart & Winston, New York.

Betz, M. (1986). Cost and quality: primary and team nursing compared. *Nursing and Health Care,* 1, 150–157.

Biley, F. C. (1992). Some determinants that effect patient participation in decision-making about nursing care. *Journal of Advanced Nursing,* 17, 414–421.

Birch, J. A. (1979). The anxious learner. *Nursing Mirror,* 148, 17–22.

Bond, S., Bond J., Fowler, P. and Fall, M. (1991). Evaluating primary nursing: part 3. *Nursing Standard,* 5(38), 36–39.

Bouman, N. P. G. and Landeweerd, J. A. (1992). Social support and coping behaviour in nursing. *Work and Stress,* 6, 191–202.

Bouman, N. P. G. and Landeweerd, J. A. (1993). Leadership in the nursing unit: relationships with nurses' well being. *Journal of Advanced Nursing,* 18, 767–775.

Bowman, G. S. and Thompson, D. R. (1989). Key areas of change needed in nursing. *Nursing Standard,* 21(3), 25–27.

Bowman, G. S., Thompson, D. R. and Sutton, T. W. (1983). Nurses' attitudes towards the nursing process. *Journal of Advanced Nursing,* 8, 125–129.

Bowman, G. S., Thompson, D. R. and Sutton, T. W. (1986). The influence of a positive environment on the attitudes of student nurses towards the nursing process. *Journal of Advanced Nursing,* 11, 583–587.

Bowman, G. S., Meddis, R. and Thompson, D. R. (1990). Independence and status: two different work methods. *Nursing Practice,* 3(2), 18–20.

Bowman, G. S., Webster, R. A. and Thompson, D. R. (1991). The development of a classification system for nurses' work methods. *International Journal of Nursing Studies,* 28, 175–187.

Bowman, G. S., Webster, R. A. and Thompson, D. R. (1992). The reactions of 40 patients unexpectedly admitted to hospital. *Journal of Clinical Nursing,* 1, 335–338.

Bowman, G. S., Meddis, R. and Thompson, D. R. (1993). An item analysis of a classification system for nurses' work methods. *Journal of Clinical Nursing,* 2, 75–80.

Bray, D. W, Campbell, R. J. and Grant, D. L. (1974). *Formative Years in Business: A Long Term AT&T Study in Managerial Lives.* John Wiley, New York.

Broadbent, D. E. (1985). The clinical impact of job design. *British Journal of Clinical Psychology,* 24, 33–44.

Brooking, J. (1991). Doctors and nurses: a personal view. *Nursing Standard,* 6(12), 24–28.

Bryman, A. (1985). *Leadership and Organizations* Routledge & Kegan Paul, London.

Bryman, A. (1989). Leadership and culture in organizations. *Public Money and Management,* Autumn, 35–41.

Buchan, J. (1993). Posting notice about skill mix exercises. *Nursing Standard,* 7(21), 37.

Burns, J. M. (1978). *Leadership.* Harper & Row, New York.

Calder, J. M. (1974). *The Story of Nursing.* Methuen, London.

Callan, V. J. (1993). Individual and organizational strategies for coping with organizational change. *Work and Stress,* 7, 63–75.

Carlsen, R. and Malley, J. D. (1981). Job satisfaction of staff registered nurses in primary and team delivery systems. *Research in Nursing and Health,* 4, 251–260.

Carr-Hill, R., Dixon, P. and Gibbs, I. (1992). *Skill Mix and the Effectiveness of Nursing Care.* Centre for Health Economics, University of York.

Chavasse, J. (1981). From task assignment to patient allocation: a change evaluation. *Journal of Advanced Nursing,* 6, 137–145.

Chavigny, K. and Lewis, A. (1984). Team or primary nursing care. *Nursing Outlook,* 32, 322–327.

Cooper, R. (1973). Task characteristics and intrinsic motivation. *Human Relations,* 26, 387–408.

Dennis, K. E. (1987). Dimensions of client control. *Nursing Research,* 38, 151–155.

Department of Health (1989). *A Strategy for Nursing.* HMSO, London.

Department of Health (1992). *The Health of the Nation: A Strategy for Health in England.* HMSO, London.

Department of Health (1993). *Report of the Taskforce on the Strategy for Research in Nursing, Midwifery and Health Visiting.* HMSO, London.

Department of Health and Social Security (1969). *Report of the Working Party on Management Structures in the Local Authority Nursing Service* (Mayston Report). HMSO, London.

Department of Health and Social Security (1972). *Report of the Committee on Nursing* (Briggs Report). HMSO, London.

Department of Health and Social Security (1983). *NHS Management Enquiry* (Griffiths Report). HMSO, London.

Department of Health and Social Security (1989). *Caring for People: Community Care in the Next Decade and Beyond.* HMSO, London.

Dignam, J. T. and West, S. G. (1988). Social support in the workplace: tests of six theoretical models. *American Journal of Community Psychology*, 16, 701–724.

Dimond, B. (1987). Your disobedient servant. *Nursing Times*, 83(4), 28–31.

Donabedian, A. (1966). Evaluating the quality of medical care. *Milbank Memorial Fund Quarterly*, 44, 166–174.

Dunne, L. M. (1991). Defining quality assurance. In Dunne, L. M. (ed.) *How Many Nurses Do I Need?*, pp. 123–128. Wolfe, London.

Dyer, W. G. (1984). *Strategies for Managing Change*. Addison-Wesley, New York.

Escriba-Aguir, V., Perez-Hoyos, S. and Bolumar, F. (1993). Effects of work organisation on the mental health of nursing staff. *Journal of Nursing Management*, 1, 3–8.

Evans, A. and Griffiths, P. (1994). *The Development of a Nursing-led In-patient Service*. King's Fund Centre, London.

Farrell, G. A. (1991). How accurately do nurses perceive patients' needs? A comparison of general and psychiatric settings. *Journal of Advanced Nursing*, 16, 1062–1070.

Follett, M. P. (1982). Primary nursing assignment. In Gillies, D. A. (ed.) *Nursing Management: A Systems Approach*, pp. 232–240. W. B. Saunders, Philadelphia.

Fretwell, J. E. (1980). Hospital ward routine – friend or foe? *Journal of Advanced Nursing*, 5, 625–636.

Game, A. and Pringle, R. (1983). *Gender at Work*. Pluto Press, London.

Gillies, D. A. (1982). *Nursing Management: A Systems Approach*. W. B. Saunders, Philadelphia.

Giovanetti, P. (1986). Evaluation of primary nursing. *Annual Review of Nursing Research*, 4, 127–151.

Gray, C. (1987). What do nurses want? *Canadian Medical Association Journal*, 136, 978–987.

Hackman, J. R. and Oldham, G. R. (1976). Motivation through the design of work: test of a theory. *Organizational Behavior and Human Performance*, 16, 250–279.

Hardy, G. (1981). *William Rathbone and the Early History of District Nursing*. G. W. & A. Hesketh, Ormskirk.

Heenan, A. (1991). Uneasy partnership. *Nursing Times*, 87(10), 25–27.

Hegyvary, S. T. (1982). *The Change to Primary Nursing*. C. V. Mosby, St Louis.

Hernandez, S. R., Kaluzny, A. D., Parker, B., Chae, Y. M. and Brewington, J. R. (1988). Enhanced nursing productivity: a social psychologic perspective. *Public Health Nursing*, 5, 52–63.

Hersey, P. and Blanchard, K. H. (1982). *Management of Organizational Behavior*. Prentice-Hall, Englewood Cliffs, NJ.

Hertzberg, F. (1968). *Work and the Nature of Man*. Staples Press, London.

Heslin, K. (1987). Nursing unit changes from team to total patient care. *Nursing Dimensions*, 64(3), 27–29.

House, J. S. (1986). Barriers to work stress: 1. Social support. In Gentry, W. D., Benson, H. and de Wolfe, Ch. J. (eds) *Behavior Medicine: Work, Stress and Health*. Martinus Nijhoff, Dordrecht.

Katzman, E. M. and Roberts, J. I. (1988). Nurse–physician conflicts as barriers to the enactment of nursing roles. *Western Journal of Nursing Research*, 10, 576–590.

Keddy, B., Jones, G. M., Jacobs, P., Burton, H. and Rogers, M. (1986). The doctor–nurse relationship: an historical perspective. *Journal of Advanced Nursing*, 11, 745–753.

Kinston, W. (1987). *A Stronger Nursing Organization*. BIOSS, Brunel University, Uxbridge.

Klein, D. (1976). Some notes on the dynamics of resistance to change: the defender role. In Bennis, W. G., Benne, K. D., Chin, R., Corey K. E. (eds) *The Planning of Change*, pp. 117–124. Holt, Rinehart & Winston, New York.

LaRocco, J. M., House, J. S. and French, J. P. R. (1980). Social support, occupational stress, and health. *Journal of Health and Social Behavior*, 21, 202–218.

Lathlean, J. (1987). Are you prepared to be a staff nurse? *Nursing Times*, 83(36), 25–27.

Lazarus, R.S. (1985). The psychology of stress and coping. *Issues in Mental Health Nursing*, 7, 399–418.

Likert, R. (1979). From production and employee-centredness to systems 1–4. *Journal of Management*, 5, 147–156.

MacGuire, J. (1989a). An approach to evaluating the introduction of primary nursing in an acute medical ward for the elderly. I: before and after a change to primary nursing. *International Journal of Nursing Studies*, 26, 243–251.

MacGuire, J. (1989b). An approach to evaluating the introduction of primary nursing in an acute medical ward for the elderly. II: operationalizing the principles. *International Journal of Nursing Studies*, 26, 253–260.

MacGuire, J. M. (1991). Quality of care assessed: using the Senior Monitor index in three wards for the elderly before and after a change to primary nursing. *Journal of Advanced Nursing*, 16, 511–520.

McGrath, A., Reid, N. and Boore, J. (1989). Occupational stress in nursing. *International Journal of Nursing Studies*, 26, 343–358.

Maggs, C. (1982). Nurse recruitment to four provincial hospitals 1881–1921. In Davies, C. (ed.). *Rewriting Nursing History*, pp. 18–40. Croom Helm, London.

Manthey, M. (1988). Can primary nursing survive? *American Journal of Nursing*, 88, 644–647.

Marks-Maran, D. (1978). Patient allocation v task allocation in relation to the nursing process. *Nursing Times*, 74, 413–416.

Marram, G. D. (1976). The comparative cost of operating a team and primary nursing unit. *Journal of Nursing Administration*, 6(4), 21–28.

Maslow, A. H. (1970). *Motivation and Personality* Harper & Row, New York.

Menzies, I. E. P. (1960). A case study in the functioning of social systems as a defence against anxiety. *Human Relations,* 13, 95–121.

Ministry of Health (1947). *Working Party on the Recruitment and Training of Nurses* (Wood Report). HMSO, London.

Ministry of Health (1966). *Report of the Committee on Senior Nursing Staff Structure* (Salmon Report). HMSO, London.

Moores, B., Singh, B. B. and Tun, A. (1982). Attitudes of 2325 active and inactive nurses to aspects of their work. *Journal of Advanced Nursing,* 7, 483–489.

Morgan, G. (1990). *Images of Organization.* Sage, London.

Naish, J. (1992). A vision of the future. *Nursing Standard,* 6(48), 22–23.

NHS Management Executive (1993). *A Vision for the Future: The Nursing, Midwifery and Health Visiting Contribution to Health and Health Care.* Department of Health, London.

Oldham, G. R. (1976). The motivational strategies used by supervisors: relationships to effectiveness indicators. *Organizational Behavior and Human Performance,* 15, 66–86.

Pearson, A. (1988). *Primary Nursing.* Croom Helm, London.

Pearson, A., Punton, S. and Durant, I. (1992). *Nursing Beds: An Evaluation of the Effects of Therapeutic Nursing.* Scutari Press, London.

Peralla, M. and Hentinen, M. (1989). Primary nursing: opinions of nursing staff before and during implementation. *International Journal of Nursing Studies,* 26, 231–242.

Pierce, J. L. and Newstrom, J. W. (1983). The design of flexible work schedules and employee responses. *Journal of Occupational Behavior,* 4, 247–262.

Porter, S. (1991). A participant observation study of power relations between nurses and doctors in a general hospital. *Journal of Advanced Nursing,* 16, 728–735.

Rafferty, A. M. (1993). *Leading Questions: A Discussion Paper on the Issues of Nurse Leadership.* King's Fund Centre, London.

Reed, S. E. (1988). A comparison of nurse-related behaviour, philosophy of care and job satisfaction in team and primary nursing. *Journal of Advanced Nursing,* 13, 383–395.

Robertson, I. T. and Smith, M. (1985). *Motivation and Job Design.* Institute of Personnel Management, London.

Royal College of Nursing (1942). *Nursing Reconstruction Committee* (Horder Report). Royal College of Nursing, London.

Royal College of Nursing (1964). *A Reform of Nursing Education* (Platt Report). Royal College of Nursing, London.

Schroeder, R. E., Rhodes, A. and Shields, R. E. (1984). Nurse acuity services: CASH vs GRASP (a determina-

tion of nurse staff requirements). *Journal of Nursing Administration,* 21(2), 72–77.

Sellick, K. J., Russell, S. and Beckmann, J. L. (1983). Primary nursing: an evaluation of its effects in patient perception of care and staff satisfaction. *International Journal of Nursing Studies,* 20, 265–273.

Shaw, J. T. and Bosenquet, N. (1993). *A Way to Develop Nurses and Nursing.* King's Fund Centre, London.

Shukla, R. K. (1982). Primary or team nursing? Two conditions determine the choice. *Journal of Nursing Administration,* 12(11), 12–15.

Sjoberg, K. B., Heiren, E. L. and Jackson, M. R. (1971). Unit assignment: a patient-centred system. *Nursing Clinics of North America,* 6, 333–342.

Stanley, I. (1983). Accountability in nursing – 7. Where do we stand with doctors? *Nursing Times,* 79(38), 46–48.

Stein, L. (1967). The doctor–nurse game. *Archives of General Psychiatry,* 16, 699–703.

Stewart, R. (1990). *Leading in the NHS.* Macmillan, London.

Thomas, L. H. and Bond, S. (1990). Towards defining the organization of nursing care in hospital wards: an emperical study. *Journal of Advanced Nursing,* 15, 1106–1112.

United Kingdom Central Council (1987). *Paper 9: The Final Proposals* (Project 2000). UKCC, London.

United Kingdom Central Council (1992). *Code of Professional Conduct,* 3rd edn. UKCC, London.

United Kingdom Central Council (1993). *PREP: The Council's Proposed Standards for Post-registration Education.* UKCC, London.

Vaughan, B. and Gough, P. (1993). Taking a lead. *Nursing Times,* 89(8), 38–40.

Watson, G. (1970). Resistance to change. In Bennis, W. G., Benne, K. D. and Chin, R. (eds). *The Planning of Change,* pp. 488–498 Holt, Rinehart & Winston, New York. .

Watts, V. H. and O'Leary, J. (1980). The components of primary nursing. *Nursing Dimensions,* 7(4), 90–95.

Webster, R., Thompson, D., Bowman, G. and Sutton, T. (1988). Patients and nurses' opinions about bathing. *Nursing Times,* 84(7), 54–57.

White, R. (1978). *Social Change and the Development of the Nursing Profession.* Henry Kimpton, London.

White, A. (1993). *Management for Clinicians.* Edward Arnold, London.

Wilson, J. (1991). Resource management: an overview. In Dunne, L. M. (ed.) *How Many Nurses Do I Need?,* pp. 9–15. Wolfe, London.

Wilson, N. M. and Dawson, P. (1989). A comparison of team nursing in a geriatric long term care setting. *International Journal of Nursing Studies,* 26, 1–13.

Zaleznik, A. (1981). Managers and leaders: are they different? *Journal of Nursing Administration,* 11(7), 25–31.

Further reading

Abel-Smith, B. (1960). *A History of the Nursing Profession.* Heinemann, London. An authoratitive and readable account of the history of nursing.

Baly, M. (1976). *Nursing and Social Change.* Heinemann, London. Contains a wealth of material pertaining to government legislation.

Bennis, W. G., Benne, K. D., Chin, R. and Corey, K. E. (1976). *The Planning of Change.* Holt, Rinehart & Winston, New York. A standard work on institutional change.

Dunne, L. M. (1991). *How Many Nurses Do I Need?* Wolfe, London. One of the few available resources on the subject of skill mix.

Hardy, G. (1981). *William Rathbone and the Early History of District Nursing.* G. W. & A. Hesketh, Ormskirk. This account of the early days of district nursing offers details omitted in most nursing history books.

Leathard, A. (1990). *Health Care Provision: Past, Present and Future.* Chapman & Hall, London. Gives a clear insight into why health policy has needed to change.

Marriner-Tomey, A. (1992). *Guide to Nursing Management.* C. V. Mosby, St Louis. A well written and detailed account of nursing management issues.

Stewart, R. (1990). *Leading in the NHS.* Macmillan, London. A clear account of leadership needs in the NHS handled in a simple and commonsense way.

Vaughan, B. and Pillmore, M. (1989). *Managing Nursing Work.* Scutari Press, London. This offers a good insight into current thinking on issues of management pertinent to nurses.

11

ACHIEVING EFFECTIVE WORK AS A PROFESSIONAL ACTIVITY

Christopher Johns

Introduction

This chapter is concerned with the conditions under which effective work can be achieved by practitioners as the essential professional activities of commitment, autonomy, responsibility and expertise.

The potential of guided reflection as the means for practitioners to develop and sustain effective and desirable work is then explored together with a description of techniques and dynamics within guided reflection. This includes an exploration of the conditions under which reflective practice will flourish or flounder, in particular arguing for a participative management style of managing nursing.

The development of reflective performance review offers the practitioner a useful way to take responsibility for demonstrating his or her effectiveness in practice in the belief that methods for managing quality need to be devolved to point-of-service delivery as an essential aspect of everyday practice.

The terms nurse and practitioner are used exchangeable. The issues outlined in this chapter are equally applicable to health visitors and midwives.

Setting the context

Effectiveness and quality

In developing the central theme of effective work, it is necessary first to consider what effective work is and how it might be recognised, developed and judged. Effectiveness is central to any discussion of quality (Maxwell, 1984; Shaw, 1986; Ellis, 1988). Yet quality remains an elusive concept despite the attention it has attracted in the health-care literature. Besides effectiveness, which can be defined as successfully achieving what is intended, other key factors that constitute an understanding of quality include efficiency, equity, accessibility, acceptability, and appropriateness (Maxwell, 1984).

Efficiency is using available resources to achieve the most effective work, or what Ellis (1988) comments on as 'value for money'. This explicitly recognises that budgets are finite and that quality is that which can be afforded. The other quality factors reflect how effectiveness needs to be viewed within wider social, political and cultural contexts. These quality factors appear to be entrenched in political issues which nursing, because it is a major contributor to health-care provision, should be involved in determining. Different professionals within health-care settings will define quality differently to reflect their own values and self-interests. In this sense quality is always a contextual and political issue. Who controls the dominant expression of quality is a reflection of the power relationships between professionals and management.

As such, it is no great surprise to see how little nursing is expressed in 'quality' terms within business plans, as this reflects nursing's traditional weakness in power terms. A prerequisite to developing and achieving effective work is to be certain of the meaning of nursing and its contribution to health-care provision. Are nurses able to control their vision of what effectiveness is, or is this objective imposed on nursing, irrespective of nurses' own beliefs and knowledge?

Defining nursing

It is impossible to 'know quality' unless it can be recognised in some way. Many nurses will intuitively or instinctively recognise 'good nursing' when they experience it, as if what determines good nursing is a universal tacit knowledge.

It has become an explicit English National Board for Nursing, Midwifery, and Health Visiting requirement for practice areas used to educate pre-registration nurses to have a written 'philosophy' of their collective beliefs and values about the nature of the nursing. The aim of developing a philosophy of care is presumably to give meaning and direction to nursing practice and to make it more likely that patients and families receive congruent and consistent care from those who work together whilst giving a vision of what nursing might be [Johns (1994a) – this work is an example of the author's own practice in developing a philosophy for practice and the impact of this work on developing practice].

Of course, the two are not the same thing. There will always be contradictions between practitioners' shared beliefs and values and actual practice. Grounding a definition of nursing in beliefs and values challenges the functional traditional world-view of nursing as defined through its tasks:

The philosophical   ⟶   The functionalist
approach   approach
– nursing defined in   – nursing defined in
term of practitioners'   terms of
beliefs and values   tasks it does and roles

The functionalist approach epitomises nurses as doers, usually directed by others, either other nurses in some hierarchical relationship, or by doctors within the stereotyped handmaiden role. The functionalist approach is further epitomised within the 'task' system of managing the delivery of care – characterised as nurses doing things to or at patients (Alfano, 1971), organised using nursing process which directs work towards specific outcomes.

The emergence of nursing models reflects the philosophical approach, underpinned with explicit and implicit assumptions that reflect the beliefs and values of the model's author. It is a measure of the dominance of the functionalist approach that these assumptions are often 'lost' in comparison with the utility value of the model's assessment strategy.

A major influence on nurses' belief systems is the increasing significance of the ideological impact of nursing as being synonymous with human caring.

Nursing as caring

It is not difficult to build up an overwhelming sense from the nursing literature that caring is the essential core of nursing. McKenna (1993) notes that

> The literature reveals that nursing and caring are historically intertwined. Caring appears to be the central core, or the fundamental underpinning, for all that is nursing (p. 72).

Leininger (1988) has stated that caring is 'the central and unifying domain for the body of knowledge and practices in nursing'.

Armstrong (1983) notes that it is

> a deeply held assumption that the role of caring, which has been so long the heart of nursing has meant a close relationship between the nurse and the patient. ... (p. 457).

This pervasive caring ideology makes it likely that nurses hold similar beliefs and values about the nature of nursing. Yet, these may differ depending on influences and experiences, and the contexts in which they practice nursing. Defining exactly what is 'caring' is of crucial significance for nursing if it is to claim 'caring' as its 'central and unifying domain'. For example, the need to distinguish professional caring with lay caring (Kitson, 1987). Morse *et al.*'s (1991) analysis of major nurse theorists approach to conceptualisations of caring identify different philosophical roots to caring definitions – caring as a human trait, caring as a moral imperative, caring as an affect, caring as interpersonal interaction, and caring as a therapeutic intervention. Other nurse theorists have challenged caring as the core of nursing, instead claiming that the central focus for nursing is human becoming (Parse, 1992).

Exploring the nursing 'caring' literature, it becomes evident that a universal practical definition of nursing is an illusion, although it is possible to reach a consensus on what constitutes nursing. Indeed recent approaches to quality assurance tools have been founded on just such premises, such as QUALPACS (Wandelt and Ager, 1974) and Monitor (Goldstone *et al.*, 1983).

If nurses were able to interpret and adapt these tools to reflect their own beliefs and values, and self-assess as the basis for negotiation and agreement, then perhaps this approach to monitoring quality may be realistic. As it is, the use of these tools risks de-powering nurses by imposing a definition of what ought to be and using this criteria to judge effective nursing practice.

I shall assume that defining and demonstrating effective work is nursing's fundamental *professional activity*, and as such, must become everyday activities concerned with developing and maintaining effectiveness within negotiated resources.

Professional activity

Strauss (1963) identifies four factors that constitute professional activity, or in other words, the attributes and values that members of a profession should demonstrate in relation to their work:

- commitment
- autonomy
- responsibility
- expertise.

Commitment

As a noun, commitment can mean 'a declared attachment to a doctrine or cause' although it can also mean 'an obligation undertaken' (*Chambers Twentieth Century Dictionary*, 1972). Obligation refers to carrying out an expected sense of duty (van Hooft, 1987). It represents the major ethical principle of deontology – that a person acts from a perceived sense of duty with good intention (Seedhouse, 1988), irrespective of the outcomes of adhering to these duties – for example, the duty always to tell a patient the truth irrespective of the

fact that it might be more compassionate to mask the truth, or that it might lead to conflict with the patient's family.

From a sense of commitment, the practitioner acts from a set of firmly held beliefs and values about caring that implicitly leads him or her to consider every situation on its merits prior to taking appropriate action (Cooper, 1991; Packard and Ferrara, 1987; Yarling and McElmurray, 1986; Johns, 1993a). This position recognises how care situations are deep human encounters that cannot easily be predicted in advance or from outside the situation. This approach doesn't dismiss the significance of considering ethical principles within health-care situations, but reduces them to a source of information to inform the deliberative process (Seedhouse, 1988). For example, consider concepts of care based on fairness and equity. In deciding how to use time most appropriately, the nurse may need to prioritise her time to spend with one patient that may be less than equitable for other patients. Similarly fairness suggests that the nurse is able to bracket her feelings of liking or disliking particular patients. The risk is that the nurse is always struggling to conform to some stereotype as to how she should behave rather than responding appropriately to the situation. As Jourard notes (1971), this may lead to a sense of self-alienation with the result that the nurse becomes unavailable to use herself as a therapeutic agent in caring.

Praxis

Carr and Kemmis (1986) discuss the concept of praxis as 'informed and committed action' (p. 46). Commitment manifests itself through concern for others and with the practitioner's self-challenge and striving to be most effective in his or her work. This can only be a reflective stance on experience – 'Have I been effective?', 'How do I know this?', 'Could I have acted in more effective ways?'.

Caring as commitment

Van Hooft (1987) critiques the nursing literature on caring and surfaces the tension between caring as unconditional giving of the self and as a conditioned professional response to situations. Van Hooft argues to support a view of caring as a professional response to the patient's health needs rather than to the person. What is without doubt, is that the nature of the response necessitates a personal response from the nurse (Hall, 1964). If nurses do *believe* that nursing is concerned with working with patients as people with unique needs, then the consequences and ability to work in these ways need to be understood and developed. As James (1989) notes in her research focused on emotional work with patients (labour)

Emotional labour is hard work and can be sorrowful and difficult. It demands that the labourer gives personal attention which means that they must give something of themselves, not just a formulaic response (p. 19).

It is this notion of 'giving something of themselves' that reflects the practitioner's commitment to act out his or her beliefs and values even in situations of personal stress. The contrast with 'a formulaic response' as highlights the distinction between involvement and detachment by the practitioner within her professional relationships. Forrest (1989), in her phenomenological study of nurses' lived experiences of caring, supports this involvement with patients as central to a concept of caring

For practising nurses, caring is first and foremost a mental and emotional presence that evolves from deep feelings for the patient's experience (p. 818).

The distinction between personal or professional relationships with patients has been described to me by practitioners (unfinished PhD research) who talk about maintaining professional distance as a coping mechanism with patients and families that present as an emotional threat. Personal relationships are characterised by a sense of commitment and a willingness to be involved, whereas professional relationships are characterised by a sense of obligation and as consequence remain detached.

If effective work is defined in holistic concepts, as indeed most nurses would aspire to, then maintaining a 'distance' clearly limits nurse's ability to work with patients and to achieve effective work. The reasons for this seem to lie more directly with the conditions under which nurses have been socialised, rather than any great loss of belief in caring as being central to nursing practice, i.e. conditions which, for whatever reason, do not value, encourage, and support nurses to become involved in therapeutic relationship with patients and families. This issue is supported by Holden (1991), who drew on Menzies-Lyth's (1988) seminal work on nursing's social defence systems on anxiety, in recognising the critical conflict between establishing 'appropriate levels of emotional attachment versus detachment in the context of the nurse–patient relationship (p. 893).

Rawnsley (1990) suggests the metaphor of instrumental friendship as a term to describe the nature of the nurse–patient relationship.

The personal warmth and affection of friendship seems alien to the artificiality of the legal bonding that defines the association between professionals and clients (p. 46).

Rawnsley suggests that the word 'professional' needs careful interpretation and understanding when applied to nursing **if** nursing is defined within a caring philosophy. As such, **effective caring** will be enhanced by commitment and personal involvement in relationships with patients and families. If this is true, then development of effectiveness must focus on developing and sustaining these aspects of work.

It is important to acknowledge Argyle's belief (1974) of a probable relationship between satisfaction and productivity for those workers who are involved deeply with their work. This suggests that creating the conditions to enable practitioners to become 'deeply involved' with their work will lead to more satisfying and productive work. Once practitioners (within my PhD research study) were able to recognise that they could effectively act out their beliefs and values of caring in day-to-day practice, the sense of satisfaction that resulted from this knowledge was inspirational.

This understanding reflects Benner and Wrubel's (1989) profound statement concerning the consequences of the loss of connection between caring and practice:

It is a peculiarly modern mistake to think that caring is the cause of burnout and that the cure it to protect oneself from caring to prevent the disease called 'burnout'. Rather the loss of caring is the sickness.

The person experiencing burnout needs to be reconnected to sustain relationships and meanings to overcome the alienation and anomie of burnout (p. 373).

Clearly Benner and Wrubel value caring as the core of nursing and see caring as giving nursing its distinct identity. They highlight the need to pay attention to creating the necessary environment to enable caring to flourish rather than flounder. The committed practitioner's satisfaction is the fulfilment of her beliefs and values in action. This feedback is essential to help sustain that work. As such, there always needs to be mechanisms in place whereby effective work can be recognised and used as the basis for learning.

Yet, do nurse practitioners want deep involvement and is deep involvement a necessary requisite for person-centred work such as nursing? Dunlop (1986) highlights the ambivalence within nursing towards this issue resulting in some simultaneously held contradictory beliefs

> In a very un-theoretical way, nursing sought to teach me to maintain both separation and linkage in my practice: separation – 'You must remember that the other is a stranger', and linkage – 'You must think and act as if he were not'. Thus one achieves something like 'caring' in its emergent sense as it is applied in the public world – a combination of closeness and distance, which always runs the risk of tipping either way (p. 664).

The nursing literature generally supports the relationship between caring and a sense of commitment (Harrison, 1990; Watson, 1985; Morse, 1991; Kitson, 1987). These theoretical descriptions are useful pointers to help practitioners reflect on and challenge their existing practice, and to expose the contradictions between practice and desirable goals of nursing which are often based on concepts of human caring.

Summary
Without a sense of commitment, the nurse's ability to care is limited within the widely held belief that caring is central to nursing's ideology. Similarly a sense of commitment is a necessary requisite for the nurse to strive towards achieving effective work and accepting responsibility for this work. As such, commitment is the root of all professional activity.

Autonomy

Autonomy has been identified as the key professional attribute (Friedson, 1971). It refers to the degree of discretion the practitioner has to make nursing decisions that concern practice. A distinction has been made between structural autonomy, i.e. defined through job descriptions that set boundaries or limits to discretionary-decision making, and attitudinal autonomy – defined as the amount of freedom a practitioner believes she has (Batey and Lewis, 1982).

The development of interest in this country of primary nursing is portrayed in the literature as

enhancing the autonomy of nurses (Ersser and Tutton, 1991). They note how

> Traditionally authority and autonomy for decision making are invested in the role of the ward sister. In primary nursing, authority and autonomy are devolved to the primary nurse. The primary nurse needs to have achieved a level of competence in which she can use her authority and autonomy to benefit the patient (p. 7).

The redistribution of authority and power that Ersser and Tutton suggest is implicit within primary nursing in contrast with more traditional forms of organising nursing, must inevitably lead to a revision in relationships between roles. My own work has indicated that the most reported source of anxiety at work for practitioners in primary nursing or district nurse roles was interpersonal conflict as they struggled to work with other practitioners and health-care workers in asserting their decision making and control of the work environment (Johns, 1993b).

However, most nurses based in hospitals do not work within primary nursing settings and may feel they have very little discretion for decision making in their day-to-day work. Wards sisters may feel they have difficulty in asserting their beliefs and values in care settings dominated by the medical model of nursing where there are unequal power relationships between themselves and doctors.

Practitioners socialised into these 'traditional' power relationships often internalise and espouse the dominant values of medicine and the organisation rather than assert nursing as caring. Freire (1972) believes that such people are promoted because they fit-in with the prevailing dominant world-view and thus act to maintain the *status quo* of power relations and the subordination of nursing as a largely oppressed group of workers.

It is ironic that ward sisters are promoted because they are the most clinically competent – with competence being measured largely in terms of technical ability rather than caring skills. The internalisation of medical values has resulted in technical skills or tasks being highly valued and rewarded, whilst caring skills are generally viewed as of low status and needing little skill, and capable of being delegated to untrained staff and nursing students, or dismissed as being merely an extension of women's innate caring skills (Lawler, 1991; James, 1989).

Hence to assert nursing's autonomy by

expressing and asserting an ideology of nursing based on caring values becomes a challenge to internalised medical dominance. It is not doctors who are likely to resist this process, but nurses themselves who have attained positions of power within medical hegemony.

The barrier of medical hegemony to nursing autonomy

Hegemony refers to the meaning systems of the dominant groups that are embedded within the health-care culture to the extent that they are uncritically accepted as normal consciousness (Grundy, 1989). In focusing on nursing values and the conditions under which this can be achieved, the awareness and assertion of nursing's autonomy and the freedom of individual practitioners to make nursing decisions become critical components to challenge hegemony.

Yet asserting nursing values within a traditionally dominant medical ideology, at least within acute care settings, is not necessarily easy to achieve. Medical dominance is embedded in the very fabric of health-care institutions – in every ritual, in every procedure, in the way people talk and respond with each other, which, as Foucault (1979) suggests, are 'regulatory controls' to ensure that nursing remains a relatively docile workforce.

Yet, the 'very taken for grantedness' of hegemony (Grundy, 1989) renders its nature difficult to access, and its existence within each nurse means that it is not an outside objective entity but something that each individual nurse needs to reach inside herself to deal with – **if** she believes in fulfilling her therapeutic potential as a nurse.

However, it is very evident that this manifestation of power is misplaced, because, as Foucault would argue, it should also ensure maximum efficiency in performance. However, this is only true if nursing, as reflected in caring values, is valued and seen as significant. Where the critical indicators of effective work are identified in terms of medical outcomes, and nursing's primary role as contributing to these, then the failure of nursing to achieve caring practices is invisible. However, to assert anything requires a clear understanding of what that something is. Hence the need for a well articulated, understood and practical definition of nursing which has meaning for practitioner and to which they feel committed towards.

The impact of professional and hierarchical modes of management

A major influence on the ability of practitioners to perceive themselves as 'free' to make decisions about nursing is the way nursing is organised and the way nursing is managed. The way nursing is organised will largely determine the degree of structural autonomy through role definition, whilst the way nursing is managed will largely determine the degree of attitudinal autonomy. Whilst it could be expected that the way nursing is organised would determine a preferred a management style, this cannot be assumed considering the way nurses have traditionally been managed within bureaucratic and overtly hierarchical systems.

Just because new structures, such as team and primary nursing in hospitals, are implemented and practitioners think differently about a situation, this doesn't necessarily lead to changed behaviour, **even when we understand the way we behave and the need to change our patterns of behaviour to become congruent with new roles**.

Hence a key question is 'how to break free from socio-cultural factors that act as restraints to developing effective work?'.

The movement towards ways of organising nursing that enhance professional autonomy can be viewed within a tension of professional versus hierarchical modes of organisation. The attribution theory of motivation suggests that behaviour is determined by a combination of perceived internal and external forces (Heider, 1958; cf. Mullins, 1989, p. 326) and work performance is linked to practitioners' locus of control, that is whether practitioners perceive outcomes as controlled by themselves or by external factors.

Mullins notes that:

> Employees with an internal control orientation are more likely to believe that they can influence their level of performance through their own abilities, skills or efforts. Employees with an external control orientation are more likely to believe their level of performance is determined by external factors beyond their influence (p. 327).

Cherniss (1980) focused the locus of control within a bureaucratic–professional tension and the nature of relationships that stem from a 'professional–collegial' or 'bureaucratic–hierarchical' orientation.

He noted how relationships within a bureaucratic–hierarchical orientation are characterised by the following:

- important decisions are made by those near the top
- subordinates wait for instructions and are expected to carry them out without question or hesitation
- personal characteristics of subordinates are of no importance – one's responsibility, discretion, and obligations are determined by one's position in the organisation (adapted from Cherniss, 1980).

Cherniss is vague in defining 'collegial' except to note that professional–collegial relationships are characterised by workers internalising a sense of values and who are largely self-monitoring. This implies this type of relationship mutually respect the internal control (autonomy) of their colleagues. Cherniss found that bureaucratic styles of management made it difficult for practitioners to

> provide effective, humane, and responsible service while adhering to the plethora of regulations imposed by faceless and seemingly insensitive bureaucrats (p. 71).

Cherniss' study offers important insights for the careers of newly qualified professionals, which included community nurses. Cherniss further draws comparisons with Kramer's (1990) work on the impact of bureaucracy:

> routine and boredom tend to occur more often when work is bureaucratically organised. In the bureaucratic mode of organisation, work is divided as much as possible into limited and often meaningless tasks with an emphasis on efficiency and fairness. Opportunity for an individual's discretion, creativity, and flexibility is minimised in an effort to maximise predictability and uniformity (p. 66).

Both Cherniss and Kramer suggest the significance of a work environment that facilitates and supports practitioner autonomy as crucial for the development of caring practices and to sustain practitioner commitment to such practices.

The locus of control theory suggests that practitioners will have different orientations to work. Mullins (1989) believes that the majority of people come to work with the original intention of wanting to do a good job and performing to the best of their abilities. Where performance fails to meet this ideal it is largely a result of how practitioners perceive they are treated by management.

Clearly an approach to management is required that creates the conditions whereby individuals can be motivated to perform well and meet both their own and the organisation's objectives, or in other words enhance their sense of autonomy. Indeed, through a participative style of management, individual and organisations' goals can merge, particularly apposite in work such as nursing which is implicitly people-centred – in that it perceives and responds to practitioners as people (Likert, 1961). If nurses are to respond to patients and families as human beings, then it would seem necessary they must be treated in like ways. Where nurses feel they are unable to make decisions, i.e. their decisions are controlled by others, then similarly patients' actions are likely to be controlled by the nurse; the nurse adopts a reactionary position of doing things to the patient in contrast of working with them.

The styles of management work as described by Likert (1961) and Blake and Mouton (1985) [both discussed in Mullins (1989)] offer useful perspectives for nursing to consider how achieving effective nursing can best be managed through valuing the development of commitment and autonomy. For example, Blake and Mouton identified seven management styles (Fig. 11.1) based on the manager's degree of concern for people and degree of concern for production.

The configuration of high concern for people and production characterises the 'team manager' who encourages collegial relationships and a belief that accomplishing effective work requires committed people who share an organisational purpose. Yet, in reality, this doesn't appear to be the case. However, the grid offers a useful tool to make management style visible, and to reflect on the impact of style on achieving desirable and effective work. Where practitioners feel manipulated through opportunistic or paternal/maternal styles of management they can only respond in defensive ways, wary and cynical about variable good intention. Existing ways of organising and managing nursing are counter-productive to developing autonomy and commitment and achieving effective work.

Frustration and alienation

The practitioner's failure to take action based on her beliefs and values to achieve desired work is likely to lead to frustration, at least until the practitioner learns to become detached from her work, and in this process to become detached or alienated from herself (Jourard, 1971). Seedhouse (1988) highlights Sartre's (1969) concept of 'bad faith' to describe people who are not true to

The Leadership Grid Figure

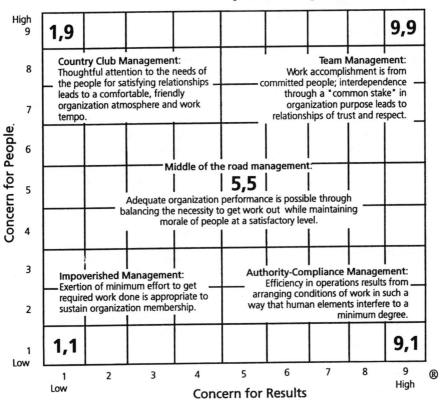

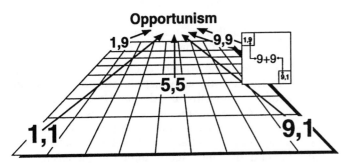

In Opportunistic Management, people adapt and shift to any Grid style needed to gain the maximum advantage. Performance occurs according to a system of selfish gain. Effort is given only for an advantage for personal gain.

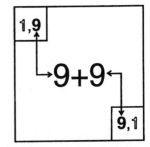

9+9: Paternalism/Maternalism
Reward and approval are bestowed to people in return for loyalty and obedience; failure to comply leads to punishment.

Fig. 11.1. *The managerial grid (Blake and Mouton, 1985). Source: The Leadership Grid® figure, Paternalism Figure and Opportunism from* Leadership Dilemmas – Grid *Solutions, by Robert R. Blake and Anne Adams McCanse, Gulf Publishing Company, Houston (Grid Figure: p. 29, Paternalism Figure: p. 30, Opportunism Figure: p. 31). Copyright 1991 by Scientific Methods, Inc. Reproduced by permission of the owners.*

themselves and adhere to a role rather than being oneself. The implication of bad faith is that the professional self can never be split from the 'personal' self, except as a form of denial of the self.

Seedhouse believes that self-denial limits the ability of the practitioner to act morally. The autonomous person is a person who acts from a true sense of self. Acting out a role is not autonomy because it involves a sense of conforming to expectations of how one should act rather than from who one is.

Coping with prolonged frustration inevitably leads to a sense of alienation – the detachment of the person from his or her work role (Mullins, 1989, p. 338). Mullins draws on the work of Blauner (1964) to highlight the four dimensions of alienation as powerlessness, meaninglessness, isolation, and self-estrangement, or in other words a state of 'burnout'.

Cherniss (1980) notes that:

Unfortunately, as long as new professionals expect their work to be stimulating and fulfilling and find it to be otherwise, the potential for burnout in this group is likely to be great ... the frustrated quest for meaning and fulfilment in work leads to the kind of psychological stress that increases the likelihood of burnout – when nurses expect and desire meaning, intellectual stimulation, and self-actualisation through work and their efforts to fulfil this need are thwarted, the frequent result is frustration and anxiety (p. 69).

Protecting self by detaching oneself from the situation is likely to make things worse because it leads to less effort and involvement, and the less effort one puts into work, the less fulfilment one is able to get from it. The result is a downward spiral until a minimal level of performance is reached. This may be characterised by lack of involvement and concern for patients, resistance to any staff development that requires either effort or involvement, resistance to new ideas and change, high sickness rates and low self-esteem reflected in moodiness and sullenness. Whilst this paints an extreme picture, it does highlight the consequences of persistent lack of autonomy in work when work processes and outcomes are frustrated.

Practitioners may resist accepting autonomy because they may be uncomfortable and expose traditional ways of coping with anxiety that are not conducive to caring values, for example by depersonalising patients, and diffusing responsibility for personal action within the nursing team (Menzies-Lyth, 1988). This suggests that practitioners will need to construct new ways of defending themselves from anxiety in ways that can sustain desired and effective work. This requires recognising and managing anxiety as a legitimate active daily work activity (Marshall, 1980) and the task of 'good management' [Menzies-Lyth, cited in Holden (1991)].

Benner and Wrubel (1989) consider that the most effective coping resources are the uncovering of the primacy of caring and a societal and personal valuing of caring, together with societal and organisational changes that support and value nursing care with status, pay and working conditions.

The expression of caring beliefs is essential work for a number of factors:

- it enables practitioners to express their personal valuing of caring
- it enables a public statement to be made about 'what nursing is and intends to be', and sets up the conditions towards achieving increasing societal recognition
- it sets up the conditions whereby the meaning of caring concepts can be considered and their implications for practice can be anticipated
- it creates a vision of a new world of practice and in doing so creates an expectation of change and ultimate fulfilment that can motivate people to take action
- it enables the difference between anticipated new ways of working and actual practice to become visible and a focus for action
- it focuses on the role of clinical leadership to facilitate this development
- it focuses commitment to care.

However, the primacy of caring can only ever be experienced through action and reflection on action in order that the desired beliefs and values can become a reality in practice. Its validation is lived experience. By envisaging everyday nursing action as political action, then every contact with patients becomes action aimed at increasing the significance of nursing with patients and relatives, and with doctors and management. The key is to demonstrate that nursing does make a significant difference to peoples' well-being (Johnson, 1974).

This significant difference can only be at the level of human caring because technical work is perceived merely as an extension of doctor's work and reinforces the handmaiden role. This is not to say that technical work is not an important aspect of nursing's role, clearly it is and should not be diminished. The issue is to put this into a caring perspective that subordinates the technical role to the primacy of caring. Paying attention to fulfilling caring beliefs in our everyday work will lead to more satisfying experiences for both nurses and their patients which will reinforce the ways in which nurses and patients value caring beliefs and values.

Unfortunately outcomes are generally seen in through-put terms rather than caring processes. As a consequence, staffing levels, skill mixes, and grading are often a soft target for minimum levels, that act to undermine the growth of nursing as human caring. Political action involves helping patients who experience poor caring to take action through complaint and voice their need for human caring often at a time of great distress. The will to empower patients and relatives to take action is an expression of professional commitment and personal integrity.

Limits to rationality

I have made an assumption that through reflection on experience the practitioner can develop self-understanding in relation to practice. This can form the basis for an increasing self-determination to make rational decisions about the manner in which he or she wishes to practice on the basis of self-understanding (Fay, 1977). As Fay emphasises – this leads to increased **autonomy**, which, as we have seen, is a crucial component of professional activity and achieving effective performance.

Whilst evidence is accruing that demonstrates the reality of this situation (Johns, 1993b), it is important to understand the limits of rationality as the basis for action. Fay highlighted these limits of rationality to take desired action as embodiment, embeddedness, and power relationships.

Embodiment recognises how our bodies act in largely habitual learnt ways in responding to the environment. We don't usually have to stop and think 'how shall I act?'.

The body has skilled knowledge of action. This becomes evident when we try to learn new skills or change learnt skills to act differently. The implication of embodiment is that 'just because I think differently about something it will not result in radically different behaviour'.

Embeddedness recognises that as people we live in a background of social norms and practices that predetermine our actions (Heidegger, 1962). It challenges a concept of the autonomous person, or the radically free person, as someone who has

free choice. Free choice must always be set against a background of historically derived social practices. We are who we are for reasons and our freedom to act is always a 'situated freedom' (Heidegger, 1962) in the sense that our choices in situations are always conditioned by our backgrounds. However, these reasons can be accessed and understood by analysing the way we act by reflecting – 'why did I act in that way?'.

This background sets up the conditions under which we live and work. Yet it is not static, it is always changing in response to social conditions, and can be altered through the actions of nurse practitioners.

Power relationships are a particular form of embeddedness, that implies that truth and knowledge are merely manifestations of the interests of those with power to retain and extend their power.

As Foucault puts it (quoted in Dreyfus and Rabinow, 1982):

> each society has its own regime of truth, its general politics of the truth ... there is a combat for the truth (p. 117).

I have already suggested how nurses may perceive themselves as having relatively little power in contrast with other health-care workers such as doctors and managers. Vested interests cause dominant groups to resist challenge. It is naive to think otherwise because of the way such people are socialised into a psychological patterns of dependency, passivity, subservience (Oakley, 1984).

As the majority of nurses are women, it is not surprising that caring has been seen largely as women's work (Watson, 1990; James, 1989) and as a consequence is not valued, even by nurses themselves. Watson (1990), in her challenge to the 'moral failure of the patriarchy', asserts that

> caring as a core value cannot be forthcoming until we uncover the broader more fundamental politic of the male-oriented world-view at work and in our lives and the lives of the people we serve (p. 62).

Hence, developing autonomy in nursing can be seen as synonymous with the wider issues of challenging patriarchy. Autonomy involves making caring visible and valued as nurses' and women's work, rather than subordinate to the work of doctors and men.

Overcoming these barriers to rationality to achieve effective work will always be a struggle. It requires ways of learning that can enable practitioners to understand these factors, and feel empowered and supported to take necessary action.

Limits to autonomy?

I have assumed that developing autonomy is a necessary condition to promote commitment and effective caring within nursing. However, a distinction needs to drawn between autonomy for nursing as opposed to autonomy for nurses. In providing continuity of care for patients in both hospital and community settings nurses are dependent on their colleagues to make decisions and take appropriate actions in response to their encounters with the patient. Practitioners with responsibility for care management cannot expect other workers simply to follow planned care that involves ethical and emotional factors because it denies them the opportunity to explore the meaning of these situations for themselves.

Understanding these issues suggests that the image of autonomy for individual nurses based on concepts such as self-reliance and control may be flawed. Indeed, this has been shown to be alien for women and possibly incompatible with caring values, in contrast with a more appropriate image

towards group responsibility, or attachment (Gilligan, 1982). Gilligan's work 'corrects' Kohlberg's bias towards men in establishing levels of moral development where women fail to develop morally to the same extent as men. Gilligan's great achievement was to recognise that women develop **differently** to men with an emphasis on caring and responsibility in contrast to justice and ethical rule following.

The implications of Gilligan's work can be extended to challenge the basis of autonomy as being an acceptable criteria for the nurse practitioner. Figure 11.2 outlines a number of comparisons between the two concepts that favour attachment as an ideal characteristic for the nurse practitioner.

However, the **image** of autonomy is centred on the independent practitioner as a self-sufficient and self-reliant decision maker. In response to this responsibility the practitioner may strive to maintain personal control through attempts to control her work environment, which includes the actions of other nurses in her absence and resisting the involvement of colleagues in decision making (Johns, 1992). These characteristics may limit the nurse's ability to learn through feedback. Feedback becomes restricted to reinforcing self-reliance rather than developing more effective ways of working (Argyris and Schon, 1974). Indeed the culture of

Autonomy	Attachment
Promotes self as independent practitioner	Promotes primary responsibility to colleagues and team functioning
Emphasises self as unilateral decision maker	Emphasises decision making based on shared interests
Emphasises self-reliance	Emphasises mutual support systems with colleagues
Encourages competitiveness and ownership of work (Johns, 1992) → limited communication	Encourages open and honest communication
Responds to moral issues by applying rules and rational thought	Responds to moral issues by careful deliberation of situational factors and emotional involvement

Fig. 11.2. *Contrasting 'autonomy' with 'attachment'.*

nursing makes it difficult for this practitioner to seek help within the traditional norms of maintaining a facade of competence and coping. As one ward sister noted in a primary nursing situation

> They feel that if they have to ask it's showing they are not good primary nurses (Johns, 1989, p. 18).

It is not as if traditional norms are going to disappear as nurses move into autonomous roles. Indeed, because these norms facilitate coping, they will be reinforced as new roles arouse anxieties about competence. Without doubt, practitioners are not prepared for autonomous roles, socialised as they are into dependent and hierarchical ways of working. Rather than responding to their colleagues in collaborative ways, it is more likely that they will respond with overt hierarchical behaviour towards junior nurses and care assistants.

Whilst this expectation of supporting colleagues can be stated as a structural part of the practitioner's role, the reality is that effective mutual support systems do not exist in cultures that emphasise self-reliance and that 'good nurses cope'. I have written elsewhere about how the 'harmonious' team (Johns, 1992) acts as a social defence system within primary nursing systems to limit the expression of feelings and to avoid conflict. The result is a facade of harmony that masks real feelings. Hence it becomes difficult both to seek and receive valid feedback and obtain support from within the team – particularly where another colleague has been the source of the stress. This is a significant point because the major source of stress in primary and district nurse settings is attributed to interpersonal conflict with other workers (Johns, 1993b).

To be mutually supportive to sustain effective work requires practitioners to be open and authentic with her colleagues. Forrest (1989) notes, in her phenomenological study of the lived experiences of staff nurses, how

> The capacity to be caring is sustained through the comfort and support found in one's immediate co-workers and in the collective spirit that arises from teamwork (p. 818).

Summary
Commitment is a necessary requisite for autonomy and both are necessary for achieving effective work. Effective work is dependent on enhancing continuity of care between practitioners and mutual support systems to sustain caring work, which may not be easily reconciled to an image of autonomy for nurses as being independent practitioners.

Responsibility

To achieve desirable and effective work, these conclusions become the conditions of professional responsibility. Responsibility is accepting the task of carrying out a specified role, the conditions of which may be either explicit or part of the culture of nursing. Bergman (1981) suggests that in accepting responsibility **responsibly** the practitioner matches her knowledge against the job specification. Each practitioner has a sense of personal capability, and where the practitioner exceeds this in accepting a new role it is likely to lead to anxiety (Argyris and Schon, 1974).

In recognising that many practitioners are unlikely to have the knowledge base and skills to respond effectively to roles where autonomy is clearly developed as a structural component (such as primary nurses), it is essential that practitioners have a period of time where they are able to develop appropriate knowledge, skills and ways of being in the role compatible with desirable and effective work. As such, the individual's responsibility is always to strive to develop expertise to achieve effective work.

This responsibility is outlined within 'the key principles set out in clause 9 of The Scope of Professional Practice' (UKCC, 1992) which emphasise the knowledge, skill, responsibility and accountability based on the revised UKCC Code of Conduct (1992).

The expectations within this clause presents a formidable challenge for the practitioner to achieve within the scope of 'normal' practice. This challenge not only highlights the need for commitment to respond but also raises the question as to how this can be sensibly and meaningfully accomplished.

Expertise

It is relatively uncontroversial to assert that the practitioner who cares deeply about her practice will be committed to developing her expertise. Winter (1989) puts it like this:

> The critical function of the professional is directed to the inevitable limits of her own knowledge and understanding. In this way the professional role may be defined as the form of activity where the improvement of effective practice coincides with the development of understanding (p. 193).

Extract from the revised UKCC Code of Conduct (1992).

The registered nurse, midwife or health visitor:

9.1 **must be satisfied** that each aspect of practice is directed to meeting the needs and serving the interests of the patient or client.

9.2 **must endeavour always** *to* achieve,. maintain and develop knowledge, skill, and competence to respond to those needs and interests.

9.3 **must honestly acknowledge** any limits of personal knowledge and skill and take steps to remedy any relevant deficits in order to effectively and appropriately meet the needs of patients and clients.

9.4 **must ensure that** any enlargement or adjustment of the scope of personal professional practice must be achieved without compromising or fragmenting existing aspects of professional practice and care and that the requirements of the Council's Code of Professional Conduct are satisfied throughout the whole area of practice.

9.5 **must recognise and honour** the direct or indirect personal accountability borne for all aspects of professional practice.

9.6 **must**, in serving the interests of patients and clients and the wider interests of society, **avoid** any inappropriate delegation to others which compromises those interests.

Winter recognises that the professional's level of knowledge is always limited and, as a consequence, the development of this knowledge must be an on-going process. This knowledge can never simply be applied to different cases because it needs always to be interpreted within the context of the particular situation. How can this expertise be developed? Reflective practice offers considerable potential because the practitioner's sense of commitment and level of expertise are always evident within narratives of her experiences. Hence through sharing, exploring, and learning through these narratives, practitioners can develop commitment and expertise in contextual and reflective ways towards achieving desirable and effective work.

Reflective practice

It is not easy to understand the meaning of reflective practice. Papers are already appearing in nursing journals that attempt to make sense of the diverse theoretical literature about reflective practice, largely from sources outside nursing. For example, Atkins and Murphy (1993) claim a meta-theory of reflective practice from analysing and reducing attributes from different theories into a model. No doubt they believe they are doing the majority of practitioners a favour – to help them make theoretical sense of reflective practice. Unfortunately Atkins and Murphy merely add to the rhetoric surrounding the meaning of reflective practice by offering interpretations of interpretations because becoming a reflective practitioner is not prescribable. Diverse frameworks reflect different intentions and proposed outcomes of the different theorists. Just as the sensible practitioner will choose an appropriate model of nursing to help her achieve more meaningful nursing practice, so the sensible would-be reflective practitioner will consider what she intends to achieve by becoming a reflective practitioner. This emphasises how the reflective practitioner views all knowledge with a healthy scepticism – she must always ask herself 'What is the value of this theory or this piece of research for my practice?', 'How can I interpret this work to suit my own practice?'

The reflective practitioner uses theory and research finding as sources of information to inform practice. This type of knowledge is generally regarded as 'scientific knowledge' or 'research findings', and it is what is referred to when nurses are urged, from the Briggs Report (HMSO, 1972) onwards, to become a research-based profession. It is the type of knowledge that nurses have generally been socialised into viewing as a 'higher form of knowing', in contrast to knowledge derived from culture, custom, and anecdotes that emerge from reflecting on and talking about experience.

Whilst a 'scientific' approach may have credibility within a world of natural sciences, its acceptance assumes that such an approach is also valid for the human sciences, in other words it assumes that people can be reduced to objects whose behaviours and actions can be predicted and prescribed for in given situations. Such an approach denies the humanness of the encounter between the nurse and the patient. It encourages the nurse to set aside her own humanness and the humanness of her patients and see herself merely as a technician applying specific rules to 'fit' specific situations; what James (1989) sees as formulaic responses. Human encounters can only ever be interpreted within the context of the immediate situation. Failure to recognise and value this can only lead to distress for both nurse and patient. However, such is the pervasive dominance of this positivist approach within medicine, and the failure of nurses to assert nursing values, that this fact is not widely appreciated or acted upon. As Schon (1983, 1987) has shown, this approach to expertise ignores the fact that to be meaningful, all knowledge has to be embedded in the culture of the practice setting.

The context-free nature of much research means that practitioners always need to interpret what this means 'for me in my practice'. For example, statistically significant evidence may exist to indicate that patients are anxious prior to surgery and that giving certain information to them reduces their anxiety post-operatively. This information is clearly useful to the practitioner when admitting a patient for surgery. Yet her own experience in working with patients may have already informed her of this fact, and she will have developed personal theories for working with anxious patients, drawing on other sources of information.

Polanyi (1962, cited by Street, 1992) coined the expression 'connoisseurship' to describe how the practitioner combines

> technical know-how with her practical knowledge to provide a perceptual knowing that is context specific, which recognises the qualitative judgements involved in clinical knowledge, a perceptual, intuitive grasp of the whole situation, which can never be reduced to sets of rules technically applied in the situation (p. 196).

The caring and reflective practitioner can develop this 'intuitive grasp' by tuning into the person being admitted and asking 'Who is this person?', 'How is this person feeling?', 'How can I help?'.

These are common-sense questions that reflect a natural concern for the other person. In recognising her own humanness, the practitioner will monitor the feelings she is using in the caring process. It is important to recognise how our own concerns interfere with seeing, knowing, and being available to work with the patient. The recognition and understanding of these factors leads to the development of reflective nursing models (Johns, 1991) that enable the practitioner to express her beliefs and values in practice situations. Such models encourage the practitioner to be creative within shared beliefs and values to 'see' and respond appropriately to the person in need of caring.

Nursing is at a crossroads with regard to its valid knowledge base. On one hand there is this view of knowledge based on 'empirics' identified by Carper (1978) as

> Knowledge that is systematically organised into general laws and theories for the purpose of describing, explaining and predicting phenomena of special concern to the discipline of nursing (p. 14).

And on the other hand there is this 'reflective' view of nursing knowledge that rejects the dominance of the 'empirical' approach. It is useful to note how Belenky *et al.* (1986) analysed women's experiences in depicting a pattern of knowing culminating in 'constructed knowledge', i.e. the integration of public theories with personal ways of knowing. Developing constructed knowledge in this sense, is always the intention of reflective practice, whereby the practitioner comes to assimilate critically external sources of knowledge into a personal way of knowing which become available within her or his repertoire of actions to be applied to practice. Work by Benner (1984) and Benner *et al.* (1991) highlights how 'expert' practitioners make decisions intuitively – in contrast with analytic rule following, and in doing so, draw on tacit or personal knowledge. Tacit knowledge (Polanyi, 1962) is embodied knowledge that enables accurate intuitive responses to practice situations. Schon (1983) notes how

> we often cannot say what it is that we know. When we try to describe it we find ourselves at a loss, or we produce descriptions that are obviously inappropriate. Our knowing is ordinarily tacit, implicit in our patterns of action and in our feel for the stuff with which we are dealing. It seems right to say that out knowing is in our doing (p. 49).

Benner (1984) drew on the Dreyfus model of skill acquisition to highlight the essential nature of the expert practitioner and to distinguish expert performance from other levels. This is important work because it draws attention to the fact that expertise is always intuitive and largely tacit. Hence, ways of developing expertise are dependent on ways of learning through experience. It is only through paying attention to experience that tacit knowledge can be accessed and intuition developed. Phillips (1987) has highlighted the significance of intuition in decision making by how:

> hot or risky decision making is characterised by unpleasant emotional arousal and high ego involvement when the nurse's values, competence and self-esteem are on the line – as a result the nurse is unable to rationally weigh the alternatives and logically justify a course of action (p. 64).

Phillips' research gives support for intuitive decision making especially in situations of emotional arousal or human involvement that characterise much of nursing's work. As such, methods of learning that focus on accessing and developing tacit knowledge become crucial for developing expertise.

Practitioners' reflections on experiences lead to a rich description of nursing practice that is imperative in the development of theories of nursing embedded in practice (Benner, 1984). Although contextually dependent, these become available to other practitioners to consider within the context of their own similar experiences. The fragile knowledge-base upon which nursing is currently practised challenges nurses to find appropriate research methods to access this type of knowledge upon which to build contextually meaningful and rigorous theories of nursing knowledge.

Barriers against an epistemology of nursing based on reflective knowledge

The movement of nurse education into higher education promises to reinforce the high value of positivist-type knowledge because of its established cultural value within these institutions (Schon, 1983, 1987). Accepting reflective practice as a valid and equally significant form of knowledge would seem to demand a paradigm shift (Kuhn, 1970). Whilst this is obvious and rational, changing viewpoints are not so easily achieved. Is it because practitioners have been socialised to see themselves as passive recipients of knowledge as opposed to critical constructors of personal knowledge? Indeed the theory of positivist knowledge assumes that the role of theory is to provide answers to the questions of practice, irrespective of the fact that so far it has singularly failed to do so (Schon, 1987). The socialisation of nurses into passive recipients of knowledge is a reflection of a traditional behaviourist approach to the nurse curriculum and nursing practice, where the nature of practice has been prescribed in largely unproblematic and ideal terms, to the extent that students have divorced the curriculum with the real world of practice.

If nurses wish to pursue an ideology of nursing grounded in human caring values then they face the challenge of re-valuing caring as the core of nursing practice. Even with an acknowledged commitment to nursing as caring, how is this to be achieved?

The Scope of Professional Practice (UKCC, 1992) draws parallels between practice and education. Paragraph 3 states how:

Just as practice must remain dynamic, be sensitive, relevant and responsive to the changing needs of patients and clients, so too must education for practice ... we regard adequate and effective provision of quality education as a prerequisite of quality care.

Consider Rawnsley's comment that

Caring may be a desirable image for nursing, but is it meaningful? Is there congruence between the lived experience of nursing practice and the intellectual pursuit of caring as nursing's professional crest? When living the reality of their practice, nurses need ways through which they can connect the conceptual concerns of the discipline with the raw data of experience (p. 42).

Rawnsley's sense of connection is the very nature of reflective practice. Reflection-on-experience enable the practitioner to access a description of his or her work experiences in order to explore, understand, and develop the meaning of practice and to expose the contradictions between what he or she aims to achieve and the way he or she practices. Through this understanding and the conflict of contradiction, the practitioner can become empowered to take the necessary action to resolve these contradictions, and as a result, achieving more desirable and effective work, and more satisfying experiences for both the nurse and his or her patients. The practitioner's sense of commitment to care drives both the will to care and the effort of reflection.

The experiences that practitioners are aware of are those experiences which cause anxiety and uncertainty. They are also a reflection of the practitioner's concern as the more concerned the practitioner is then the more things matter to her, especially in situations of suffering and conflict which characterise much of nursing practice. The moment of reflection is often a response to a vague sense of unease prior to deploying appropriate defence mechanisms to neutralise this sense of anxiety. Hence the practitioner's willingness to learn through reflection may be ambivalent – on the one hand the desire to fulfil her therapeutic potential, whilst, on the other hand, the need to protect herself. All practitioners will, at times, experience frustration, helplessness and despair.

This is particularly so for those new in the profession (Cherniss, 1980) or with those accepting radically new roles, for example in primary nursing.

The practitioner may have difficulty 'seeing' the contradictions within her practice or ways of taking action to resolve these contradictions. This suggests that being reflective is not easy work (Gray and Forsstrom, 1991; Emden, 1991), and needs guidance (Cox *et al.*, 1991). There are many reasons why reflective practice should be **guided** to ensure its effective use as a development tool (Johns, 1994).

Guidance helps the practitioner to put these issues into perspective and to engender a sense of empowerment to take appropriate action based on new understandings.

Guided reflection

Guided reflection is a formal opportunity for a practitioner to share and learn through work experiences with a person designated to facilitate and sustain the practitioner's achievement of effective work, either on an individual basis or within a group.

The notion of guidance is synonymous with clinical supervision. The 'Vision for the Future' (NHSME, 1993) defines supervision as

> a term used to describe a formal process of professional support and learning which enables individual practitioners to develop knowledge and competence, assume responsibility for their own practice and enhance consumer protection and safety of care in complex situations, It is central to the process of learning and to the expansion of the scope of practice and should be seen as a means of encouraging self-assessment and analytical and reflective skills (p. 3).

This statement promotes supervision as the answer to fulfil the expectations of professional activity I have previously outlined. It also suggests that whilst supervision creates a sense of expectation and the space in which therapeutic competence can be developed, reflection gives it shape and coherence through a structured approach.

It is probably true to say that most people feel they reflect from time to time during their day. In this sense 'reflection' may appear to have deceptively simple ring to it. Yet in practice, practitioners struggle to reflect in meaningful ways because it is such a different way of perceiving practice. The technical difficulty of reflection may be aided by using a model of structured reflection (Johns, 1994). A model developed from my own research is shown in Fig. 11.3.

The analysis of the supervision process indicates that practitioners commence reflection at a very descriptive level and may take six to eight months to move into a reflective mode. However, a word of caution. The model is **merely** an heuristic device because of the danger and intention of all formal models to frame reality. The model offers cue questions that aim to tune the practitioner into her experience. The wider intention of the model is to enable the practitioner to learn to internalise reflection as a way of viewing her world of practice

The following cues are offered to help practitioners access, make sense of, and learn through experience:	
1.	**Description**
1.1	Write a description of the experience
1.2	What are the key issues within this description that I need to pay attention to?
2.	**Reflection**
2.1	What was I trying to achieve?
2.2	Why did I intervene as I did?
2.3	What were the consequences of my actions: • for the patient and family • for myself • for the people I work with.
2.4	How did I feel about this experience when it was happening?
2.5	How did the patient feel about it?
2.6	How do I know how the patient felt about it?
3.	**Influencing factors**
3.1	What internal factors influenced my decision making and actions?
3.2	What external factors influenced my decision making and actions?
3.3	What sources of knowledge did or should have influenced my decision making and actions?
4.	**Alternative strategies**
4.1	Could I have dealt better with the situation?
4.2	What other choices did I have?
4.3	What would be the consequences of these other choices?
5.	**Learning**
5.1	How can I make sense of this experience in light of past experience and future practice?
5.2	How do I **now** feel about this experience?
5.3	Have I taken effective action to support myself and others as a result of this experience?
5.4	How has this experience changed my ways of knowing in practice? • empirics • ethics • personal • aesthetics (Carper, 1978)

Fig. 11.3. *Model of structured reflection: ninth edn, July 1993.*

and to transcend the model as personal knowledge. In this way the model aims to enable imagination and creativity rather than conformity and thus a stifled way of viewing practice. Using the model to reflect on experience prior to sharing the experience in supervision prepares the practitioner to make best use of supervision time. Where the practitioner does not do this, then the dialogue in supervision inevitably tends to reflect the supervisor asking the sorts of questions set out within the model of structured reflection.

Guided reflection involves a contracted relationship between a designated supervisor and the practitioner that deals with mutual expectations and ground rules of the relationship, for example confidentiality of disclosed experiences. Meetings are usually planned for one hour every two or three weeks.

As the 'vision' definition of supervision suggests, expectations should be based on the three key functions identified as significant within clinical supervision:

- formative   concerned with developing skills and knowledge to achieve effective and desirable work
- restorative concerned with sustaining therapeutic work.
- normative   concerned with monitoring performance against standards

[Procter (undated) cited in Faugier and Butterworth (undated)].

Choosing the supervisor

Drawing on my experience and analysis of working as a line manger supervisor, and as an external supervisor, I would advocate the practitioner's line manager as supervisor. This creates the opportunity for the practitioner and line manager to work actively towards a collegial relationship and enhancing the conditions whereby commitment, autonomy and responsibility can be developed and sustained. The fact that a practitioner may not find it easy to relate to the line manger is all the more reason why these two people should get together to forge an effective relationship, if effective work is the desired outcome.

This reinforces an acknowledged participative style of management and creates the opportunity to 'role model' desirable collegial relationships in moving openly away from hierarchical relationships (as considered essential in professional roles). Bureaucratic–hierarchical socialisation presents as a major barrier to the practitioner taking action to become more effective in work. By working with her line manager the practitioner is immediately dealing with this major barrier.

It offers the line manager a structured way to fulfil role responsibility towards facilitating the development of practitioners into effective roles. The nature of learning in becoming effective is discussed later.

It establishes the role of the line manager as clinical expert. Becoming a supervisor forces a re-evaluation of one's clinical role in the face of an increasing managerial focus. The concept of 'expert', in this sense, refers to the specialist context-related knowledge of the practice setting, in contrast to transferable skills the practitioner has developed. This may be a significant issue with the focus on clinical leadership within the 'Vision for the Future' document (NHSME, 1993).

The line manager knows the practitioner's practice and patients. This prevents the practitioner avoiding the reality of situations or 'pulling the wool over the supervisor's eyes'. The practitioner may have good reasons for wanting to avoid the reality of certain experiences. This obviously needs to be respected but can usefully become a focus for reflection. Knowing the practitioner's practice also enables the supervisor to bring cues from outside supervision into the guided reflection session. For example, the practitioner may talk about a certain experience with one patient which prompts the supervisor to share her own observations of the practitioner's and her own work with this patient.

Knowing the practitioner's practice also enables the supervisor to re-examine norms of everyday practice that have become taken for granted and are not perceived as 'problematic'. This technique has been particularly useful when the practitioner has no specific experiences to share or wishes to avoid responsibility for guided reflection work. My approach is to say something like 'Let's run through your patients ... tell me about Mrs Jackson and her husband'. As the practitioner begins to share this work – the key is to make what is said problematic – 'Why do you think she felt sad?', 'How else could you have responded?'.

This process enables the line manager to get feedback about the practitioner's performance and make intuitive judgements about the practitioner's effectiveness. This is an important dimension in being responsible for the overall quality of care within the unit. It also enables the line manger to monitor informally the practitioner's development and what aspects of practice the practitioner needs to focus further reflection. This exposes a potential tension between the formative/restorative functions with the normative function where the practitioner may develop a sense of being judged. Two points are significant. Firstly, it is essential that the supervisor emphasises the formative/restorative functions in order to offset the practitioner's perception of being judged with consequent defensive behaviour. The key issue is to give the practitioner valid feedback to enable him or her to fulfil a sense of professional responsibility for monitoring her own effectiveness. Giving valid feedback also enables the line manger to acknowledge the practitioner's achievements – an important factor for the practitioner in developing a sense of self-worth and confidence. Without doubt, the line manager is an important and influential person in the practitioner's work-life.

Judging effectiveness is intended to become a mutual, shared process. However, this may take some time due to the previous hierarchical orientation of both supervisor and practitioner.

Sharing 'difficult' or 'emotional' experiences may not be easy for the practitioner, especially if she believes that 'good nurses cope' or attempts to maintain a facade of competence. Sharing such experiences is a consequence of trusting the supervisor and breaks down previously learnt norms, whilst enabling the line manger to offer appropriate support. Without doubt, the process of reflection may challenge the practitioner's normal coping mechanisms in dealing with work anxiety and stress. Equally the process of focusing on stress may enable the practitioner actively to confront it and work through it.

It enables the line manager to support the practitioner and at the same time challenge her towards developing self and practice. The balance of support and challenge presents the optimum learning environment (Borders and Leddick, 1987) which leads to increasing performance (OPDC, undated). The learning milieu of supervision of high challenge–high support links with Blake and Mouton's (1985) managerial grid of high support = concern for people, and high challenge = concern for production (see Fig. 11.1).

Most committed practitioners can sustain a challenge for a period of time but without effective support this can lead to exhaustion and burnout. In contrast high support but without challenge leads to 'comfort' work and feelings of frustration by practitioners. Supervisors have noted how they have felt practitioners are under enough pressure without them adding to it (unpublished research data). The idea of challenge may appear threatening to both the practitioner and the supervisor with the risk of exposing conflict. In such situations both the supervisor's 'maternal' attitudes and the practitioner's 'pressure' become a focus for reflection and action. Without doubt, threat is counter-productive to learning through reflection. Where threat is experienced it will only engender a defensive response. It is the supervisor's key task to create a milieu of psychological safety through ensuring the practitioner controls which experiences to share.

Situations of low challenge and low support are incompatible with developing effective work leading to apathy and minimal performance (OPDC, undated). Managers responsible for resources should create an environment of high challenge–high support in acting responsibly. I believe the fact that nursing managers do not do this is a reflection of how little nursing work is valued and the misguided belief that nursing is expensive and costs must be contained, irrespective of outcome. Hence you don't invest in resources which are generally seen as expendable.

External supervisors

In comparison, an 'external' supervisor, i.e. a supervisor outside the practice setting, may be more skilled in guided reflection skills, or the practitioner may feel safer with an outsider. The supervisor should be determined by considering the situation rather than be prescribed within a specific model.

Parallel processes

This relationship between supervisor and practitioner recreates parallel aspects of the practitioner's relationship with patients, the dynamics of which can be revealed within guided reflection. For example, the supervisor 's approach and response to the practitioner aims to reflect a desirable way of approaching and responding to the patient. Hence the supervisor always asks 'Who is this person?', 'What are her needs?', 'How is she feeling?', 'How does she make me feel?', 'How can I best help her?'.

This parallel can be revealed and used to explore the practitioner's approach and response to patients whilst simultaneously role-modelling good practice.

How the practitioner feels about a patient may be recreated in how he or she responds to the supervisor. The skilled supervisor 'surfaces' these unspoken dynamics and makes them available to work through with the practitioner in ways the practitioner can use in her practice.

Both the 'supervision' relationship and the 'nurse–patient' relationship aim to be therapeutic, i.e. the supervisor or practitioner aim to act in the best interest of the other person within such a relationship. However, there is always a parallel tension between being prescriptive and being reflective in therapeutic interactions, with the risk of the supervisor or practitioner imposing their viewpoints on the other because they feel they should act from a position of authority or feel pressured to achieve results.

Framing

Framing means making sense of situations by either constructing or utilising a meaning system. The supervisor can use a range of framing techniques to help the practitioner make sense and learn through their shared experiences. As Brookfield (1987) meaningfully comments

> In trying to find meaning in our lives and to make sense of the things that happen to us, we seek frameworks of understanding that we can impose on the bewildering chaos of our existence (p. 45).

Five types of 'framing' have emerged from an understanding of the supervision process:

- ideological framing
- problem framing
- reality perspective framing
- theoretical framing
- temporal framing.

Ideological framing

Socialisation of the practitioner into the unit's value system is an important aspect of supervision work. This socialisation is agreed as desirable work and is achieved by exploring the contradictions between actual practice and espoused beliefs and values. I have labelled this as 'ideological framing'. Where beliefs and value are implied within descriptions of experience, they can be made explicit to the practitioner.

Problem framing

Problem framing enables the practitioner to break down complex experiences in order to make sense and understand what is going on prior to reviewing or contemplating action. The model of structured reflection (Fig. 11.3) explicitly encourages this framing by challenging the practitioner to identify the issues within the described experience that are significant for reflection.

Reality perspective framing

Reality perspective framing enables the practitioner to see the 'real world' and the barriers that limit desired action. It is supportive to counter the practitioner's sense of frustration at not being able to take desired or effective action.

Theoretical framing

Theoretical framing refers to helping the practitioner make sense of her experiences within theoretical frameworks and research findings in a way that can be immediately applied to practice situations, creating the conditions where the practitioner can meaningfully assimilate instrumental knowledge or empirics (Carper, 1978) into her practice.

Temporal framing

Temporal framing enables the practitioner to make sense of the shared experience in terms of past experiences and future practice. It aims to establish a sense of continuity between experiences and between supervision session, for example by picking up issues from previous sessions and challenging the practitioner to review alternative ways of dealing with clinical situations and their consequences. Temporal framing has this anticipatory intention of preparing the practitioner for future experiences.

Developing effectiveness through reflection

An analysis of practitioners' experiences in guided reflection has identified key aspects of practice necessary for practitioners to become effective in achieving desired practice. These have been arranged in a distinct pattern of learning based on 'ways of knowing' (Fig. 11.4) that progresses through each of the ways of knowing.

'Knowing self'

This learning involves a process of unlearning learnt norms that emerge as barriers to achieving effective work, and moving towards new norms compatible with this aim. Many examples of this learning have already been described in this chapter, for example, norms that encourage managing a facade of competence and discourage seeking appropriate help.

'Knowing therapeutic work'

This learning is concerned with becoming effective in therapeutic work with patients and families. It includes dimensions such as making ethical decisions and taking ethical action, using the self therapeutically in working with patients, and with aesthetic action – taking appropriate and skilled actions in response to grasping, interpreting and envisioning clinical situations (Carper, 1978). [For example see Johns (1993a, b) for a description of practitioner development in this aspect of practice.]

'Knowing responsibility' and 'knowing others'

This learning recognises that individual therapeutic work between the practitioner and the patient takes place against a wider background of many patients and shared practices with nurses and other health-care workers. It involves learning to give and receive valid feedback to colleagues to fulfil responsibility to patients for ensuring effective and consistent care. It also involves ensuring the practitioner receives effective support to sustain effective work. This work is highlighted in the following example.

> **Reflective point**
> Reflect on the dialogue* given below of a practitioner's shared experience within supervision.

*This dialogue is taken from a guided reflection that forms part of my PhD study.

In particular note:
- the ways of knowing evident within this dialogue
- your perception of Maggie's sense of commitment, autonomy and responsibility as reflected within this experience
- the different framing techniques
- how this experience relates with your own work experiences
- how you have learnt from this description in context of your own practice

(you may want to record a number of your own work experiences in a diary to assist this learning process).

Maggie Bryant. Paternalism versus advocacy – clash of values and conflict

In Gayle's sixth supervision session she blurts out her discomfort in working with Maggie Bryant, the hospital-based social worker.

Gayle: ... I want to go out with Maggie Bryant and then she might talk to me properly!

Jane, her supervisor responded: That was a throw-away comment – I would like to pick-up on that.

Gayle disclosed: It was a couple of comments she said. I understood her to be coming to the hospital. I didn't confirm it. She was put out – patronising in the way she spoke to me. I think she doesn't respect my work. I try hard to ... it may stem from the fact I don't appreciate what she does – yet I think I do. I think I'll go out with her and develop our relationship. She has so

Focus of experience	Aim of work
Intrapersonal – Self in context of the environment	'Knowing' self
Interpersonal – Self in context of the patient	'Knowing' therapeutic work
Intrapersonal – Self in context of therapeutic work with others	'Knowing' responsibility
Interpersonal –	'Knowing' others

Fig. 11.4. *Learning through reflection.*

much information she doesn't tell me. She lets me know bits slowly.

Jane asked: You feel you respect her work?

Gayle replied: Yes I do. She has expertise with benefits, peoples' different social situations, facilities available. I think I must come across as not having a clue. I do know some things but she uses it as a position of power.

Jane helps Gayle to frame this point: 'Knowledge can be powerful – perhaps she sees herself on a higher plane than you as a nurse – all the professions see themselves in a hierarchy?

However Gayle proudly exclaimed: But today I won!

Jane cautiously responded: It was a case of winning?

Gayle said: It was with Hector; I told them about how much worse he was since coming in here. He used to be able to hold his head up and fasten his buttons and now he can't. I don't want him to get worse. At the multidisciplinary social meeting I said – 'he should go home' but she said 'No'. Three times I said it – and then I brought Hector up and he told them definitely. I acted as his advocate. He doesn't want to be here. He doesn't identify with anyone. She and the GP didn't want to know. They thought they knew him better.

Jane helped put this into context: Perhaps they do know him better overall but not at this time and in this context and that makes the difference. Knowing him has caused an issue of ownership.

Gayle responded: They are very involved, but like relatives not as professionals.

Jane used this distinction to challenge Gayle: What do you see as the differences between personal and professional involvement?

Gayle: It's about allocation of time – I know this sounds quite cold but it's not meant to be. I hadn't thought about it until now, it is about accepting responsibility. At work you plan care – you're personally available – with personal involvement you are emotional about them all the time. Professional responsibility takes over from personal involvement – at a level where you can rationalise you're involvement. ... I can't find the right vocabulary but with Maggie ... it's like she's talking about her dad – she really gets angry ... you may get angry but you have to accept your limitations ... you can stand back and look.

Jane: Perhaps one of the limitations of standing back is becoming detached?

Gayle: I don't think so. You shouldn't take your work home. It's a fine line. They see Hector as a relative rather than acting as trained people ... they have a personal commitment.

Jane: It could be – it seems very materialistic – they have the power, take no risks, the patients are helpless.

Gayle: They make the decisions for the person rather than helping someone to make their own decisions and respecting their choices whatever they are.

Jane: So there's a different philosophy?

Gayle: I think it's important that patients go to meetings. I know some say it is difficult and don't know what to do. But if they know there is a group of people who will decide for them then they will decide to go if you support them.

Jane: So there is a role for the primary nurse in preparing patients for these meetings?

Gayle: Yes – they need to know what is going on and to identify with a person – to think about the problems and not to be brought in cold. ...

Issues

This experience is centred in the conflict of values and ownership between Jane and Maggie that resembles a battle – personified by the concept of 'I won'.

(At least) three major conflicts are evident:

1. The role of health-care workers as advocates versus paternalism.

Advocate – enabling others to take action	⟵⟶	Paternalism – taking action on behalf of others

Gayle advocates for the patient's rights to be involved in decision making whilst Maggie (and unidentified others) decide they know best for him. Gayle's challenge to this blatant paternalism is profound. However, this experience illustrates the gulf of values that divides them and the real threat this poses for therapeutic work.

2. The sense of conflict polarises roles and sets up the conditions for competition as to who owns the patient and can thus claim legitimate responsible for making decisions. This reduces situations to games of win–lose and the potential for stoking the conflict between them – as someone has to lose.

3. The conflict within roles – between professional and personal involvement.

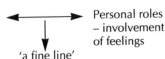

Professional roles ←————→ Personal roles
– detachment   – involvement
of feelings   of feelings
            'a fine line'

Gayle's involvement with Hector is clearly evident. Gayle attacks Maggie for a different and unacceptable paternal type of professional involvement. However, Gayle is uncertain of her role of 'involvement'. She talks about 'a fine line' between personal and professional involvement – 'you shouldn't take your work home'. Gayle seems to assume that 'involvement' means loss of emotional control. The art of involvement is not to take it home with you! However, this needs to be learnt.

The experience highlights the significance of Gayle 'knowing' her role responsibility within the context of desirable work and the crucial need to 'know' others who clearly impact on her ability to achieve effective work. Failure to work to mutual goals within shared understandings of beliefs and roles becomes a failure to achieve therapeutic work and a source of considerable conflict and frustration.

Besides these domains of 'knowing', Fig. 11.5 illustrates Maggie's self-perceived development and my review comments along four developmental themes – themes that reflect the ability to confront issues, become assertive, deal with conflict, accept personal involvement, acknowledge and share feelings, cope more effectively, and be available to colleagues for mutual support – all significant in achieving effective work. This covers a period of 15 months after Maggie commenced work in her first primary nurse post. Prior to this appointment she was experienced as a staff nurse within a 'team nursing' situation on an acute medical ward.

Failure to develop this learning represents a failure to achieve work that is both effective and satisfying. Yet how much attention do line managers pay to staff morale and ways of enabling practitioners to achieve effective work? From a human resource perspective it is gross mismanagement not to maximise the potential of the most expensive resource in health-care: nursing personnel. This point returns to the issue of managing quality and the ways in which it can be demonstrated through practitioner accountability compatible with professional activity. The remainder of this chapter explores the development of reflective performance reviews, as a means of demonstrating professional accountability.

Performance review

Performance at work is always subject to evaluation as part of some strategy of labour control; the only issues is how this is done (Thomason, 1988).

The NHS individual performance review (revised edition, 1987) aims to minimise the sense of oppression usually associated with performance review by enabling practitioners to set and agree objectives and negotiate rating of them, overseen by a 'grandparent' or equity assessor to ensure fair play. The term 'grandparent' is unfortunate because it suggests either the practitioner or the manager are children or parents, and given the hierarchical organisation of the health service, it is not beyond the imagination to suppose the manager is the parent, and the practitioner is the child. The grandparent is the wise old man giving his son good advice and curbing the manager's tendencies to bully his children.

People hanker after feedback on their performance in order to feel secure and well motivated, and to acknowledge their progress and development. Yet the fear of bad news may make people uncertain (Torrington *et al.*, 1987).

Fitzgerald (1989) notes how

> appraisal is seen by nurses to be of little value. Indeed some have suggested that it is time-wasting, punitive, and sometimes destructive.

Within bureaucratic–hierarchical organisations, performance review is a form of worker surveillance aimed at eradicating professional resistance to the management culture (Elliott, 1989) that reinforces dominant values and demands conformity. Heron (1981) believes that external rewards and punishments lead the practitioner to conform to what is expected of them, or in other words they are driven by expectations from others, rather than from their own expectations of desired work. Heron argues that this approach:

> can lead to vocational alienation – the person exercises his vocational role in a way that is cut off from his real needs, interests, concerns, and feelings, and hence uses the role in his human relations with his client somewhat defensively and rigidly (p. 5).

The illusion of equity created by such documents as the NHS individual performance review ignores the extent to which workers can be expected to act

274   *Christopher Johns*

Maggie's developmental theme review
[the visual analogue line is 10 cm long – Maggie was asked to mark her development along this line]

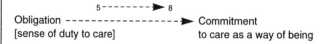

Obligation ------------------➤ Commitment
[sense of duty to care]   to care as a way of being

Maggie quickly demonstrated her commitment to therapeutic work despite the barriers of lack of support and previous learnt hierarchy of work.
She also was willing to confront the distinction between professional and personal roles necessary to be available and work with her patients and families in holistic ways.

Dependence ----------------➤ Responsibility
within hierarchy for role
[sense of subordination]

The lack of leadership and support Maggie experienced when she commenced work quickly confronted her ability to take responsibility for her role. Much of this work was new for her – most notably working with respite care families. She demonstrates her responsibility to improve her effectiveness of this care. She is less successful in carrying out her responsibility to patients by giving feedback to others when this was necessary to ensure therapeutic work, and in fulfilling supportive roles to her colleagues.

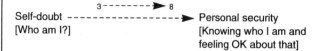

Self-doubt ------------------➤ Personal security
[Who am I?]   [Knowing who I am and
                                                 feeling OK about that]

Maggie's work in guided reflection is a catalogue of coming to terms with herself in the context of her work both individually with her patients and with her colleagues. She was well defended and self-reliant, yet she is able to challenge herself to feel more secure of herself in new [therapeutic ways]. She is on the threshold of mutual therapeutic ways of working with her colleagues although this has still to be attained. She certainly feels more self-assured.

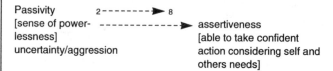

Passivity
[sense of power-   ------------➤ assertiveness
lessness]   [able to take confident
uncertainty/aggression   action considering self and
                                              others needs]

Maggie felt she was not an assertive person and found it difficult to assert herself in certain difficult situations. Yet she demonstrated a growing ability to be assertive, for example in William Richardson's care plan, although she less aware of the possible consequences of this type of action for others.
    She has had to battle through a dilemma of win–lose relationships which are naturally aggressive by nature. She also retains her own sense of ownership of patients – with limited involvement of other workers in care planning, for example lack of communication with night associate nurse regarding William's sleeping in the chair.
    To be assertive needs mutual responses from colleagues – it is difficult to be assertive in conditions where colleagues are unable to reciprocate. Yet Alice begins to demonstrate a willingness to respond to Lyall in ways that are helpful to him rather than to just 'win'.

Fig. 11.5. *Maggie's developmental theme review.*

from a position of inequity with managers socialised in hierarchical ways. Its success requires a participative style of management with clearly defined roles to help the line manager and the practitioner to recognise and focus on the practitioner's areas of weakness and strength within his or her role. Such recognition has a number of intended positive outcomes:

1. to enable the practitioner and the manager to experience a greater sense of satisfaction with work
2. to lead to improved performance in terms of nursing actions and achievement of desired outcomes for patients and families.
3. to maintain effective communication channels between the manager and those she manages and enable negotiation of shared expectations.

Young and Hayne (1988) note that the evaluation of an employee's performance has four objectives

1. to provide an opportunity **for reflection** and feedback on work performance and the work environment for a given period of time between an employee and supervisor
2. to acknowledge and encourage appropriate and above standard performance
3. to identify and remove distracters, dissatisfiers, and obstacles, as well as ineffective behaviours
4. to identify areas of growth for the employee and the organisation.

This last point is often dealt with by identifying and managing a number of objectives (Drucker, 1968; McGregor, 1987). The aim is simply for the manager and practitioner to agree a set of verifiable objectives to be achieved over a pre-determined period. Setting negotiated goals in performance review is significant within a goal theory of motivation. Mullins (1989) notes how

> people strive to achieve goals in order to satisfy their emotions and desires and how research studies have provided strong support for the theory that practitioners' goals or intentions play an important part in determining behaviour (p. 325).

However, adopting such an approach in nursing leads to a difficulty with identifying meaningful and measurable outcomes that reflect the qualitative dimensions of caring – such as respect, comfort, meeting psychological needs, and responding to relative's distress.

Competence

Traditionally, in nursing, the best clinical nurses were promoted and then assumed that since they knew 'good' nursing practice they were qualified to evaluate their staff, i.e. see it in others. This approach leads to a particular view of what good practice is and is limited by the extent to which the person is an 'expert'. Hence a key issue in appraisal is knowing the competencies that practitioners should exhibit and ways in which these can be monitored (Furnham, 1990).

There is another view of performance appraisal that sees it as providing milestones, feedback, guidance and monitoring (Torrington *et al.*, 1989, p. 310). When the responsibility for demonstrating effectiveness is devolved to the practitioner, these become intertwined. Such an approach requires neither objectives nor competencies to be set or against which to judge the practitioner. It presupposes a receptive and open organisation in which participants have the opportunity and feel able to challenge all practices, because it is only within an organisation which respects and practices freedom that the possibility exists to challenge traditional meaning systems (Grundy, 1989, p. 91).

Reflective performance review

Such an approach exists within the possibilities of reflective performance review. This approach is built on the beliefs that

- participative management is essential
- practitioners have devolved authority for managing work with subsequent autonomy to act
- that reflective practice has been utilised as a staff development and support method.

Reflective reviews involve the practitioner 'looking back' over his or her reflected experiences, over an agreed period of time (say six months), in order to demonstrate the growth of effective practice. Reflected experiences are analysed to identify key areas of the practitioner's practice which are supported through a series of experiences to illustrate how the practitioner has changed reflexively towards achieving effective work within clinical situations. This review becomes the focus for negotiation and agreement of effective performance and establishing focus for future reflection.

Reflective review – Shirley Rivet

1. What did I want to achieve over the last 6 months?

The following list shows the areas where I wanted to improve/achieve:

1. Find a support network within my profession, a 'back-up' system. District nursing can be an isolated profession and I was feeling this effect.
2. To be acknowledged as a fully qualified district nurse – to feel my professional decisions were accepted/ correct. I also wanted to be challenged at times.
3. Help to address the 'wider' issues of district nursing such as attending appropriate meetings, role as a teacher, implications of 'community care' ...
4. Focus on my role to become more effective and develop a greater depth of understanding within this role.
5. Time – to evaluate /assess myself – to become a reflective practitioner.
6. Promote my teaching role; support nursing auxiliaries by developing my management role such as introducing IPR for the auxiliary within our team.
7. To improve quality nursing by doing a caseload review with a colleague.
8. To improve my knowledge base by attending specific workshops – doppler training, multicultural awareness.

2. What have I achieved over the last six months?

1. Through supervision I have now learnt not to get so involved with patients and carers. It has helped me to set up coping mechanisms by not taking this work home so much. I have learnt to identify how to detach myself by using/working with other professionals and by being proactive in difficult situations rather than reacting to them.*
2. Starting to learn and understand my problems when faced with conflict and how to deal with this.
3. Reflecting on the supervision notes, I see how much I have to got to know myself better.
4. I have acknowledged that relationships with GPs were difficult and sometimes humiliating. I still need to set up more coping mechanisms but I feel that with my colleague we are very slowly making an impact.
5. Supervision, as a reflective process, has enabled me to 'see' the stress building up in me and how to handle specific issues slowly and to deal with each one to achieve a better decision.†
6. On the subject of 'wider' issues, such as involvement in the changes in the NHS – I have found that I do not address them. I sometimes feel 'swamped' by the demands as a manager and I cannot take them all in.‡
7. Other management achievements have been to increase the nursing auxiliary support network; set up a teaching programme for auxiliaries in group 5; and set an IPR date with Greer [auxiliary within my team].
8. I am also managing to attend study days without feeling unduly pressurised/ guilty. These have been useful and I plan to attend the three 'diabetic' study days in January. By being involved I have spoken with the diabetic liaison sister who has offered to set me set up a 'refresher' programme for M team.
9. The case load review has not yet been achieved due to working schedule constraints. I feel it will take some time to set up a monitoring tool and with caseload pressures, I haven't felt like tackling it just yet.
10. Looking back on the reflective process, I am still learning and have along way to go. I do feel I have used it in situations of conflict with patients and it has assisted me in making decisions at the time.

3. What have been the consequences of my achievements?

(a) For myself –

I am definitely more aware of myself, how I react and try not to be drawn into patient's personal problems. I am recognising that a patient has to take control of the problem.

I am learning to be more proactive and plan action when faced with a problem – making life easier for myself. I am 'diving' in so quickly when assessing situations and feel less stressed when dealing with patients cases.

(b) For patients –

I am not allowing personal feelings to interfere as much with professional decisions which leads to more rational decision making.

Patients are more involved in setting own goals.

They are cared for by a more relaxed and self-controlled professional.

(c) For people I work with –

I require less peer support which in turn reduces the pressure on my colleagues.

The nursing auxiliary feels included in the team. She is more valued. Indeed the whole team feels stronger now.

For my colleague – Kristen (district nurse) – I have come to realise how initially I had not fully accepted her as a replacement for Ann (staff nurse). By understanding this situation we now work as a team and communication has improved.

4. How do I know what the consequences have been?

(a) For myself –

I recently had a situation when a patient and family wanted me to make a very important decision for them – should his wife stop working not knowing how long he may live (1–2 years or a few months!). In the past I would have reacted too fast. Now, I stopped and thought – then offered advice by suggesting they do a list and analyse every issue and then make a decision. I strongly said that such a decision could not be made by me.

Another example is a patient with a pressure area problem related to his chronic illness. He always refused a 'research based, professional judgement' which led to the pressure sore occurring. I was constantly worrying about his non-compliance and couldn't accept it. Recently I wrote with him a care plan highlighting the need for compromise as a problem. In the last week, when the sore worsened, he accepted the suggestion of a particular treatment. He had decided himself.

(b) For patients –

By being proactive I have channelled a difficult situation – a patient's wife has been criticising 'behind us' alternatively the hospital staff and our care – she cannot accept her husband's prognosis. The situation was becoming more difficult since everyone was feeling manipulated and I was anxious of the patient's return home. I decided to reduce the conflict by promoting a very high verbal and written communication between all professionals and the wife.
Information/advice was given to the wife about the future community care her husband would receive. This information was made clear and realistic so she could make her own decisions. Since by being proactive, they were able to make their own decision without feeling pressured by my own 'hang-ups' if a conflict had resulted from the initial situation of manipulation. The case at home is working well and his wife is feeling well supported.

*A major focus of Shirley's shared experiences highlighted how she got so involved with the families she worked with that it blurred her responsibilities and her ability to help these families. Shirley was becoming angry and guilty in her work. The learning focus was to be available to these families without diminishing her sense of concern for them but without becoming 'over-involved' (Morse, 1991).

†Eighty percent of Shirley's shared experiences were concerned with situations of anxiety and uncertainty.

‡Shirley's response to these demands is shared with all the practitioners in the study. It was as if one thing after another was being passed down onto them without time to explore the significance of these issues. It also took time away from being with patients which Shirley saw as her prime concern.

Figure 11.6. *Reflective review – Shirley Rivet.*

Recording experiences

Data for the review are available from guided reflection sessions notes, which are accurately recorded (Johns, 1994). The practitioner is also encouraged to keep a reflective diary to record experiences, although this has been shown to be a haphazard and arduous activity for many practitioners, especially in the early stages of supervision.

The responsibility is on the practitioner to produce the review. However I would negotiate study leave for the practitioner to achieve this whilst emphasising her or his responsibility to demonstrate achieving and maintaining effective work. This responsibility can be written into the job specification.

The initial approach to developing and introducing reflective reviews was based around adapting the model of structured reflection. The cue questions can be reduced to three basic questions:

1. what sense can I make of my recent work experiences in terms of achieving effective work?
2. where do I need to focus future effort in order to develop increased effectiveness?
3. how can this be best achieved? (Reflective practice being one useful method.)

An example of a performance review using this approach is shown in Fig. 11.6. The practitioner in this example is a district nurse. Shirley has been in guided reflection for a year when she wrote this review. Initially she found it difficult to perceive how to do this task – because she was not used to taking her responsibility for demonstrating her own effectiveness and controlling her own professional development.

Besides the work shown in Fig. 11.6, the review also included (but omitted in this example):

5. what factors have influenced what I have achieved?
6. how do I feel about my achievements?
7. what have I learnt from doing this activity? Shirley noted 'I am quite amazed by what my achievements have been' and 'I need to pursue reflection since it is still not an automatic process'
8. what do I want to achieve over the next 6 months?

To summarise this approach, reflective reviews are an extension of on-going, individual development within an open participative approach to organising and managing nursing work. They enable the practitioner to look back and make sense of experience over time and to fulfil role responsibility for demonstrating the achievement of effective work and identifying the conditions that limit this achievement and lead to a mutual acknowledgement of achievement. By focusing on key areas of development, they enable the manager to be certain that staff development is appropriately focused.

Conclusion

This chapter has focused on understanding, developing and monitoring effective work, using the concept of professional activity in order to understand the critical factors involved. If nursing as caring is to be a force in health care it requires all practitioners to take personal responsibility for professional activity and for using innovative and practical ways such as reflective practice to make this a reality.

References

Alfano, G. (1971). Healing or caretaking – which will it be? *Nursing Clinics of North America*, 6(2), 273–280.

Argyle, M. (1974). *The Social Psychology of Work*. Penguin Books, Harmondsworth.

Argyris, C. and Schon, D. A. (1974). *Theory in Practice: Increasing Professional Effectiveness*. Jossey-Bass, San Francisco.

Armstrong, D. (1983). The fabrication of nurse–patient relationships. *Social Science and Medicine*, 17(8), 457–460.

Atkins, S. and Murphy, K. (1993). Reflection: a review of the literature. *Journal of Advanced Nursing*, 18, 1188–1192.

Batey, M. V. and Lewis, F. M. (1982). Clarifying autonomy and accountability in nursing service: part 1. *The Journal of Nursing Administration*, 12(9), 13–18.

Belenky, M. F., Clinchy, B. M., Goldberger, N. R. and Tarule, J. M. (1986) *Women's Ways of Knowing*. Basic Books, New York.

Benner, P. (1984). *From Novice to Expert: Excellence and Power in Clinical Nursing Practice*. Addison-Wesley, Menlo Park, California.

Benner, P. and Wrubel, J. (1989). *The Primacy of Caring: Stress and Coping in Health and Illness*. Addison-Wesley, Menlo Park, California.

Benner, P., Tanner, C. and Chelsa, C. (1991). From beginner to expert: Gaining a differentiated clinical world in critical care nursing. *Advances in Nursing Science*, 14(3), 13–28.

Bergman, R. (1981). Accountability – definition and dimensions. *International Nursing Review*, 28(2), 53–59.

Blake, R. B. and Mouton, J. S. (1985). *The Managerial Grid III*, 3rd edn. Gulf Publishing, Houston.

Blauner, R. (1964). *Alienation and Freedom*. University of Chicago Press, Chicago.

Borders, L. D. and Leddick, G. R. (1987). *Handbook of Counseling Supervision*. Association for Counselor Education and Supervision, Virginia.

Briggs Committee (1972). *Report of the Committee on Nursing*. HMSO, London.

Brookfield, S. D. (1987). *Developing Critical Thinkers*. Open University Press, Milton Keynes.

Carper, B. (1978). Fundamental patterns of knowing in nursing. *Advances in Nursing Science*, 1(1), 13–23.

Carr, W. and Kemmis, S. (1986). *Becoming Critical*. The Falmer Press, Lewes.

Cherniss, G. (1980). *Professional Burnout in Human Service Organizations*. Praeger Publishers, New York.

Cooper, M. C. (1991). Principle-oriented ethics and the ethic of care: A creative tension. *Advances in Nursing Science*, 14(2), 22–31.

Cox, H., Hickson, P. and Taylor, B. (1991). Exploring reflection: knowing and constructing practice. In Gray, G. and Pratt, R. (eds) *Towards a Discipline of Nursing*, pp. 373–390. Churchill Livingstone, Melbourne.

Dreyfus, H. L. and Rabinow, P. (1982). *Michel Foucault: Beyond Structuralism and Hermeneutics*. Harvester Wheatsheaf, New York.

Drucker, P. F. (1968). *The Practice of Management*. Pan Books.

Dunlop, M. J. (1986). Is a science of caring possible? *Journal of Advanced Nursing*, 11, 661–670.

Elliott, J. (1989). Knowledge, power, and teacher appraisal. In Carr, W. (ed.) *Quality in Teaching*, pp. 201–219. Falmer Press, Lewes.

Ellis, R. (1988). Quality assurance and care. In Ellis, R. (ed.) *Professional Competence and Quality Assurance in the Caring Professions*. Croom Helm, London.

Emden, C. (1991). Becoming a reflective practitioner. In Gray, G. and Pratt, R. (eds), *Towards a Discipline of Nursing*, pp. 373–390. Churchill Livingstone, Melbourne.

Ersser, S. and Tutton, E. (1991). Primary nursing – a second look. In Ersser, S. and Tutton, E. (eds) *Primary Nursing in Perspective*, pp. 3–30. Scutari Press, London.

Faugier, J. and Butterworth, T. (undated). *Clinical Supervision: A Position Paper*. School of Nursing Studies, University of Manchester.

Fay, B. (1977). How people change themselves: the relationship between critical theory and its audience. In Ball, T. (ed.) *Political Theory and Praxis: New Perspectives*. University of Minnesota Press, Minneapolis.

Fay, B. (1987). *Critical Social Theory*. Polity Press, Cambridge.

Fitzgerald, M. (1989). Performance planning and review. In Vaughan, B. and Pilmoor, M. (eds) *Managing Nursing Work*. Scutari Press, London.

Forrest, D. (1989). The experience of caring. *Journal of Advanced Nursing*, 14, 815–823.

Foucault, M. (1979). *Discipline and Punish; The Birth of the Prison* (translated by Sheridan, A.) Vintage/Random House, New York.

Foucault, M. (1981). *The History of Sexuality*, Vol. 1. Penguin Books, Harmondsworth.

Freire, P. (1972). *Pedagogy of the Oppressed*. Penguin Books, Harmondsworth.

Friedson, E. (1971). *Professional Dominance*. Atherton Press, Chicago.

Furnham, A. (1990). A question of competency. *Personnel Management*, 22(6), 37.

Gilligan, C. (1982). *In a Different Voice: Psychological Theory and Women's Development*. Harvard University Press, Cambridge, MA.

Goldstone, L. A., Ball, J. A. and Collier, M. M. (1983). Monitor: an index of the quality of nursing care for acute medical and surgical wards. Newcastle upon Tyne Polytechnic Products.

Gray, J. and Forsstrom, S. (1991). Generating theory from practice: the reflective technique. In Gray, G. and Pratt, R. (eds) *Towards a Discipline of Nursing*, pp. 373–390. Churchill Livingstone, Melbourne.

Grundy, S. (1989). Beyond professionalism. In Carr, W. (ed.) *Quality in Teaching*, pp. 79–100. Falmer Press, Lewes.

Hall, L. (1964). Nursing – what is it? *Canadian Nurse*, 60(2), 150–154.

Harrison, L. L. (1990). Maintaining the ethic of caring in nursing. *Journal of Advanced Nursing*, 15, 125–127.

Heidegger, M. (1962). *Being and Time* (translated by Macquarrie, J. and Robinson, E.). Harper & Row, New York.

Heider, F. (1958). *The Psychology of Interpersonal Relations*. John Wiley, New York.

Heron, J. (1981). *Assessment*. British Post-graduate Medical Federation, London.

Holden, R. J. (1991). An analysis of caring: attributions, contributions, and resolutions. *Journal of Advanced Nursing*, 16, 893–898.

James, N. (1989). Emotional labour. *The Sociological Review*, 37(1), 151–142.

Johns, C. C. (1991). The Burford Nursing Development Unit holistic model of nursing practice. *Journal of Advanced Nursing*, 16, 1090–1098.

Johns, C. C. (1992). Ownership and the harmonious team: barriers to developing the therapeutic nursing team in primary nursing. *Journal of Clinical Nursing*, 1, 89–94.

Johns, C. C. (1993a). On becoming effective in taking ethical action. *Journal of Clinical Nursing*, 2, 307–312.

Johns, C. C. (1993b). Professional supervision. *Journal of Nursing Management*, 1(1), 9–18.

Johns, C. C. (1994). *Guided Reflection*. In Palmer, A., Burn, S. and Bulman, C. (eds). *Reflective Practice in Nursing*. Blackwell Scientific, Oxford.

Johnson, D. E. (1974). Development of theory: a requisite for nursing as a primary health care profession. *Nursing Research*, 23(5), 373–377.

Jourard, S. (1971). *The Transparent Self*. Van Nostrand, Norwalk, NJ.

Kitson, A. (1987). A comparative analysis of lay caring and professional nursing caring relationships. *International Journal of Nursing Studies*, 24(2), 155–165.

Kramer, M. K. (1990). Holistic nursing: implications for knowledge development and utilization. In Chaska, N. L. (ed.) *The Nursing Profession: Turning Points*, pp. 245–254. C. V. Mosby, St Louis, MO.

Kuhn, T. (1970). *The Structure of Scientific Revolutions*, 2nd edn. University of Chicago Press, Chicago.

Lawler, J. (1991). *Behind the Screens: Nursing, Somology, and the Problem with the Body*. Churchill Livingstone, Melbourne.

Leininger, M. (1988). *Care: The Essence of Nursing and Health*. Wayne State University Press, Detroit.

Likert, R. (1961). *New Patterns of Management.* McGraw-Hill.

Marshall, J. (1980). Stress amongst nurses. In Cooper, C. L. and Marshall, J. (eds) *White Collar and Professional Stress,* pp. 19–62. John Wiley, Chichester.

Maxwell, R. J. (1984). Quality assessment in health. *British Medical Journal,* 288(1), 470–471.

McGregor, D. (1987). *The Human Side of Enterprise.* Penguin Books, Harmondsworth.

McKenna, G. (1993). Caring is the essence of nursing practice. *British Journal of Nursing,* 2(1), 72–75.

Menzies-Lyth, I. (1988). *Containing Anxiety in Institutions.* Free Association Books, London.

Morse, J. M. (1991). Negotiating commitment and involvement in the nurse–patient relationship. *Journal of Advanced Nursing,* 16, 455–468.

Morse, J. M., Bottorff, J., Neander, W. and Solberg, S. (1991). Comparative analysis of conceptualizations and theories of caring. *Image: Journal of Nursing Scholarship,* 23(3), 119–126.

Mullins, L. J. (1989). *Management and Organizational Behaviour,* 2nd edn. Pitman, London.

NHS Management Executive (1993). *Vision for the Future.* London.

NHSTA (1987). *Guide and Model Documentation for Individual Performance Review,* revised edn. Training and Development Publications, London.

Oakley, A. (1984). The importance of being a nurse. *Nursing Times,* 80(50), 24–27.

OPDC (undated). Supervision. OPDC, Taunton (unpublished).

Packard, J. S. and Ferrara, M. (1988). In search of the moral foundation of nursing. *Advances in Nursing Science,* 10(4), 60–71.

Parse, R. R. (1992). Human becoming: Parse's theory of nursing. *Nursing Science Quarterly,* 5(1), 35–42.

Phillips, L. R. (1987). Critical points in decision making. In Hannah, K. J., Reimer, M., Mills, W. C. and Letourneau, S. (eds). *Clinical Judgement and Decision Making: The Future with Nursing Diagnosis.* John Wiley, New York.

Polanyi, M. (1962). *Personal Knowledge.* Routledge & Kegan Paul, London.

Proctor, B. (undated). Supervision: a co-operative exercise in accountability. In Marken, M. and Payne, M. (eds) *Enabling and Ensuring.* Leicester National Youth Bureau and Council for Education and Training in Youth and Community Work.

Rawnsley, M. (1990). Of human bonding: The context of nursing as caring. *Advances in Nursing Science,* 13(1), 41–48.

Satre, J. P. (1969). *Being and Nothingness.* University Paperbacks, Methuen, London.

Schon, D. A. (1983). *The Reflective Practitioner.* Avebury, Aldershot.

Schon, D. A. (1987). *Educating the Reflective Practitioner.* Jossey-Bass, San Francisco.

Seedhouse, D. (1988). *Ethics: The Heart of Health Care.* John Wiley, Chichester.

Shaw, C. D. (1986). *Introducing Quality Assurance.* King's Fund Project Paper 64. King's Fund, London.

Strauss, G. (1963). Professionalism and occupational associations. *Industrial Relations,* 20(5), 8.

Street, A. F. (1991). *Inside Nursing.* State University of New York Press, New York.

Thomason, G. (1988). *A Textbook of Human Resource Management.* Institute of Personnel Management, London.

Torrington, D., Weightman, J. and Johns, K. (1989). *Effective Management: People and Organization.* Prentice-Hall, Hemel Hempstead.

UKCC (1992). *The Scope of Professional Practice.* UKCC, London.

Van Hooft, S. M. (1987). Caring and professional commitment. *The Australian Journal of Advanced Nursing,* 4(4), 29–38.

Wandelt, M. and Ager, J. (1974). *Quality Patient Care Scale.* Appleton-Century-Crofts, New York.

Watson, J. (1985). *Nursing: Human Science and Human Care.* Appleton-Century-Crofts, Norwalk, CT.

Watson, J. (1990). The moral failure of the patriarchy. *Nursing Outlook,* 38(2), 62–66.

Winter, R. (1989). Teacher appraisal and the development of professional knowledge. In Carr, W. (ed.) *Quality in Teaching,* pp. 183–200. Falmer Press, Lewes.

Yarling, R. R. and McElmurray, B. J. (1986). The moral foundation of nursing. *Advances in Nursing Science,* 8(2), 63–73.

Young, L. C. and Hayne, A. N. (1988). *Nursing Administration: From Concepts to Practice.* W. B. Saunders, Philadelphia.

INDEX